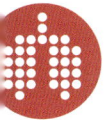
ERS|p

CW01460603

Handbook

Invasive Mechanical Ventilation

Editors
Leo Heunks and
Marcus J. Schultz

PUBLISHED BY

THE EUROPEAN RESPIRATORY SOCIETY

CHIEF EDITORS

Leo Heunks and Marcus J. Schultz (Amsterdam, the Netherlands)

ERS STAFF

Caroline Ashford-Bentley, Alice Bartlett, Matt Broadhead, Alyson Cann, Sarah Cleveland, Rachel Gozzard, Jonathan Hansen, Catherine Pumphrey, Elin Reeves, Claire Marchant, Ben Watson

©2019 European Respiratory Society

Cover image: Tyler Olson, shutterstock

Design by Claire Marchant and Ben Watson, ERS
Typeset by Nova Techset
Printed in the UK by Page Bros (Norwich) Ltd.
Indexed by Merrall-Ross International

CONTACT, PERMISSIONS AND SALES REQUESTS:
European Respiratory Society, 442 Glossop Road, Sheffield, S10 2PX, UK
Tel: +44 114 2672860 Fax: +44 114 2665064 e-mail: books@ersnet.org

Print: ISBN: 978-1-84984-121-4
Online ISBN: 978-1-84984-122-1

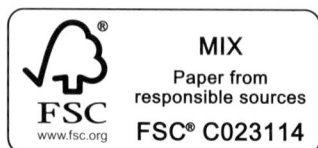
MIX
Paper from
responsible sources
FSC® C023114
FSC
www.fsc.org

Table of contents

Contributors

Chief Editors

Leo Heunks
Dept of Intensive Care Medicine,
Amsterdam UMC location VUmc,
and Amsterdam Cardiovascular
Sciences Research Institute,
Amsterdam, The Netherlands
l.heunks@amsterdamumc.nl

Marcus J. Schultz
Nuffield College, Oxford University,
Oxford, UK; Mahidol-Oxford
Research Unit (MORU), Mahidol
University, Bangkok, Thailand; Dept
of Intensive Care and Laboratory
of Experimental Intensive Care
and Anesthesiology, Amsterdam
University Medical Centers, location
AMC, Amsterdam, The Netherlands.
marcus.j.schultz@gmail.com

Authors

Hernán Aguirre-Bermeo
Unidad de Cuidados Intensivos,
Hospital Vicente Corral Moscoso,
Cuenca, Ecuador
hermar0699@gmail.com

Jean-Michel Arnal
Service de réanimation, Hôpital
Sainte Musse, Toulon, France;
Medical Research and New
Technologies, Hamilton Medical AG,
Bonaduz, Switzerland
jean-michel@arnal.org

Antonio Artigas
Intensive Care Unit, Hospital
Universitario Sagrado Corazón,
Barcelona, Critical Care Center,
ParcTaulí Hospital Universitari,
Institut d'Investigació i Innovació
Parc Taulí I3PT, Universitat
Autònoma de Barcelona, Sabadell,
and CIBER Enfermedades
Respiratorias, Instituto de Salud
Carlos III, Madrid, Spain
aartigas@tauli.cat

Carmen Sílvia Valente Barbas
INCOR, University of São Paulo
Medical School and Staff Physician
Adult ICU, Hospital Israelita Albert
Einstein, São Paulo, Brazil
carmen.barbas@gmail.com

Tobias Becher
Dept of Anaesthesiology and
Intensive Care Medicine, University
Medical Centre Schleswig-Holstein,
Kiel, Germany
tobias.becher@uksh.de

Thomas Bein
Dept of Anesthesiology, University
Hospital, Regensburg, Germany
thomas.bein@ukr.de

Giacomo Bellani
University of Milan-Bicocca, Dept
of Experimental Medicine; and
San Gerardo Hospital, Dept of
Perioperative Medicine and Intensive
Care, Monza, Italy
giacomo.bellani1@unimib.it

Alexandra Beurton
Service de médecine intensive-
réanimation, Hôpital de Bicêtre,
Hôpitaux universitaires Paris-Sud,
AP-HP, and Inserm UMR S_999,
Université Paris-Sud, Le Kremlin-
Bicêtre, France
alex.beurton@gmail.com

Lluís Blanch
Critical Care Center, ParcTaulí
Hospital Universitari, Institut
d'Investigació i Innovació Parc
Taulí I3PT, Universitat Autònoma
de Barcelona, Sabadell, and CIBER
Enfermedades Respiratorias,
Instituto de Salud Carlos III, Madrid,
Spain
LBlanch@tauli.cat

Lieuwe D. Bos
Dept of Intensive Care, Respiratory
Medicine, and Laboratory for
Experimental Intensive Care and
Anesthesiology (L·E·I·C·A), University
of Amsterdam, Amsterdam, The
Netherlands
l.d.bos@amc.uva.nl

Laurent Brochard
Interdepartmental Division of Critical
Care Medicine, University of Toronto
and Keenan Research Centre and
Li Ka Shing Knowledge Institute, St
Michael's Hospital, Toronto, Canada
BrochardL@smh.ca

Christian S. Bruells
Dept of Anesthesiology, University
Hospital of the RWTH Aachen,
Aachen, Germany
cbruells@ukaachen.de

Luigi Camporota
Dept of Adult Critical Care, Guy's and
St Thomas' NHS Foundation Trust,
King's Health Partners, London, UK
luigi.camporota@gstt.nhs.uk

Irene Cavalli
Alma Mater Studiorum – Università
di Bologna, Dipartimento di Scienze
Mediche e Chirurgiche, Anesthesia
and Intensive Care Medicine,
Policlinico di Sant'Orsola, Bologna,
Italy
irenee.cavalli@gmail.com

Lu Chen
Keenan Research Centre and Li
Ka Shing Institute, Dept of Critical
Care, St Michael's Hospital; and
Interdepartmental Division of Critical
Care Medicine, University of Toronto,
Toronto, Canada
ChenL1@smh.ca

Davide Chiumello
SC Anestesia e Rianimazione,
Ospedale San Paolo – Polo
Universitario, ASST Santi Paolo e
Carlo, Milan, Italy
chiumello@libero.it

Rebecca F. D'Cruz
Lane Fox Clinical Respiratory
Physiology Research Centre, Guy's
and St Thomas' NHS Foundation
Trust; Centre for Human and
Applied Physiological Sciences,
King's College London; National
Institute for Health Research (NIHR)
Biomedical Research Centre at Guy's
and St Thomas' NHS Foundation
Trust and King's College London,
London, UK
rebecca.dcruz@gstt.nhs.uk

Candelaria de Haro
Critical Care Center, Hospital
Universitari Parc Taulí, Institut
d'Investigació i Innovació Parc
Taulí I3PT, Universitat Autònoma
de Barcelona, Barcelona; and
Biomedical Research Networking
Center in Respiratory Diseases
(CIBERES), Instituto de Salud Carlos
III, Madrid, Spain
cdeharo@tauli.cat

Frans de Jongh
Dept of Neonatology, AMC Hospital,
Amsterdam, The Netherlands
f.h.dejongh@amsterdamumc.nl

Gustavo Faissol Janot de Matos
University of São Paulo Medical
School and Staff Physician Adult ICU,
Hospital Israelita Albert Einstein, São
Paulo, Brazil
gjanot@gmail.com

Alexandre Demoule
AP-HP, Groupe Hospitalier Pitié-
Salpêtrière Charles Foix, Service de
Pneumologie, Médecine Intensive et
Réanimation (Département "R3S")
and Sorbonne Université, INSERM,
UMRS1158 Neurophysiologie
respiratoire expérimentale et
clinique, Paris, France
alexandre.demoule@aphp.fr

Heder J. de Vries
Dept of Intensive Care Medicine,
Amsterdam UMC location VUmc,
and Amsterdam Cardiovascular
Sciences Research Institute,
Amsterdam, The Netherlands
h.vries@amsterdamumc.nl

Martin Dres
AP-HP, Groupe Hospitalier Pitié-
Salpêtrière Charles Foix, Service
de Pneumologie et Réanimation
Médicale du Département R3S,
and Sorbonne Université, INSERM,
UMRS1158 Neurophysiologie
Respiratoire Expérimentale et
Clinique, Paris, France
martin.dres@aphp.fr

José Aquino Esperanza
Critical Care Center, Hospital
Universitari Parc Taulí, Institut
d'Investigació i Innovació Parc
Taulí I3PT, Barcelona; Biomedical
Research Networking Center in
Respiratory Disease (CIBERES),
Instituto de Salud Carlos III, Madrid;
and Universitat de Barcelona,
Facultat de Medicina, Barcelona,
Spain.
jaquino@tauli.cat

Antonio M. Esquinas
Intensive Care Unit, Hospital
Morales Meseguer, Murcia, Spain
antmesquinas@gmail.com

Ricardo Estêvão Gomes
Pulmonology Dept, Hospital Garcia
de Orta, Almada, Setúbal, Portugal
ricardoegomes@gmail.com

Eddy Fan
Interdepartamental Division of
Critical Care Medicine, University of
Toronto; and Division of Respirology,
Dept of Medicine, University Health
Network and Mount Sinai Hospital,
Toronto, Canada
eddy.fan@uhn.ca

Bernard Fikkers
Radboudumc, Dept of Intensive
Care, Nijmegen, The Netherlands
Bernard.Fikkers@radboudumc.nl

Christoph Fisser
Dept of Internal Medicine II,
University Hospital, Regensburg,
Germany
christoph.fisser@ukr.de

Tim Frenzel
Dept of Intensive Care Medicine,
Radboud UMC, Nijmegen, The
Netherlands
Tim.Frenzel@radboudumc.nl

Inéz Frerichs
Dept of Anaesthesiology and
Intensive Care Medicine, University
Medical Centre Schleswig-Holstein,
Kiel, Germany
inez.frerichs@uksh.de

Louis-Marie Galerneau
Médecine Intensive Réanimation
CHU Grenoble, Université de
Grenoble, Grenoble, France
lmarie.galerneau@chu-grenoble.fr

Marcelo Gama de Abreu
Pulmonary Engineering Group,
Dept of Anaesthesiology and
Intensive Care Medicine, University
Hospital Carl Gustav Carus,
Dresden, Germany
mgabreu@uniklinikum-dresden.de

Marco Giani
University of Milan-Bicocca, Dept
of Experimental Medicine; and
San Gerardo Hospital, Dept of
Perioperative Medicine and Intensive
Care, Monza, Italy
marco.giani@unimib.it

Rik Gosselink
Faculty of Movement and
Rehabilitation Sciences, Dept
Rehabilitation Sciences KU Leuven,
and Division of Critical Care
Medicine, University Hospitals
Leuven, Leuven, Belgium
rik.gosselink@kuleuven.be

Claude Guérin
Médecine Intensive Réanimation
CHU Lyon France, Université de
Lyon, Lyon, France
claude.guerin@chu-lyon.fr

Nicholas Hart
Lane Fox Clinical Respiratory
Physiology Research Centre, Guy's
and St Thomas' NHS Foundation
Trust; Centre for Human and
Applied Physiological Sciences,
King's College London; National
Institute for Health Research (NIHR)
Biomedical Research Centre at Guy's
and St Thomas' NHS Foundation
Trust and King's College London,
London, UK
nicholas.hart@gstt.nhs.uk

Robert Huhle
Pulmonary Engineering Group, Dept
of Anaesthesiology and Intensive
Care Medicine, University Hospital
Carl Gustav Carus, Dresden,
Germany
robert.huhle@tu-dresden.de

Christina Iezzi
Speech and Language Therapy Dept,
Critical Care, Guy's & St Thomas'
NHS Foundation Trust, London, UK
Christina.Iezzi@gstt.nhs.uk

Annemijn H. Jonkman
Dept of Intensive Care Medicine,
Amsterdam UMC location VUmc,
and Amsterdam Cardiovascular
Sciences Research Institute,
Amsterdam, The Netherlands
ah.jonkman@amsterdamumc.nl

Georgios Kaltsakas
Lane Fox Clinical Respiratory
Physiology Centre, Guy's and St
Thomas' NHS Foundation Trust;
Centre for Human and Applied
Physiological Sciences, King's
College, London, UK
georgios.kaltsakas@gstt.nhs.uk

Cenk Kirakli
University of Health Sciences, Dr.
Suat Seren Chest Diseases and
Surgery Training and Research
Center, Intensive Care Unit, Izmir,
Turkey
ckirakli@hotmail.com

Federico Longhini
Anesthesia and Intensive Care Unit,
University Hospital Mater Domini,
Dept of Medical and Surgical
Sciences, Magna Graecia University,
Catanzaro, Italy
longhini.federico@gmail.com

Cong Lu
Dept of Paediatric Intensive Care,
Beijing Children's Hospital, Capital
Medical University, Beijing, China;
and Keenan Research Centre and Li
Ka Shing Institute, Dept of Critical
Care, St Michael's Hospital, Toronto,
Canada
conglu.bch@icloud.com

Rudys Magrans
Biomedical Research Networking
Center in Respiratory Diseases
(CIBERES), Instituto de Salud Carlos
III, Madrid, Spain
rmagrans@tauli.cat

Jordi Mancebo
Servei de Medicina Intensiva,
Hospital de la Santa Creu i Sant Pau,
Barcelona, Spain
jmancebo@santpau.cat

Luis Morales-Quinteros
Intensive Care Unit, Hospital
Universitario Sagrado Corazón,
Barcelona, Spain
luis.morales@quironsalud.es

Elise Morawiec
AP-HP, Groupe Hospitalier Pitié-
Salpêtrière Charles Foix, Service de
Pneumologie, Médecine Intensive et
Réanimation (Département "R3S"),
Paris, France
elise.morawiec@aphp.fr

Stefan Muenster
Dept of Anesthesiology and
Intensive Care Medicine, University
Hospital Bonn, Bonn, Germany
Stefan.Muenster@ukbonn.de

Paolo Navalesi
Anesthesia and Intensive Care Unit,
University Hospital Mater Domini,
Dept of Medical and Surgical
Sciences, Magna Graecia University,
Catanzaro, Italy
pnavalesi@unicz.it

Guilherme Benfatti Olivato
Dept of Critical Care Medicine,
Hospital Israelita Albert Einstein, São
Paulo, Brazil
guilherme.olivato@einstein.br

Ezgi Ozyilmaz
Dept of Chest Disease, Faculty of
Medicine, Çukurova University,
Adana, Turkey
ezgiozyilmaz@hotmail.com

Sunil Patel
Respiratory and Intensive Care
Medicine, Royal Brompton Hospital
and Imperial College London,
London, UK
sunilpatel@doctors.org.uk

Nicole Philips
Keenan Research Centre and Li
Ka Shing Institute, Dept of Critical
Care, St Michael's Hospital; and
Interdepartmental Division of Critical
Care Medicine, University of Toronto,
Toronto, Canada
n.philips@hotmail.com

Lise Piquilloud
Adult Intensive Care and Burn Unit,
Lausanne University Hospital and
Univerity of Lausanne, Lausanne,
Switzerland
Lise.Piquilloud@chuv.ch

Lara Pisani
Respiratory and critical care unit,
Alma Mater Studiorum, University
of Bologna, Sant'Orsola Malpighi
Hospital, Bologna, Italy
larapisani81@gmail.com

Christian Putensen
Dept of Anesthesiology and
Intensive Care Medicine, University
Hospital Bonn, Bonn, Germany
Christian.Putensen@ukbonn.de

V. Marco Ranieri
Alma Mater Studiorum – Università
di Bologna, Dipartimento di Scienze
Mediche e Chirurgiche, Anesthesia
and Intensive Care Medicine,
Policlinico di Sant'Orsola, Bologna,
Italy
m.ranieri@unibo.it

Louise Rose
King's College London, London, UK
louise.rose@kcl.ac.uk

Michela Rauseo
University of Toronto,
Interdepartmental Division of Critical
Care Medicine, Dept of Anesthesia,
Toronto, Canada and Dept of
Anesthesia and Intensive Care Unit,
Azienda Ospedaliero Universitaria
"Ospedali Riuniti di Foggia" and
University of Foggia, Foggia, Italy
michela.rauseo@hotmail.it

Leonardo Sarlabous
Critical Care Center, Hospital
Universitari Parc Taulí, Institut
d'Investigació i Innovació Parc
Taulí I3PT, Universitat Autònoma
de Barcelona, Barcelona; and
Biomedical Research Networking
Center in Bioengineering,
Biomaterials and Nanomedicine
(CIBER-BBN), Instituto de Salud
Carlos III, Madrid, Spain
Lsarlabous@tauli.cat

Annia Schreiber
University Health Network, Division
of Respirology, Dept of Medicine,
Toronto, ON, Canada
anniafleur.schreiber@gmail.com

Ary Serpa Neto
Dept of Critical Care Medicine,
Hospital Israelita Albert Einstein,
and Cardio-Pulmonary Dept,
Pulmonary Division, Instituto do
Coração, Hospital das Clinicas
HCFMUSP, Faculdade de Medicina,
Universidade de São Paulo, São
Paulo, Brazil; and Dept of Intensive
Care, Academic Medical Center,
Amsterdam, The Netherlands
ary.neto2@einstein.br

Giuseppe Francesco Sferrazza Papa
Casa di Cura del Policlinico,
Dipartimento di Scienze
Neuroriabilitative, Milan; and
Dipartimento di Scienze della Salute,
Università degli Studi di Milano,
Milan, Italy
francesco.sferrazza@gmail.com

Zhong-Hua Shi
Dept of Intensive Care Medicine,
Amsterdam UMC location VUmc,
and Amsterdam Cardiovascular
Sciences Research Institute,
Amsterdam, The Netherlands
hua.shi@outlook.com

Michael Sklar
Interdepartmental Division of Critical
Care Medicine, University of Toronto
and Keenan Research Centre and Li
Ka Shing Knowledge Institute,
St Michael's Hospital, Toronto,
Canada
michaelcsklar@gmail.com

Peter Somhorst
Dept of Intensive Care, Erasmus
MC University Medical Center,
Rotterdam, The Netherlands
p.somhorst@erasmusmc.nl

Irene Telias
Interdepartamental Division of
Critical Care Medicine, University of
Toronto; Keenan Research Center
and Li Ka Shing Knowledge Institute,
St. Michael's Hospital; and Division
of Respirology, Dept of Medicine,
University Health Network and
Mount Sinai Hospital, Toronto,
Canada
telias.irene@gmail.com

Nicolas Terzi
Médecine Intensive Réanimation
CHU Grenoble, Université de
Grenoble, Grenoble, France
nterzi@chu-grenoble.fr

Nic Tjahjadi
Dept of Intensive Care Medicine,
Amsterdam UMC location VUmc,
Amsterdam, The Netherlands
n.tjahjadi@amsterdamumc.nl

Tommaso Tonetti
Dept of Anesthesia and Intensive
Care, Parma University Hospital,
Parma, Italy
tommaso.tonetti@gmail.com

Pieter R. Tuinman
Dept of Intensive Care Medicine,
Amsterdam UMC location VUmc,
Amsterdam, The Netherlands
p.tuinman@amsterdamumc.nl

Francesco Vasques
Dept of Adult Critical Care, Guy's and
St Thomas' NHS Foundation Trust,
King's Health Partners, London, UK
francesco.vasques@gstt.nhs.uk

Norbert Weiler
Dept of Anaesthesiology and
Intensive Care Medicine, University
Medical Centre Schleswig-Holstein,
Kiel, Germany
norbert.weiler@uksh.de

Jakob Wittenstein
Pulmonary Engineering Group,
Department of Anaesthesiology and
Intensive Care Medicine, University
Hospital Carl Gustav Carus, Dresden,
Germany
jakob.wittenstein@uniklinikum-
dresden.de

Preface

"读万卷书不如行万里路"
"First read plenty of books, then travel plenty of places"
Confucius, 551–479 BC

Thank you for picking up this *ERS Practical Handbook of Invasive Mechanical Ventilation*. In doing so you are probably interested in artificial ventilation in general, and "invasive ventilation" in particular, but you also appear interested in reading a medical book. The former is not surprising if you are a doctor or nurse treating patients in need of ventilatory support: artificial ventilation is the cornerstone of the treatment of acute respiratory failure. The interesting question is, why would you still read a medical book in 2020? Many people have unrestricted access to hundreds of medical journals online, in addition to a variety of apps, podcasts and online videos. All these "electronic" services provide an endless amount of useful, if not practical information, and such media undoubtedly will become even more important now artificial intelligence and machine learning have entered our profession. New sources of information are a fantastic achievement, which have not only increased, and continue to increase access to information, but have probably also improved patient care, and thus patient outcomes.

However, with so much information at hand one may not see the wood for the trees. Indeed, during our daily rounds or when teaching trainees, we noticed that trainees were very aware of the most recently published RCTs on ventilatory support but frequently lacked a basic knowledge of ventilator modes, patient–ventilator interaction and ways to monitor invasively ventilated patients.

For instance, we are all aware of the RCTs that have shown survival benefit when using a low *versus* a high V_T in patients with ARDS. But does it matter whether a low V_T is delivered in a controlled mode, in a partially supported mode, or maybe in an automated, artificial intelligence-driven mode? Is a low V_T always protective? Does a low V_T, maybe, affect patient–ventilator interactions, respiratory muscle function, or even haemodynamics? To answer these questions, a fundamental understanding of the basics of invasive ventilation is required.

But there are several other topics to be discussed at the bedside. How should we act when hypoxaemia becomes refractory? When should we consider prone positioning and how does prone positioning improve outcome? What are the effects on ventilation/perfusion ratios? Is there still a role for inhalation therapies, lung recruitment manoeuvres and extracorporeal oxygenation and decarboxylation? What are their indications, and how are they best applied in clinical practice? What are the principles of artificial ventilation in patients with obstructive lung diseases or patients with interstitial lung diseases? This handbook provides concise information that is useful at the bedside for safe ventilation in patients with different lung diseases, written by recognised experts.

A prerequisite for safe invasive ventilation is adequate respiratory monitoring. Clinicians have several techniques available at the bedside, including pulse oximetry, chest radiography and CT, and lung ultrasound, but also more sophisticated techniques, such as electrical impedance tomography and oesophageal pressure measurements. Experts in this field describe the principles of these techniques, possible indications and pitfalls. This will help the clinician to choose the appropriate monitoring technique for invasively ventilated patients under different clinical conditions.

Last but not least, the process of liberating a patient from invasive ventilation, *i.e.* weaning, requires much attention. How can partially supported modes or automated modes help here? And what if a patient fails to wean? When can a tracheostomy be helpful? Especially in awake, spontaneously breathing patients, it could be important to monitor patient–ventilator interactions, respiratory mechanics and breathing efforts. Although many scientific papers have been published about weaning from invasive ventilation, very few provide clinical guidance about how to set the ventilator in a weaning patient. Experts in the field of ventilator weaning provide useful recommendations about how to ventilate patients during the weaning process and a practical approach to the difficult to wean patient.

All the of above is covered in the chapters in this book that all follow a similar approach: providing basic background information, helpful graphics, a summary of the evidence, and finally a list for further reading.

To finish, we would like to express our sincere gratitude to the authors that have contributed to this book – they are the experts and the knowledge-base that drives this book. Selection of authors for this book was by an invitation to the members of Assembly 2 of the European Respiratory Society (ERS), made during the ERS International Congress in Paris, France in 2018. Both early career members and senior members responded enthusiastically and spent their valuable time writing these chapters for you. We would also like to thank the ERS publications office for their support and hard work to complete this ambitious project. And thank you, dear reader, for picking up this handbook. We hope you enjoy reading it and that it helps you to improve your understanding of the basics of invasive ventilation. After reading this book, you will spend more time at the bedside applying what you learned from the nicely written chapters in this book. Choosing the correct individual settings, the best mode, closely observing how the ventilator and patient interact, and understanding what you actually monitor will certainly further improve your knowledge of invasive mechanical ventilation. To paraphrase Confucius: First read plenty of books, than observe and manage plenty of ventilated patients.

Leo Heunks and Marcus J. Schultz
Chief Editors

Get more from this Handbook

By buying the *ERS Practical Handbook of Invasive Mechanical Ventilation*, you also gain access to the electronic version of the book, as well as an accredited online CME test.

Simply visit http://ersbookshop.com/titles and add the *ERS Practical Handbook of Invasive Mechanical Ventilation* to your cart. At the checkout, enter the unique voucher code printed on the inside front cover of the book. You will then be able to download the entire book in PDF format to read on your computer or mobile device.

You'll also be able to take the online CME test. This Practical Handbook has been accredited by the European Board for Accreditation in Pneumology (EBAP) for 8 CME credits.

Also available from the ERS

ERS Practical Handbook of Noninvasive Ventilation
Edited by Anita K. Simonds

This handbook provides a concise 'why and how to' guide to NIV from the basics of equipment and patient selection to discharge planning and community care.
Leading clinicians and researchers in the field have been brought together to provide an easy-to-read guide to all aspects of NIV. Topics covered include: equipment, patient selection, adult and paediatric indications, airway clearance and physiotherapy, acute NIV monitoring, NIV in the ICU, long-term NIV, indications for tracheostomy ventilation, symptom palliation, discharge planning and community care, and setting up an NIV service.

List of abbreviations

AHI	Apnoea–hypopnoea index
AIDS	Acquired immunodeficiency syndrome
ALS	Amyotrophic lateral sclerosis
ARDS	Acute respiratory distress syndrome
ARF	Acute respiratory failure
ASB	Assisted spontaneous breathing
ASV	Adaptive servo ventilation
ASSPCV	Assisted pressure-controlled ventilation
AVAPS	Average volume-assured pressure support
BMI	Body mass index
CF	Cystic fibrosis
COPD	Chronic obstructive pulmonary disease
CPAP	Continuous positive airway pressure
ECG	Electrocardiogram
EPAP	Expiratory positive airway pressure
FEV1	Forced expiratory volume in 1 s
$F_{I}o_2$	Inspiratory oxygen fraction
FVC	Forced vital capacity
HIV	Human immunodeficiency virus
ICU	Intensive care unit
IPAP	Inspiratory positive airway pressure
IPPV	Intermittent positive pressure ventilation
IVAPS	Intelligent volume-assured pressure support
NIV	Noninvasive ventilation
NPV	Negative pressure ventilation
OHS	Obesity hypoventilation syndrome
OSA(S)	Obstructive sleep apnoea (syndrome)
$P_{a}co_2$	Arterial carbon dioxide tension
$P_{a}o_2$	Arterial oxygen tension
PAV	Proportional assist ventilation
PCV	Pressure-controlled ventilation
PEEP	Positive end-expiratory pressure
PSV	Pressure support ventilation
$P_{tc}co_2$	Transcutaneous carbon dioxide tension
$S_{a}o_2$	Arterial oxygen saturation
RCT	Randomised controlled trial
$S_{p}o_2$	Arterial oxygen saturation measured by pulse oximetry
TB	Tuberculosis
TLC	Total lung capacity
VCV	Volume-controlled ventilation
V_T	Tidal volume

Conflicts of interest

Lu Chen: None declared.

Davide Chiumello: None declared.

Rebecca F. D'Cruz: None declared.

Candelaria de Haro: None declared.

Frans de Jongh: None declared.

Gustavo Faissol Janot de Matos: None declared.

Alexandre Demoule: reports personal fees from Medtronic, Baxter, Hamilton, Getinge and Respinor, grants, personal fees and non-financial support from Philips, grants and personal fees from Fisher & Paykel, and grants from the French Ministry of Health, outside the submitted work

Heder J. de Vries: None declared.

Martin Dres: M. Dres reports travel expenses and expertise fees from Lungpacer Medical Inc.

José Aquino Esperanza: None declared.

Antonio M. Esquinas: None declared.

Ricardo Estêvão Gomes: None declared.

Eddy Fan: reports personal fees from MC3 Cardiopulmonary and ALung Technologies, outside the submitted work.

Bernard Fikkers: None declared.

Christoph Fisser: None declared.

Tim Frenzel: None declared.

Inéz Frerichs: reports grants from the European Commission (projects: WELCOME (Grant No. 611223), CRADL (Grant No. 668259) and WELMO (Grant No. 825572)), personal fees from Dräger Medical (speaking fees and reimbursement of travel costs), outside the submitted work.

Louis-Marie Galerneau: None declared.

Marcelo Gama de Abreu: reports personal fees from AMBU Medical, grants and personal fees from GlaxoSmithKline, and grants and personal fees from GE Healthcare, outside the submitted work.

Marco Giani: reports personal fees from Pfizer, outside the submitted work;

Rik Gosselink: None declared.

Claude Guérin: None declared.

Nicholas Hart: reports unrestricted grants from Philips-Respironics, Resmed, B&D Electromedical, and Fisher-Paykel outside of the area of work commented on here with the funds held by Guy's & St Thomas' NHS Foundation Trust; financial support from Philips for development of the MYOTRACE technology that has patent filed in Europe (US pending) outside the area of work commented on here; personal fees for lecturing from Philips-Respironics, Resmed, Fisher-Paykel outside the area of work commented on here; N. Hart is on the Pulmonary Research Advisory Board for Philips outside the area of work commented on here with the funds for this role held and administered by Guy's & St Thomas' NHS Foundation Trust.

Robert Huhle: None declared.

Christina Iezzi: None declared.

Annemijn H. Jonkman: None declared.

Georgios Kaltsakas: None declared.

Cenk Kirakli: None declared.

Federico Longhini: has a patent HFNC+CPAP - Intersurgical SpA pending.

Cong Lu: None declared.

Rudys Magrans: None declared.

Jordi Mancebo: None declared.

Luis Morales-Quinteros: None declared.

Elise Morawiec: None declared.

Stefan Muenster: None declared.

Paolo Navalesi: reports grants and personal fees from Maquet Critical Care; non-financial support from Draeger and Intersurgical SpA; personal fees from Orionpharma, Philips, ResMed, MSD Merck Sharp & Dohme and Novartis, all outside the submitted work. In addition, P. Navalesi has a patent NEXT Helmet - Intersursigal SpA with royalties paid, and a patent HFNC+CPAP - Intersurgical SpA pending.

Guilherme Benfatti Olivato: None declared.

Ezgi Ozyilmaz: None declared.

Sunil Patel: None declared.

Nicole Philips: None declared.

Lise Piquilloud: reports fees from Getinge for lectures related to NAVA.

Lara Pisani: reports personal fees from Resmed, Fisher and Paykel, and Chiesi, outside the submitted work.

Christian Putensen: None declared.

V. Marco Ranieri: None declared.

Louise Rose: None declared.

Michela Rauseo: None declared.

Leonardo Sarlabous: None declared.

Annia Schreiber: None declared.

Ary Serpa Neto: None declared.

Giuseppe Francesco Sferrazza Papa: None declared.

Zhong-Hua Shi: None declared.

Michael Sklar: None declared.

Peter Somhorst: reports personal fees from Getinge, outside the submitted work

Irene Telias: reports personal fees from Covidien, Argentina and MBMed SA, outside the submitted work.

Nicolas Terzi: reports personal fees from Boerhinger Ingelheim France, outside the submitted work.

Nic Tjahjadi: None declared.

Tommaso Tonetti: None declared.

Pieter R. Tuinman: None declared.

Francesco Vasques: None declared.

Norbert Weiler: None declared.

Jakob Wittenstein: None declared.

Mechanisms of hypoxaemia and hypercapnia

Rebecca F. D'Cruz and Nicholas Hart

The primary function of the respiratory system is maintenance of gas exchange, which is achieved through ventilation, diffusion and perfusion. These processes enable oxygenation of systemic tissue and removal of carbon dioxide, a metabolic by-product of cellular respiration. An understanding of the physiological principles that cause hypoxaemia and hypercapnia underpins effective oxygenation and ventilation strategies for patients in respiratory failure.

Hypoxaemia

Oxygen diffuses down a pressure gradient from the alveoli into the pulmonary capillaries and is transported in blood predominantly by binding reversibly to haemoglobin. Oxygenation can be quantified by measuring oxygen saturation, which represents the proportion of haemoglobin binding sites bound to oxygen, and $P_{a}O_2$, which quantifies the amount of oxygen dissolved in plasma. $S_{a}O_2$ reflects the oxygen content of arterial blood, $S_{p}O_2$ reflects oxygen content measured by pulse oximetry. Although it is difficult to define a normal range for $P_{a}O_2$ given the limited data in healthy subjects, ranges of 90–110 mmHg (12.0–14.6 kPa) can be applied, with a value of <60 mmHg (8.0 kPa) diagnostic of hypoxaemia. Hypoxaemia should be distinguished from hypoxia, which is insufficient oxygen at the cellular level, categorised as:

- hypoxic (low $P_{a}O_2$ and $S_{a}O_2$),
- anaemic (reduced oxygen-carrying capacity of blood),

Key points

- Hypoxaemia and hypercapnia are quantified with arterial partial pressures of oxygen ($P_{a}O_2$) and carbon dioxide ($P_{a}CO_2$).

- Abnormal gas exchange may be evaluated by calculating the alveolar–arterial P_{O_2} gradient ($P_{O_2(A-a)}$) and the $P_{a}O_2$ (mmHg) to fraction of inspired oxygen ($F_{I}O_2$) ratio ($P_{a}O_2/F_{I}O_2$).

- The five principal causes of hypoxaemia are ventilation/perfusion mismatch, hypoventilation, diffusion limitation, right-to-left shunt and reduced inspired oxygen tension.

- Hypercapnia arises as a consequence of imbalance in the load–capacity–drive relationship of the respiratory muscle pump.

- circulatory (insufficient oxygen delivery), or
- histotoxic (cells cannot utilise oxygen despite normal delivery).

$P_{O_2(A-a)}$ can be used to determine the presence of abnormal gas exchange:

$$P_{O_2(A-a)} = P_{AO_2} - P_{aO_2}$$

where P_{AO_2} is the alveolar oxygen tension.

Using the alveolar gas equation:

$$P_{AO_2} = P_{IO_2} - P_{aCO_2}/R$$

where P_{IO_2} is the partial pressure of inspired oxygen and R is the respiratory exchange ratio (taken as 0.8).

Defining the alveolar–arterial gradient requires accurate quantification of P_{IO_2}. This can be achieved during invasive ventilation, but is unreliable when supplementary oxygen is delivered *via* nasal cannula or a standard facemask. Calculation of P_{aO_2} (mmHg) to fraction of inspired oxygen (F_{IO_2}) ratio (P_{aO_2}/F_{IO_2}) is more practical and may be used to define and monitor patients with ARDS. A P_{aO_2}/F_{IO_2} of ≤300 mmHg (40.0 kPa) indicates impaired gas exchange.

Hypercapnia

Carbon dioxide is transported in the blood predominantly as bicarbonate and is quantified using P_{aCO_2} (normal reference range 34–45 mmHg (4.6–6.0 kPa)). P_{aCO_2} is the gold standard to diagnose hypercapnia and should be measured prior to commencing or discontinuing invasive ventilation. In a steady clinical state with normal cardiac output, central or mixed venous samples correlate closely with P_{aCO_2}; however, peripheral venous P_{CO_2} correlates poorly and should not be used as a surrogate measure of P_{aCO_2}.

Arterial blood gases performed to obtain P_{aCO_2} are invasive and painful; therefore, alternative methods of carbon dioxide monitoring may be implemented. P_{tcCO_2} measures carbon dioxide diffusing through the skin using a heated skin probe that causes local arterialisation. Earlobe placement of a probe heated to 42°C produces P_{tcCO_2} values that correlate acceptably with P_{aCO_2}. If available, P_{tcCO_2} can be used to continuously monitor carbon dioxide trends to support monitoring of clinical progress and response to interventions.

Capnography can be used during invasive ventilation to measure carbon dioxide at the airway opening and involves an infrared absorption sensor positioned in the ventilator circuit. The capnography waveform comprises four phases:

- Phase I measures inspired gas and early expiration of anatomical dead space, where carbon dioxide is absent
- Phase II measures expired alveolar gas, therefore P_{CO_2} rises steeply
- Phase III measures the plateau of expired alveolar gas, providing a value for end-tidal P_{CO_2} (P_{ETCO_2})
- Phase IV commences at inspiration of the next breath at which carbon dioxide falls back to zero

When ventilation and perfusion are perfectly matched, P_{ETCO_2} accurately reflects alveolar and therefore arterial carbon dioxide. However, if alveolar ventilation and perfusion are mismatched, P_{ETCO_2} underestimates P_{aCO_2}. Expiratory time set on the ventilator may also cause P_{ETCO_2} to underestimate P_{aCO_2} by cutting expiration short before a representative end-tidal value is obtained. Absolute values of P_{ETCO_2} should therefore not be used as a surrogate of P_{aCO_2} to monitor clinical trajectory in critical care or during decision making for weaning from invasive ventilation. However, P_{ETCO_2} trends may be useful to monitor patients' progress and may be used by advanced ventilator modes which can adjust settings based on P_{ETCO_2}. P_{ETCO_2} is also valuable in confirmation of endotracheal tube placement and indication of return of spontaneous circulation following cardiac arrest.

Respiratory failure

Hypoxaemic type 1 respiratory failure (P_{aO_2} <60 mmHg (8.0 kPa)) represents intrinsic lung failure. Hypercapnic type 2 respiratory failure (P_{aCO_2} >45 mmHg (6.0 kPa)) represents failure of the respiratory muscle pump, in which there is imbalance in the load–capacity–drive relationship of the respiratory system. Causes of hypoxaemia are listed in table 1.

Mechanisms of hypoxaemia

Ventilation/perfusion mismatch P_{aO_2} is determined by the ratio of alveolar ventilation to pulmonary perfusion. Lung areas with a higher V'/Q' ratio (high ventilation relative to perfusion) have higher P_{AO_2} and lower alveolar carbon dioxide tension (P_{ACO_2}) and contribute minimally to arterial oxygenation. Areas with a lower V'/Q' ratio (low ventilation relative to perfusion) have lower P_{AO_2} and higher P_{ACO_2} and contribute more to gas exchange since they are better perfused. Pathological processes that increase heterogeneity of lung ventilation and perfusion increase V'/Q' mismatch, with the net effect of hypoxaemia.

V'/Q' mismatch may also lead to hypercapnia. This may be mitigated by compensatory hyperventilation triggered by chemoreceptors that increase neural respiratory drive (NRD) in response to rising hydrogen ions as a consequence of increased P_{aCO_2}. Due to the linear shape of the carbon dioxide dissociation curve, increased minute ventilation tends to normalise hypercapnia through increased carbon dioxide elimination from regions of both high and low V'/Q' ratios. Hypoxaemia may be improved but cannot be corrected by hyperventilation due to the sigmoid shape of the oxygen dissociation curve, which benefits only lung regions with a moderately low V'/Q' ratio. In obstructive lung disease, which is characterised by expiratory flow limitation, increased respiratory rate shortens the time available for adequate expiration. The consequent acute increase in end-expiratory lung volume is termed dynamic hyperinflation, which increases work of breathing, due to the elastic and threshold loads it imposes, and may impair ventilation and lead to hypercapnia, due to increased physiological dead space. Other compensatory mechanisms to mitigate the effects of hypoxaemia include increased oxygen uptake by peripheral tissue and increased cardiac output.

V'/Q' mismatch is the commonest cause of hypoxaemia and can be quantified using $P_{O_2(A-a)}$, with an increased gradient reflecting greater mismatch.

Table 1. Mechanisms of hypoxaemia

Mechanism	Causes

Ventilation/ perfusion (V'/Q') mismatch	Low V'/Q'
	  COPD
	  Asthma
	  Pulmonary oedema
	  Interstitial lung disease

	High V'/Q' Pulmonary embolism

Hypoventilation	NRD depression
	  Pharmacological
	  Cortical/brainstem ischaemia, haemorrhage or trauma

	Nerve/neuromuscular junction pathology
	  Spinal cord lesion
	  Poliomyelitis
	  Motor neuron disease
	  Guillain–Barré syndrome
	  Myaesthenia gravis

	Muscle weakness
	  Muscular dystrophy
	  Inflammatory myopathy
	  Critical illness
	  Hyperinflation (functional respiratory muscle weakness)
	  Electrolyte imbalance
	  Thyroid myopathy

	Chest wall abnormality
	  Obesity
	  Kyphoscoliosis
	  Flail chest

Diffusion limitation	Interstitial lung disease

Shunt	Anatomical
	  Intracardiac
	  Pulmonary arteriovenous malformation
	  Hepatopulmonary syndrome

	Physiological
	  ARDS
	  Pneumonia
	  Atelectasis

Reduced P_{IO_2}	Altitude

Hypoventilation P_{AO_2} is determined by alveolar ventilation and capillary uptake of oxygen. If alveolar ventilation falls, alveolar oxygen falls and carbon dioxide rises. Provided alveolar perfusion remains stable, the diffusion gradient between the alveoli and pulmonary capillaries consequently falls, giving rise to hypoxaemia and hypercapnia.

Diffusion limitation Thickening of the blood–gas barrier causes incomplete gas transfer *via* diffusion between the alveoli and pulmonary capillaries. Diffusion limitation alone is insufficient to cause resting hypoxaemia, but hypoxaemia may manifest during exercise (when increased cardiac output reduces erythrocyte time in the pulmonary circulation, which reduces the time available for adequate gas exchange) or in combination with V'/Q' mismatch, which may occur in interstitial lung diseases.

Shunt Right-to-left shunting is when blood passes from the right to left side of the heart without passing through ventilated lung. This profound V'/Q' mismatch causes hypoxaemia that cannot be corrected with 100% inspired oxygen. The degree of response in P_{aO_2} to 100% inspired oxygen depends on the shunt fraction:

$$Q_s/Q_t = (C_{cO_2} - C_{aO_2})/(C_{cO_2} - C_{vO_2})$$

where Q_s is pulmonary physiologic shunt, Q_t is cardiac output, C_{cO_2} is pulmonary capillary oxygen content, C_{aO_2} is arterial oxygen content and C_{vO_2} is mixed venous oxygen content.

Reduced inspired oxygen tension P_{IO_2} falls with barometric pressure, which occurs at altitude. Referring to the alveolar gas equation, P_{aO_2} theoretically falls at the same rate as P_{IO_2}, provided P_{CO_2} and R remain constant. In practice, hypoxia at altitude stimulates hyperventilation, which lowers carbon dioxide and increases P_{O_2} compared with at sea level.

Mechanisms of hypercapnia

Hypercapnia is a consequence of imbalance in the loads, capacity and drive of the respiratory muscle pump (figure 1).

Respiratory muscle load Loads imposed on the respiratory muscle pump may be resistive (secondary to airways obstruction, bronchospasm or secretions) or elastic as a consequence of reduced respiratory system compliance (as in obesity, scoliosis, chest wall disease, hyperinflation, pleural effusion and abdominal distension, which reduce extrinsic chest wall compliance; or pneumonia, alveolar oedema, atelectasis and interstitial lung disease, which reduce intrinsic lung compliance). If present, intrinsic positive airways pressure (PEEPi) imposes a threshold load which must be overcome to generate inspiratory flow. PEEPi is characteristic of obstructive lung disease, in which increased airways resistance limits expiratory airflow, resulting in hyperinflation. PEEPi may also occur in obesity where breathing at low V_T causes early airway closure.

Respiratory muscle loads can be quantified by measuring the transdiaphragmatic pressures required to generate airflow using gastric and oesophageal balloon catheters connected to a pressure transducer. The area under the diaphragm pressure curve defines the pressure–time product, which reflects respiratory muscle load. PEEPi is measured as the change in oesophageal pressure generated prior to the onset of inspiratory flow.

Inspiratory muscle capacity Inspiratory muscle capacity may be impaired where there is pathology of the spinal cord, peripheral nerves, neuromuscular junction or skeletal muscle (table 1), and can be quantified with maximal voluntary inspiratory manoeuvres, including sniff nasal pressure and maximum inspiratory pressure at

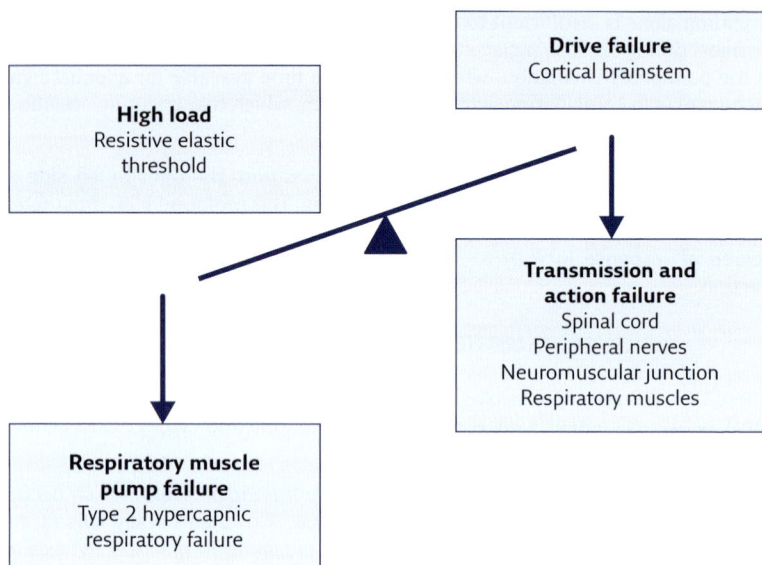

Figure 1. Type 2 hypercapnic respiratory failure is an imbalance between NRD, the load on the respiratory muscles and capacity of the respiratory muscles. Reproduced from Suh et al. *(2012),* Medicine; *40: 293–297, with permission.*

the mouth. For patients who cannot perform maximal voluntary manoeuvres, such as patients in intensive care, twitch transdiaphragmatic pressure with phrenic nerve magnetic stimulation can be performed in specialist centres.

Neural respiratory drive NRD reflects the balance between respiratory muscle load and capacity. As it is not possible to directly measure output from the central respiratory control centre, surrogate measures are applied in clinical practice. Mouth occlusion pressure in the first 100 ms of inspiration at functional residual capacity ($P_{0.1}$), measured with a pneumotachograph and one-way valve, is a simple and noninvasive marker of NRD. $P_{0.1}$ in healthy subjects is ~1 cmH$_2$O. Large differences between $P_{0.1}$ and minute ventilation indicate increased respiratory muscle load. $P_{0.1}$ is less reliable at higher operating lung volumes and with airflow resistance, particularly in patients with obstructive lung disease and PEEPi. Electromyography of the diaphragm (EMGdi, using a gastro-oesophageal multipair electrode catheter) or parasternal muscles (EMGpara, using surface electrodes) has been used as a physiological biomarker reflecting NRD. EMGpara has been used to monitor inpatient clinical trajectory during severe COPD exacerbations and can predict COPD patients who are safe to be discharged from hospital. EMGpara also reflects disease severity and exercise-induced breathlessness in COPD, asthma and cystic fibrosis.

Summary

Hypoxaemia (P_{aO_2} <60 mmHg (8.0 kPa)) is most commonly caused by V'/Q' mismatch. Hypercapnia (P_{aCO_2} >45 mmHg (6.0 kPa)) is a consequence of imbalance in the loads and capacity of the respiratory muscle pump, which can be assessed by measuring NRD. The alveolar–arterial PO_2 gradient ($PO_{2(A-a)}$) and PaO_2/FIO_2 ratio are used to evaluate gas exchange abnormalities. Management of respiratory failure must always involve identification and treatment of the underlying pathophysiology.

Further reading

- D'Cruz RF, *et al.* (2018). Positive airway pressure devices for the management of breathlessness. *Curr Opin Support Palliat Care*; 12: 246–252.

- Jolley CJ, *et al.* (2009). A physiological model of patient-reported breathlessness during daily activities in COPD. *Eur Respir Rev*; 18: 66–79.

- Wagner PD (2015). The physiological basis of pulmonary gas exchange: implications for clinical interpretation of arterial blood gases. *Eur Respir J*; 45: 227–243.

- West J (2015). West's Respiratory Physiology: The Essentials. Philadelphia, Lippincott Williams and Wilkins.

Respiratory mechanics

Guilherme Benfatti Olivato, Robert Huhle, Marcelo Gama de Abreu and Ary Serpa Neto

Invasive ventilation with positive pressure promotes relevant changes in respiratory system mechanics, and there are several variables with clinical relevance that can be measured during invasive ventilation. Currently, most ventilators display ventilatory curves, for example airway pressure, gas flow and respiratory system volume. Using modelling, data on respiratory mechanics can be derived from these signals.

Monitoring of the respiratory system mechanics should be conducted routinely on every patient submitted to invasive ventilation. Among several possibilities, its applications include:

1) diagnosis;
2) correct titration of ventilatory settings according to physiological thresholds and therapeutic goals; and
3) continuous assessment of the response to the treatment.

This chapter highlights the concepts of basic monitoring of respiratory mechanics in patients under invasive ventilation.

Resistance

Gas flow originates from a pressure gradient, from the higher pressure towards the lower. In patients undergoing invasive ventilation, this may exist between

Key points

- Monitoring of respiratory system mechanics should be conducted routinely on every patient submitted to invasive ventilation.

- Resistance of the airway (R_{aw}) is the relationship between the pressure gradient in the airways and flow ($P_{aw} - P_{plat}$/flow).

- C_{rs} is the relationship between the inspiratory volume and the variation of pressure inside the chest wall and the lungs ($V_T/P_{plat} - PEEP$).

- The mechanical power of ventilation, which can be calculated from routinely measured ventilator parameters, has been associated with pulmonary inflammation, oedema and in-hospital mortality in critical ill patients.

the trachea (P_{tr}) and the alveoli (P_{alv}). Therefore, when the tracheal and alveolar pressures are known, for an established flow, it is possible to calculate the airway resistance. The relationship between the pressure gradient in the airways and flow determine the resistance of the airway (R_{aw}). Assuming the flow during inspiration is constant, the following formula can be considered:

$$R_{aw} = \frac{P_{tr} - P_{alv}}{\text{Flow}} \tag{1}$$

For patients under invasive ventilation, the pressure is measured before the endotracheal tube; therefore, the resistance measured using proximal inspiratory pressure, mentioned as the pressure in the airway (P_{aw}), is in fact the sum of the resistances of the endotracheal tube and of the patient's airway, being referred to as the total R_{aw} of the respiratory system. This difference between the P_{aw} and the P_{alv} is called resistive pressure (P_{res}), and as P_{alv} equals the airway pressure during zero flow end-inspiration occlusion P_{plat}, the R_{aw} can therefore be summarised as (figure 1):

$$R_{aw} = R_{aw}(\text{tube}) + R_{aw}(\text{patient}) = \frac{P_{aw} - P_{alv}}{\text{Flow}} = \frac{P_{res}}{\text{Flow}} = \frac{P_{aw} - P_{plat}}{\text{Flow}} \tag{2}$$

The unit of measurement of R_{aw} is $cmH_2O \cdot s \cdot L^{-1}$ and values considered normal in humans are between 4 and 8 $cmH_2O \cdot s \cdot L^{-1}$, depending on the internal diameter of

$$R_{aw} = \frac{P_{peak} - P_{plat}}{\text{Flow}} = \frac{40 - 30}{1} = 10 \ cmH_2O \cdot s \cdot L^{-1}$$

$$C_{rs} = \frac{V_T}{P_{plat} - PEEP} = \frac{500}{30 - 5} = 20 \ mL \cdot cmH_2O^{-1}$$

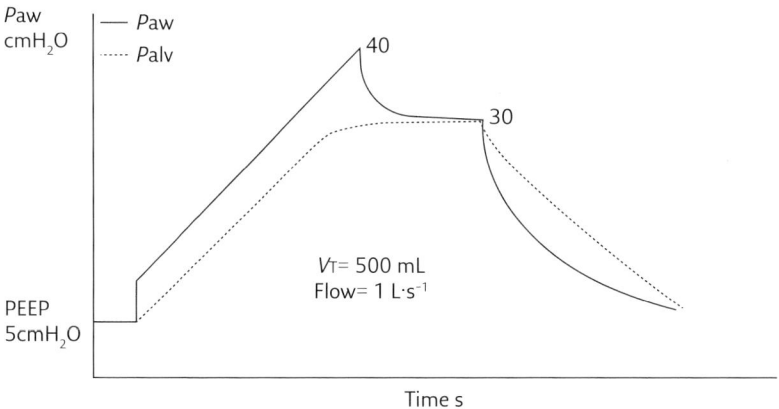

Figure 1. Calculation of R_{aw} and C_{rs} of the respiratory system in a patient under volume-controlled invasive ventilation. Knowing the V_T, with constant or rectangular inspiratory flow and measuring the P_{plat} and P_{peak}, R_{aw} and C_{rs} can be calculated. Reproduced and modified from Barbas et al. (2014), Rev Bras Ter Intensiva; 26: 89–121, with permission.

Table 1. *Expected ranges of the variables discussed*

	Raw cmH$_2$O·s·L^{-1}	Crs mL·cmH$_2$O^{-1}	Mechanical power J·min^{-1}
Normal	4–8	60–80	Not defined
ARDS	4–8	35–45	Not defined
COPD	10–30	50–70	Not defined

the tube and the presence or absence of an obstruction to the air flow in the airway (table 1). Conditions such as bronchospasm and the presence of secretions in the airway are the most common causes of elevation in R_{aw}.

Compliance

The increase in pulmonary volume during the inspiratory phase leads to pulmonary and chest wall expansion, stretching the elastic structures of the respiratory system. Similar to a spring system, the elastic structure exerts opposite forces proportional to the deformation, which is in turn equivalent to the inspiratory volume. This elastic force, diffused through the lung's surface, generates positive intrapulmonary pressure. The relationship between the inspiratory volume (ΔV) and the variation of pressure inside the chest wall and the lungs (ΔP) corresponds to the respiratory system compliance (C_{rs}):

$$C_{rs} = \frac{\Delta V}{\Delta P} \tag{3}$$

In the presence of PEEP, the difference in pressure due to the inspiratory volume, is the difference between the P_{alv} and the PEEP. The C_{rs} can therefore be summarised as:

$$C_{rs} = \frac{\Delta V}{P_{alv} - PEEP} \tag{4}$$

Compliance is the variable that evaluates the stiffness of the respiratory system. During ventilatory support, C_{rs} represents the relationship between the ΔV and the difference between P_{plat} and the pressure at the end of expiration (PEEP):

$$C_{rs} = \frac{\Delta V}{P_{plat} - PEEP} \tag{5}$$

The unit of measurement of C_{rs} is mL·cmH$_2$O^{-1} and values considered normal are around 60–80 mL·cmH$_2$O^{-1} (table 1). Its inverse is called elastance (defined as $1/C_{rs}$). C_{rs} may be reduced in clinical scenarios like tuberculosis, pulmonary fibrosis or ARDS.

While C_{rs} as described above can be determined during tidal ventilation without any additional intervention, the quasi-static compliance of the respiratory system (C_{stat})

is measured during prolonged end-inspiratory occlusion and during slow inflation manoeuvres. In contrast to the commonly used C_{rs}, the true C_{stat} is the compliance of the respiratory system with any viscoelastic stress and strain at equilibrium with zero flow. However, to date, the additional clinical value of measuring C_{stat} compared with C_{rs} has not been shown and thus it is rarely measured in clinical practice.

Resistance and compliance in clinical practice

The measurement of the P_{plat} is mandatory for the calculation of respiratory mechanics. To identify the resistive and elastic elements throughout the respiratory cycle, the inspiratory pause, that delays the opening of the expiratory valve is of unique importance. During an inspiratory pause there is no flow in the airway, therefore, the pressure measured at the end of this pause (P_{plat}) is close to the P_{alv}. In addition, the pressure measured immediately before the pause is the P_{peak}. Yet, in every respiratory cycle the ventilator measures the variation in volume, namely the V_T and the flow (figure 1). Thus, in clinical practice, R_{aw} and C_{rs} are calculated according to equations (2) and (5), defined above.

Respiratory mechanics modelled by resistance and compliance require a passive respiratory system, *e.g.* without spontaneous breathing activity. Recent results of modelling only portions of the expiratory signals suggest that an approximation is possible in assisted ventilation modes. However, care must be taken that no spontaneous breathing activity is overlapping with the analysed signal portion.

Lung compliance and transpulmonary pressure

The respiratory system has two main tissue components: the lung parenchyma, that fills the cavity formed by the chest wall, and the diaphragm. The parenchyma consists of a soft tissue containing different amounts of elastin and collagen fibres. The lung parenchyma has a higher mechanical compliance compared with the chest wall, which is formed by solid bones, and the diaphragm, the major muscle driving spontaneous breathing. The compliance of the parenchyma is subject to huge variations due to pathology and therapy during invasive ventilation (*e.g.* oedema, collapse). The compliance of the chest wall and the diaphragm may be considered as time invariant during short to medium intervals of invasive ventilation, but might be subject to externally restricted movement.

The transpulmonary pressure (P_L) can be derived as the difference between P_{alv} and the pressure in the pleura (P_{pl}), a liquid filled double membrane that connects the lung to the chest wall without restricting lung movement along the latter:

$$P_L = P_{alv} - P_{pl} \qquad (6)$$

Lung compliance (C_L) can be obtained by:

$$C_L = \frac{V_T}{P_{plat} - PEEP - (P_{plat,L} - PEEP_L)} \qquad (7)$$

where $P_{plat,L}$ is transpulmonary end-inspiratory pressure and $PEEP_L$ is transpulmonary end-expiratory pressure. P_{pl} is subject to hydrostatic alterations, depending on the body position. In the supine position, ventral pleural pressure can be up to 10 cmH$_2$O lower than dorsal pleural pressure. Similarly, in caudal regions

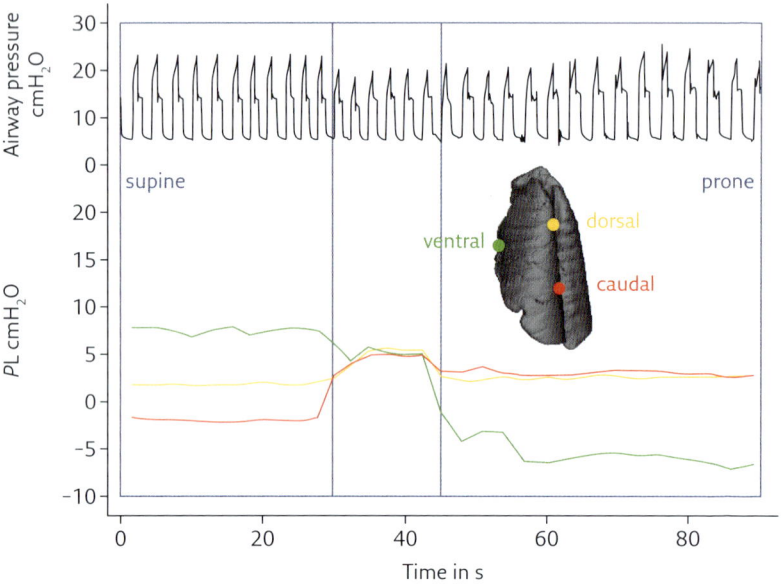

Figure 2. *Transpulmonary pressure (P*L*) in ventral (green), dorsal (yellow) and caudal (red) regions in a healthy pig during shifting from a supine to prone position during volume-controlled ventilation.*

the weight of the abdominal cavity increases P_{pl}. If P_{pl} exceeds P_{alv}, the P_L becomes negative. This essentially means that the respective alveoli collapse as the alveolus' exterior pressure exceeds its internal pressure. Therefore, dorsal and caudal lung regions are more prone to collapse in the supine position (figure 2).

As the direct local measurement of P_{pl} is highly invasive, it is not suitable for clinical application. However, a minimally invasive surrogate for the average P_{pl} of the whole lung is assessable through measurement of oesophageal pressure (P_{oes}). This is increasingly used in clinical scenarios, such as PEEP titration, assessing the amount of spontaneous breathing, and potentially muscular work and power of ventilation.

Mechanical work and mechanical power

To overcome resistive and elastic forces during tidal controlled invasive ventilation as well as during spontaneous breathing, mechanical work (MW) or mechanical energy is performed by the ventilator and/or by the respiratory muscles, respectively. The derivation of MW and mechanical power (MP) from the routinely measured respiratory signals during controlled invasive ventilation and an approximation from the respiratory mechanical parameters resistance and compliance is presented in this section.

Mechanical energy or MW during tidal ventilation is derived by integration of P_{aw} change over the respective change of V_T:

$$MW = \int_{(V_T)} \Delta P_{aw}(V)dV \qquad (8)$$

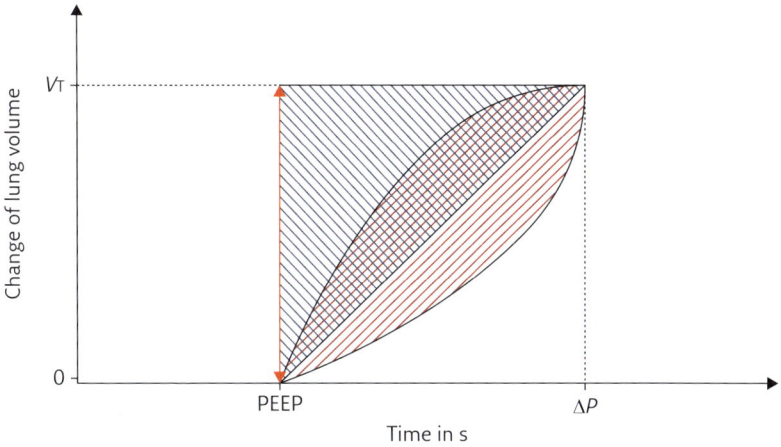

Figure 3. Change of lung volume during tidal ventilation with PEEP, driving pressure (ΔP) and tidal volume (VT). Elastic MW (blue lines), resistive MW during inspiration (red lines) and during expiration (crossed) areas are shown; airway pressure does not change from zero to PEEP during tidal ventilation and thus no PEEP-related MW is present (area is zero, indicated by the red double arrow).

Conversely, inspiratory MW can be calculated integrating the inspiratory pressure volume curve from zero to V_T. This MW is spent to overcome the elastic and resistive components of the respiratory system.

The expiratory MW is derived when integrating the expiratory pressure volume curve from V_T to zero (figure 3). While inspiratory MW is positive, expiratory MW is negative from the perspective of the ventilator, as this work is performed by the elastic recoil forces of the respiratory system. One part of this expiratory MW is spent pushing volume back into the expiratory branch of the ventilator circuit and another part is used to overcome resistive forces during expiration. As both the resistive and the elastic components of the respiratory system govern the MW, the later can be expressed as a function of dynamic respiratory system compliance (C_{dyn}) and respiratory system resistance (R_{aw}):

$$MW = \int_{(V_T)} \left(R_{aw} \cdot \dot{V} + \frac{1}{C_{dyn}} \cdot V \right) dV \tag{9}$$

Assuming constant flow, volume-controlled invasive ventilation with a rectangular inspiratory flow curve and constant resistance and compliance during inspiration:

$$MW = \left(R_{aw} \cdot \frac{1+I:E}{60 \cdot I:E} \cdot RR + \frac{1}{2 \cdot C_{dyn}} \right) \cdot V_T^2 \tag{10}$$

where I:E is inspiratory to expiratory ratio and RR is the respiratory rate.

MP may be derived from MW by multiplication with RR:

$$MP = RR \cdot V_T^2 \cdot \left(\frac{1}{2} EL_{rs} + RR \cdot \frac{(1+I:E)}{60 \cdot I:E} \cdot R_{aw} \right) \tag{11}$$

where EL_{rs} is the elastance of the respiratory system.

A minimisation of MP is discussed as a bedside tool to avoid development of VILI (table 1). MP was associated with neutrophilic inflammation in a retrospective analysis of a study in an experimental model of ARDS. MP was furthermore associated with in-hospital mortality in critical ill patients in a retrospective study.

During spontaneous breathing, all the mechanical work involved is performed by the respiratory muscles. Hence, equation (8) becomes:

$$MW = \int_{(V_T)} P_{mus}(V)dV \tag{12}$$

with intra-thoracic pressure generated by the respiratory muscles (P_{mus}) to achieve a respective V_T; however, the measurement of oesophageal and static recoil pressure of the chest wall is necessary. In assisted invasive ventilation a comparable method may be used with good agreement with equation (8).

Summary

Mechanical ventilators can continuously measure airway flow, pressure and volumes, allowing the calculation of R_{aw} and C_{rs}, and the display of volume–pressure and flow–volume loops. Whereas routine measurement of local P_{pl} is not feasible in clinical practice, measurement of its minimally invasive surrogate P_{oes} has gained increased attention and might be useful in clinical practice. However, its potential to improve clinical outcome remains uncertain. The mechanical work and power of ventilation, which can be calculated from routinely measured ventilator parameters, have been associated with pulmonary inflammation, oedema and in-hospital mortality in critical ill patients. However, further research is warranted to define their potential as targets for invasive ventilation.

Further reading

- Gattinoni L, *et al.* (2016). Ventilator-related causes of lung injury: the mechanical power. *Intensive Care Med*; 42: 1567–1575.

- Huhle R, *et al.* (2019). Power of ventilation and its relationship with neutrophilic inflammation in a double hit model of acute respiratory distress syndrome. *Am J Respir Crit Care Med*; 199: A7250.

- Kiss T, *et al.* (2019). Effects of positive end-expiratory pressure and spontaneous breathing activity on regional lung inflammation in experimental acute respiratory distress syndrome. *Crit Care Med*; 47: e358–e365.

- Marini JJ (1990). Lung mechanics determinations at the bedside: instrumentation and clinical applications. *Respir Care*; 35: 669–696.

- Sassoon CSH, *et al.* (1998). Work of breathing during mechanical ventilation. *In:* Marini JJ, *et al.*, eds. Physiological Basis of Ventilator Support. New York, Marcel Dekker; pp. 261–302.

- Serpa Neto A, *et al.* (2018). Mechanical power of ventilation is associated with mortality in critically ill patients: an analysis of patients in two observational cohorts. *Intensive Care Med*; 44: 1914–1922.

- Shapiro R, *et al.* (1998). Monitoring of the mechanically ventilated patient. *In:* Marini JJ, *et al.*, eds. Physiological Basis of Ventilatory Support. New York, Marcel Dekker; pp. 709–771.

- Stenqvist O (2003). Practical assessment of respiratory mechanics. *Br J Anaesth*; 91: 92–105.

- Tobin MJ (1990). Respiratory monitoring. *JAMA*; 264: 244–251.

- Yoshida T (2019). Guiding ventilation with transpulmonary pressure. *Intensive Care Med*; 45: 535–538.

Effects of invasive ventilation on the lungs

Irene Cavalli, Tommaso Tonetti and V. Marco Ranieri

Definition, pathophysiological and clinical features

Invasive ventilation is the supportive therapy for patients with acute respiratory failure that rests the respiratory muscle while providing adequate gas exchange. With this purpose invasive ventilation is a lifesaving technique. Extensive studies on the impact of invasive ventilation on patients with several forms of acute respiratory failure (ARDS; patients undergoing general anaesthesia; and brain death candidates subject to organ donation) have demonstrated that the inappropriate application of invasive ventilation can worsen/induce lung injury (VILI).

VILI is characterised by inflammatory cell infiltrates, hyaline membranes, increased vascular permeability and pulmonary oedema. Histologically, this damage resembles the damage that occurs in ARDS patients. However, several experimental studies have shown that injurious ventilatory regimens may alter alveolar–capillary barrier permeability inducing oedema, impair endothelial and epithelial cells, and induce an inflammatory response even in previously healthy lungs. Clinically, this damage causes impaired gas exchange and a decrease in lung and respiratory system compliance. Both increase the number of days of ventilator dependency and mortality.

VILI may occur at both high and low lung volumes. At high lung volumes, overdistension can increase alveolar–capillary permeability leading to pulmonary oedema (volutrauma). It can also cause alveolar rapture and air leak (barotrauma). By contrast, at low lung volumes the damage may be determined by the cyclic opening and closing of airways and lung units (atelectrauma), resulting in surfactant malfunction and local hypoxia. The physical forces involved in these phenomena may induce the activation of

Key points

- Invasive ventilation can cause VILI in previously damaged lung and even in healthy lungs.
- Improve protective invasive ventilation in any eligible patient.
- Target VILI using simple, available and repeatable tools such as P_{plat} and ΔP, without forgetting that other factors (such as PEEP and respiratory rate) may be equally important in determining VILI.

inflammatory mediators within the lung (biotrauma). The latter may then be released in the systemic circulation, leading to multiorgan dysfunction.

The damage caused by invasive ventilation submits the lung to non-physiological lung stress and strain. Stress represents the net force applied to the lung parenchyma, opposed by the elastic force of alveolar wall. Strain represents the deformation of a structure, defined as the change in length or volume from the initial length or volume. From a pulmonary perspective, stress is the alveolar distending pressure (alveolar pressure minus pleural pressure, *i.e.* transpulmonary pressure); and strain is the ratio of volume change (*i.e.* V_T) to functional residual capacity (FRC).

Protective invasive ventilation

The concept of VILI is now generally accepted, thus the goal of invasive ventilation is to provide gas exchange while minimising VILI.

A landmark study by the ARDS network demonstrated a significant mortality reduction (31% *versus* 39.8% of the control group) when invasive ventilation was performed according to the lung-protective ventilation protocol: low V_T (V_T of 6 mL per kg predicted body weight (PBW)), P_{plat} <30 cmH_2O and moderate PEEP. This protocol also decreased the number of days of ventilator dependency when compared with traditional invasive ventilation (V_T of 12 mL per kg PBW and P_{plat} <50 cmH_2O). A flowchart of protective invasive ventilation and the setting of PEEP/F_{IO_2} are available in figure 1 and in table 1, respectively.

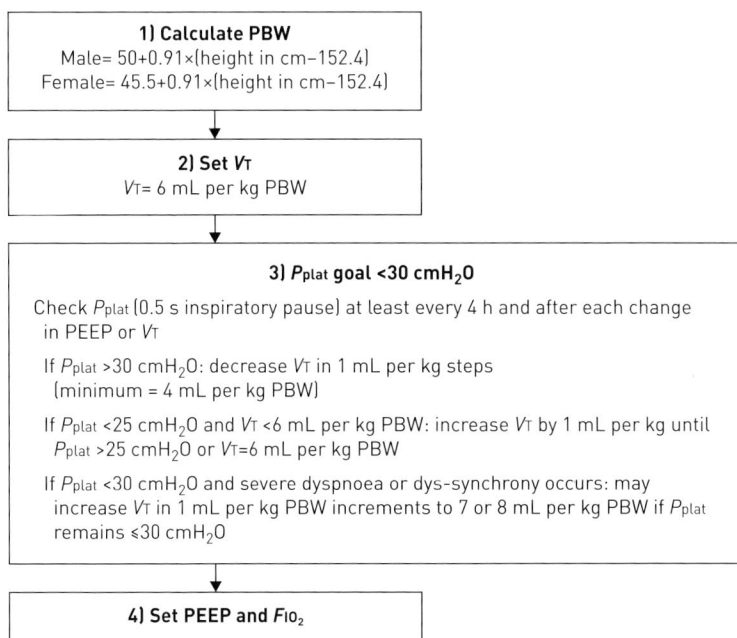

---

1) Calculate PBW
Male= 50+0.91×(height in cm−152.4)
Female= 45.5+0.91×(height in cm−152.4)

↓

2) Set V_T
V_T= 6 mL per kg PBW

↓

3) P_{plat} goal <30 cmH_2O

Check P_{plat} (0.5 s inspiratory pause) at least every 4 h and after each change in PEEP or V_T

If P_{plat} >30 cmH_2O: decrease V_T in 1 mL per kg steps (minimum = 4 mL per kg PBW)

If P_{plat} <25 cmH_2O and V_T <6 mL per kg PBW: increase V_T by 1 mL per kg until P_{plat} >25 cmH_2O or V_T=6 mL per kg PBW

If P_{plat} <30 cmH_2O and severe dyspnoea or dys-synchrony occurs: may increase V_T in 1 mL per kg PBW increments to 7 or 8 mL per kg PBW if P_{plat} remains ≤30 cmH_2O

↓

4) Set PEEP and F_{IO_2}

Figure 1. *Invasive ventilation protocol. Information from The Acute Respiratory Distress Syndrome Network, et al. (2000).*

Table 1. Setting of PEEP/F_{IO_2}

PEEP cmH$_2$O	F_{IO_2}
5	0.3-0.4
8	0.4-0.5
10	0.5-0.7
12	0.7
14	0.7-0.9
16-18	0.9
18-24	1.0

Information from The Acute Respiratory Distress Syndrome Network, *et al.* (2000).

While a reduction in V_T has shown noticeable benefits in terms of VILI reduction, the best PEEP setting is still a challenge. In fact, setting PEEP prevents the damage that occurs at low lung volume. Nevertheless, on one hand a low PEEP may be not sufficient to keep the alveoli open; while on the other hand, a higher PEEP may have haemodynamic consequences and may be associated with lung overdistension. Several studies based on a population of ARDS patients have tried to find the best PEEP able to improve oxygenation while minimising the side-effects of inappropriate PEEP level. A meta-analysis of three large RCTs comparing higher *versus* lower PEEP in the context of lung-protective invasive ventilation showed a significant reduction in mortality in moderate and severe ARDS patients when the higher PEEP strategy was used. No significant effect was found among patients with mild ARDS, in which a strategy of high PEEP levels can even be harmful. All in all, the results of the meta-analysis suggest treating patients with moderate and severe ARDS with higher rather than lower PEEP levels. Another RCT compared lung recruitment associated with PEEP titration according to the best respiratory system compliance *versus* low PEEP levels in patients with moderate and severe ARDS. In this case the routine use of lung recruitment and titrated PEEP increased mortality compared with low PEEP. These findings suggest avoiding the routine use of lung recruitment and PEEP titration in these populations. More recently, an RCT has compared PEEP titration with an oesophageal pressure-guided strategy *versus* an empirical high PEEP–F_{IO_2} strategy in a population of patients with moderate-to-severe ARDS. No significant difference in death and ventilator-free days was found comparing the two strategies. These findings do not support a PEEP titration strategy guided by oesophageal pressure instead of an empirical high PEEP–F_{IO_2} strategy. Hence, the best method to set PEEP remains uncertain in ARDS patients and is even less clear in non-ARDS patients. Different methods based on lung mechanics, imaging or transpulmonary P_{plat} have been proposed and require further investigation.

Monitoring during invasive ventilation: strategies that may reduce incidence of VILI

Despite protective invasive ventilation, accurate respiratory monitoring is necessary in order to minimise the risks, preventing further injury and allowing the lungs and airways to heal. The measurement of different pulmonary mechanical variables may be useful to guide invasive ventilation and minimise VILI.

Plateau pressure P_{plat} refers to the pressure applied to the small airways and alveoli during the end-inspiratory pause, when there is no flow and proximal airway pressure equilibrates with the alveolar pressure. An end-inspiratory occlusion manoeuvre (0.5 s) during volume-controlled ventilation (VCV) allows the measurement of P_{plat}. It has been demonstrated that a P_{plat} value <28–30 cmH$_2$O prevents lung overdistension. It is possible to keep the P_{plat} value under the threshold of 28–30 cmH$_2$O by reducing V_T.

P_{plat} is the pressure at the end of an occlusion of the airways at end-inspiration. As such, P_{plat} represents alveolar pressure, *i.e.* the elastic distending pressure of lungs and chest wall provided the patient is not actively contracting the respiratory muscles. Measuring P_{plat} therefore allows estimation of the elastic distending pressure applied to the lung during controlled-mode invasive ventilation. Clarifications are necessary if a volume-controlled or a pressure-controlled mode of ventilation is used.

During VCV (figure 2), the peak inspiratory pressure is the sum of the elastic and resistive pressure. Thus, during an end-inspiratory occlusion manoeuvre, the flow ceases and airway pressure falls until it reaches a steady state (P_{plat}) allowing quantification of the elastic recoil pressure of the respiratory system.

By contrast, during pressure-controlled ventilation (PCV) (figure 3), the preset pressure limit (P_{max}) reflects the total pressure applied to the respiratory system in its resistive and elastic components. If the inspiratory flow does not reach zero, the preset pressure does not equal the P_{plat}. Hence, the P_{max} during PCV does not reflect

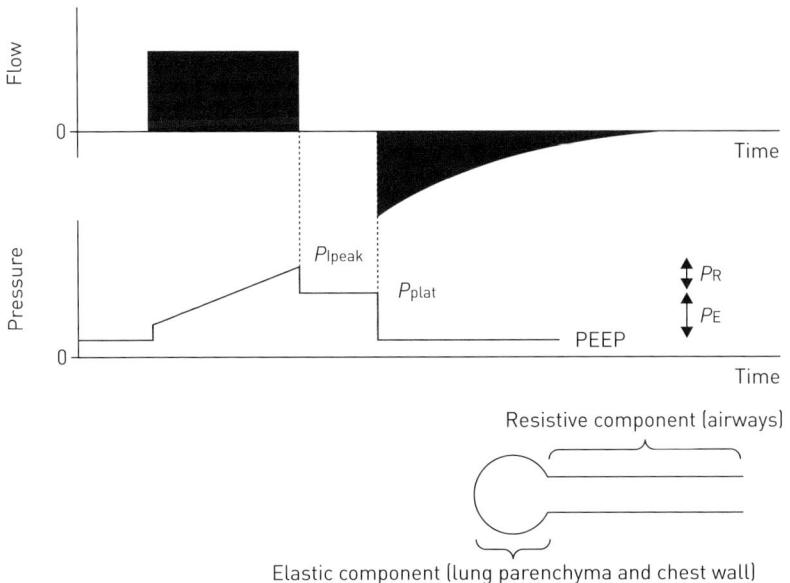

Figure 2. Airway pressure and flow waveforms during constant flow VCV. The effect of an end-inspiratory occlusion manoeuvre is shown. P$_{Ipeak}$: peak inspiratory pressure; P$_R$: resistive pressure; P$_E$: elastic pressure.

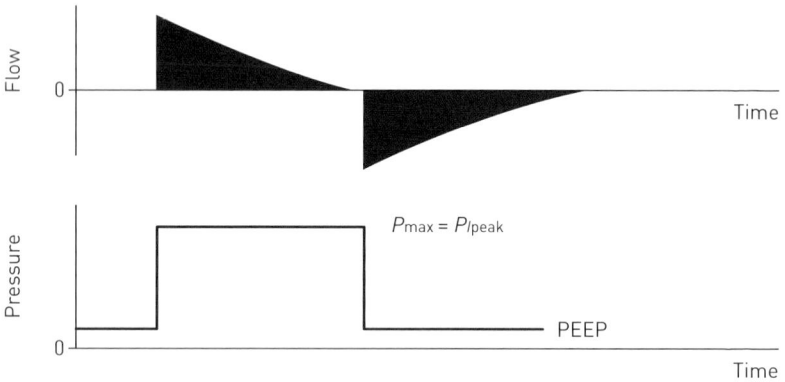

Figure 3. Airway pressure and flow waveforms during PCV.

the P_{plat}. Some mathematical corrections have been proposed in order to better estimate elastic pressure at the end of an end-inspiratory occlusion during PCV.

Stress index The stress index value (SI) describes the shape of the pressure–time curves during constant-flow V_T delivery and muscle paralysis. During VCV, at constant flow, the rate of change in pressure is related to the changes in respiratory system compliance. This is due to the fact that the contribution from airways resistance is not influenced by changes in volume during constant flow. Relying on this assumption, the airway opening pressure (P_{AO}) is a function of respiratory time (t):

$$P_{AO} = a \times t b + c \tag{1}$$

where a represents the value of the slope of the curve, c is the pressure value at time equals zero, and b is a dimensionless number that describes the shape of the pressure–time curve and represents the SI. When SI = 1 the pressure–time curve is linear, and the respiratory system compliance is constant during tidal inflation. When SI < 1 the shape of the pressure–time curve shows a downward concavity. This means that the respiratory system compliance increases during tidal inflation suggesting tidal recruitment of collapsed alveoli and potential recruitment when adding PEEP. Thus, it is recommended to increase PEEP. When SI > 1 the shape of the pressure–time curve shows an upward concavity, representing tidal hyperinflation and a decrease in compliance. In this case, it is recommended to decrease PEEP or V_T (figure 4).

Markers of injurious ventilation were minimised using ventilator settings associated with 0.9 < b < 1.1.

Transpulmonary pressure Pressure applied on the lungs, or transpulmonary pressure (P_L), is the difference between airway pressure (P_{aw}) and pleural pressure (P_{pl}):

$$P_L = P_{aw} - P_{pl} \tag{2}$$

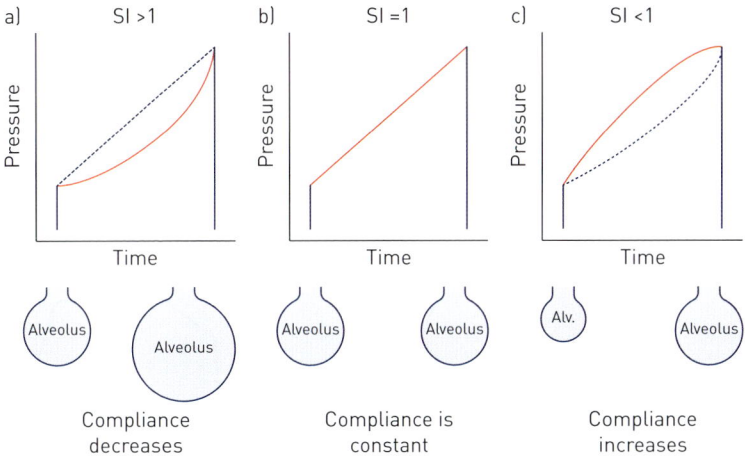

Figure 4. a) SI with overdistension, b) normal SI, and c) SI with tidal recruitment.

The P_L reflects the distending pressure of the lung. For patients not making respiratory effort and mechanically ventilated, the P_{aw} measured during a period of zero flow is called the P_{plat} and represents the alveolar pressure. The P_{plat} can be easily estimated at the end inspiration, when airflow is zero. Estimating P_{pl} is more difficult because of the lack of noninvasive techniques. However, a minimally invasive technique is represented by oesophageal pressure (P_{oes}) measurement *via* a catheter with an air-filled thin-walled latex balloon inserted nasally or orally. This measurement is considered representative of P_{pl}. Thus, equation 2 becomes:

$$P_L = P_{plat} - P_{oes} \qquad (3)$$

Other authors have shown that the absolute value of P_{oes} cannot be used as surrogate measure of the P_{pl} and they propose that the relative variations in P_{oes} and airway pressures should be used instead to estimate P_L.

P_{plat} is the most common variable used in clinical practice to identify lung overdistension. However, P_{plat} alone can misrepresent the stress on the lung parenchyma in at least two extreme (but not very rare) cases: 1) when the chest wall is stiff; and 2) when a patient with marked dyspnoea is undergoing NIV.

1) In a patient who is not making respiratory effort (figure 5), the P_{plat} represents the distending pressure of the lungs plus the chest wall. If a patient has a stiff chest wall (*e.g.* severe obesity, massive ascites, pleural effusion) much of the pressure applied by the ventilator will be used to distend the chest wall, rather than the lung. Thus, a high value of P_{plat} may overestimate the real distending pressure of the lung. A stiff chest wall is associated with increases in P_{pl}. Thus, the measurement of the P_{oes} may be useful to estimate the real P_L. For example, if the P_{aw} is 30 cmH$_2$O and the P_{oes} is 25 cmH$_2$O, the P_L will be 5 cmH$_2$O (P_L=30 cmH$_2$O – 25 cmH$_2$O=5 cmH$_2$O).

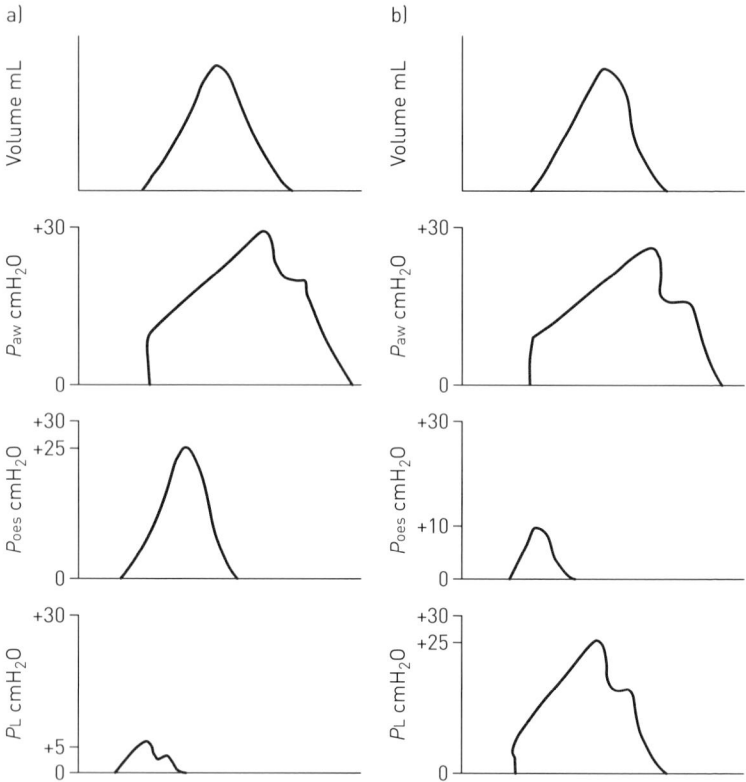

Figure 5. Controlled invasive ventilation in a) a patient with a stiff chest wall (increased elastance of the chest wall) and b) a normal anaesthetised, paralysed patient (elastance of the chest wall is constant). In a) $P_L = P_{aw} - P_{oes} = 30$ cmH$_2$O-25 cmH$_2$O$=5$ cmH$_2$O, in b) $P_L = P_{aw} - P_{oes} = 30$ cmH$_2$O-10 cmH$_2$O$=20$ cmH$_2$O.

2) When a patient has marked dyspnoea and spontaneous effort occurs (figure 6), large negative swings in P_{pl} may occur increasing the risk of lung injury. In this case P_{aw} alone may underestimate the real lung stress. For example, if P_{aw} is 10 cmH$_2$O and P_{oes} is -15 cmH$_2$O, the P_L will be 25 cmH$_2$O ($P_L = 10$ cmH$_2$O $- (-15$ cmH$_2$O$) = 25$ cmH$_2$O).

In conclusion, P_L represents the distending pressure of the lung, estimated as P_{aw} minus P_{oes}. P_{oes} allows the determination of what fraction of P_{aw} is applied to overcome lung and chest wall elastance.

Driving pressure It has been proposed that swings in pressure during invasive ventilation may be a better predictor of VILI, rather than the absolute pressure value. This swing in pressure, known as ΔP, can be calculated as P_{plat} minus PEEP ($\Delta P = P_{plat} -$ PEEP). In a patient with ARDS, an increment in ΔP (which means a decrease in respiratory system compliance if the V_T is kept constant) is associated

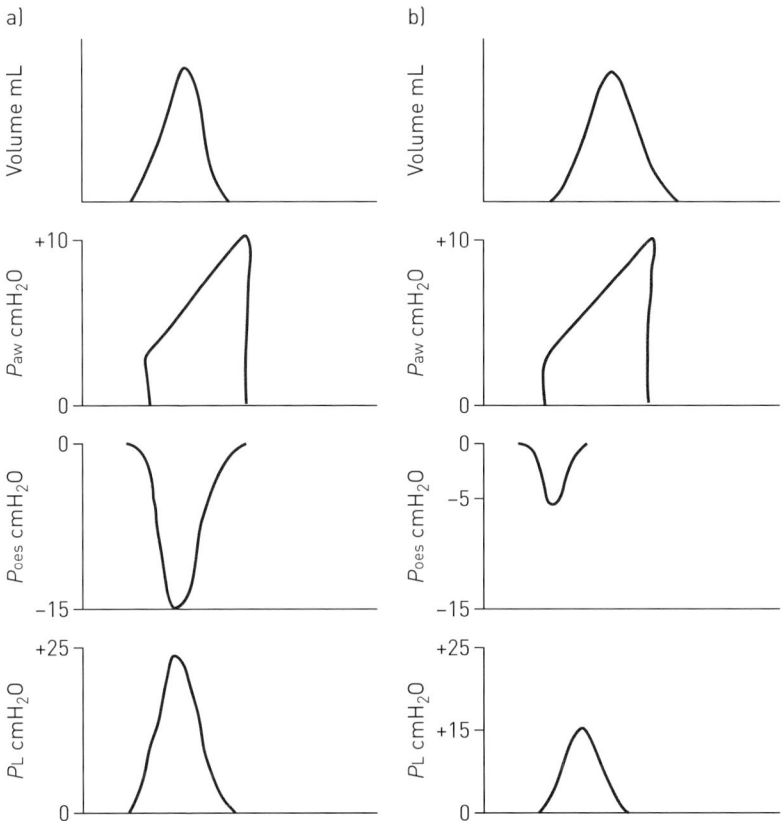

Figure 6. Pressure support ventilation in a) a patient with marked respiratory distress and b) a patient with no respiratory distress. In a) PL=Paw–Poes=10 cmH$_2$O–(–15 cmH$_2$O)=25 cmH$_2$O, in b) PL=Paw–Poes=10 cmH$_2$O–(–5 cmH$_2$O)=15 cmH$_2$O.

with increased mortality, even when protective invasive ventilation is applied. In fact, keeping the ΔP value under 14 cmH$_2$O significantly increases survival.

Mechanical power Different mechanical variables have been shown to contribute to VILI. These variables (V_T, P_{plat}, ΔP, PEEP, flow and respiratory rate) have been addressed separately in previous studies.

The mechanical power equation unifies the variables known to be related to development of VILI:

$$\text{Power}_{rs} = RR \cdot \left\{ \Delta V^2 \cdot \left[\frac{1}{2} \cdot EL_{rs} + RR \cdot \frac{(1+I:E)}{60 \cdot I:E} \cdot R_{aw} \right] + \Delta V \cdot PEEP \right\} \qquad (4)$$

where RR is the respiratory rate, ΔV is the change in volume, EL_{rs} is the elastance of the respiratory system, I:E is the inspiratory to expiratory ratio and R_{aw} is the airway resistance.

This equation focuses on the concept that changing one single variable may not be sufficient to prevent VILI if the value of mechanical power is not changing. For example, a reduction in V_T may not be sufficient if simultaneously requiring an increase of respiratory rate in order to maintain an adequate minute ventilation. Changing V_T, ΔP and inspiratory flow produce an exponential increase in mechanical power (factor = 2). A higher respiratory rate increases mechanical power value with an exponent of 1.4, while a higher PEEP produces a linear increment of mechanical power. Although, to date, the mechanical power has been mainly studied in experimental settings, it is promising and may have important clinical implications. Although a threshold value for mechanical power in humans has still to be identified and RCTs on mechanical power are lacking, this approach helps the clinician in considering the many damage factors, which are often neglected when setting protective ventilation.

Further reading

- Akoumianaki E, *et al.* (2014). The application of esophageal pressure measurement in patients with respiratory failure. *Am J Respir Crit Care Med*; 189: 520-531.

- Amato MB, *et al.* (2015). Driving pressure and survival in the acute respiratory distress syndrome. *N Engl J Med*; 372: 747-755.

- Beitler JR, *et al.* (2019). Effect of titrating positive end-expiratory pressure (PEEP) with an esophageal pressure–guided strategy vs an empirical high PEEP-F_{IO_2} strategy on death and days free from mechanical ventilation among patients with acute respiratory distress syndrome. a randomized clinical trial. *JAMA*; 321: 846-857.

- Briel M, *et al.* (2010). Higher *vs* lower positive end-expiratory pressure in patients with acute lung injury and acute respiratory distress syndrome: systematic review and meta-analysis. *JAMA*; 303: 865-873.

- Chiumello D, *et al.* (2014). The assessment of transpulmonary pressure in mechanically ventilated ARDS patients. *Intensive Care Med*; 40: 1670-1678.

- Dos Santos CC, *et al.* (2000). Invited review: mechanisms of ventilator-induced lung injury: a perspective. *J Appl Physiol (1985)*; 89: 1645-1655.

- Fan E, *et al.* (2017). An Official American Thoracic Society/European Society of Intensive Care Medicine/Society of Critical Care Medicine clinical practice guideline: mechanical ventilation in adult patients with acute respiratory distress syndrome. *Am J Respir Crit Care Med*; 195: 1253-1263.

- Gattinoni L, *et al.* (2016). Ventilator-related causes of lung injury: the mechanical power. *Intensive Care Med*; 42: 1567-1575.

- Mauri T, *et al.* (2016). Esophageal and transpulmonary pressure in the clinical setting: meaning, usefulness and perspectives. *Intensive Care Med*; 42: 1360-1373.

- Pesenti A, *et al.* (1991). The effects of positive end-expiratory pressure on respiratory resistance in patients with the adult respiratory distress syndrome and in normal anesthetized subjects. *Am Rev Respir Dis*; 144: 101-107.

- Ricard JD, *et al*. (2002). Ventilator-induced lung injury. *Curr Opin Crit Care*; 8: 12–20.

- Rittayamai N, *et al*. (2015). Pressure-controlled *vs* volume-controlled ventilation in acute respiratory failure: a physiology-based narrative and systematic review. *Chest*; 148: 340–355.

- Sahetya SK, *et al*. (2017). Setting positive end-expiratory pressure in acute respiratory distress syndrome. *Am J Respir Crit Care Med*; 195: 1429–1438.

- Silva PL, *et al*. (2015). Mechanisms of ventilator-induced lung injury in healthy lungs. *Best Pract Res Clin Anaesthesiol*; 29: 301–313.

- Slutsky AS, *et al*. (2014). Ventilator-induced lung injury. *N Engl J Med*; 370: 980.

- Terragni P, *et al*. (2016). Dynamic airway pressure-time curve profile (stress index): a systematic review. *Minerva Anestesiol*; 82: 58–68.

- Terragni PP, *et al*. (2013). Accuracy of plateau pressure and stress index to identify injurious ventilation in patients with acute respiratory distress syndrome. *Anesthesiology*; 119: 880–889.

- The Acute Respiratory Distress Syndrome Network, *et al*. (2000). Ventilation with lower tidal volumes as compared with traditional tidal volumes for acute lung injury and the acute respiratory distress syndrome. *N Engl J Med*; 342: 1301–1308.

- Writing Group for the Alveolar Recruitment for Acute Respiratory Distress Syndrome Trial (ART) Investigators, *et al*. (2017). Effect of lung recruitment and titrated positive end- expiratory pressure (PEEP) *vs* low PEEP on mortality in patients with acute respiratory distress syndrome: a randomized clinical trial. *JAMA*; 318: 1335–1345.

Effects of invasive ventilation on the respiratory muscles

Annemijn H. Jonkman, Zhong-Hua Shi and Leo Heunks

A disturbance in the balance between the capacity and loading of the respiratory muscles may result in respiratory failure. For these patients, invasive ventilation is a life-saving intervention that aims to reduce the work of breathing and improve gas exchange. While invasive ventilation can partially or completely unload the respiratory muscles, respiratory muscle function may deteriorate in ventilator-bound ICU patients. Compared to peripheral skeletal muscles, the diaphragm appears more affected by critical illness and invasive ventilation. Diaphragm weakness is associated with prolonged ventilator weaning, increased risks of ICU re-admission and hospital re-admission, and mortality. Therefore, it is of crucial importance to limit the detrimental effects of critical illness and invasive ventilation on the respiratory muscles.

While the respiratory muscle pump consists of multiple inspiratory and expiratory muscles, this chapter focuses on the diaphragm, the main muscle for inspiration. We summarise the prevalence of diaphragm muscle weakness in ventilated ICU patients and potential mechanisms causing ventilator-induced diaphragm dysfunction. Clinical implications of diaphragm dysfunction are discussed, as well as monitoring techniques and potential preventive and therapeutic strategies to limit the development of diaphragm weakness.

Definition and prevalence of diaphragm muscle weakness in ICU patients

The gold standard to assess *in vivo* diaphragm strength in ventilated patients is to measure the change in transdiaphragmatic twitch pressure induced by magnetic stimulation of the phrenic nerves ($P_{di,tw}$). This assessment provides a standardised

Key points

- Diaphragm weakness occurs rapidly during invasive ventilation and is associated with prolonged ventilator weaning and poor outcome.

- Prolonged low diaphragm activity can lead to disuse atrophy. Excessive respiratory muscle loading can cause diaphragm injury.

- A diaphragm-protective ventilation strategy enables a new opportunity to minimise, prevent or recover from the effects of invasive ventilation on the diaphragm.

measure of contractility, because it does not need the patient's cooperation. As this technique requires invasive pressure measurements of the diaphragm using gastric and oesophageal balloons, the change in twitch pressure generated at the outside tip of the endotracheal tube ($P_{et,tw}$) is proposed as a noninvasive surrogate. Using $P_{et,tw}$, diaphragm weakness has been defined as $P_{et,tw}$ <11 cmH$_2$O. With this definition, diaphragm weakness is already present within 24 h after intubation in up to 64% of ventilated patients, meaning that critical illness can impair diaphragm function at a very early stage, probably even before the patient is admitted to the ICU and exposed to invasive ventilation. At the time of initiation of ventilator weaning, incidence is even higher (63–80%).

A more feasible and readily available bedside technique to measure inspiratory muscle strength is the assessment of maximal inspiratory pressure (P_{Imax}). P_{Imax} can be measured in selected cooperative patients following a maximum inspiratory effort against a closed airway, using a hand-held device connected to the endotracheal tube or tracheostomy tube. Alternatively, in poorly cooperative patients, pressures can be assessed by performing a 20-s end-expiratory hold manoeuvre. Although P_{Imax} is poorly correlated with $P_{et,tw}$, high values for P_{Imax} exclude inspiratory muscle weakness, whereas low values might also reflect poor technique or effort.

Ultrasound can be used to evaluate diaphragm function. Thickness of the diaphragm is best visualised at the zone of apposition (lateral rib cage between the eighth and tenth ribs). During inspiration, the diaphragm contracts and thickens. The magnitude of thickening (thickening fraction (TF$_{di}$)) during tidal breathing reflects the activity of the diaphragm. The TF$_{di}$ during a maximal inspiratory effort (TF$_{di,max}$) has been used to estimate strength, in which a TF$_{di,max}$ <20% was found indicative of severe diaphragm weakness. Using this definition, studies have shown that diaphragm weakness is present in 29% of patients at the time of the first spontaneous breathing trial and in 36% of patients at the time of extubation. In addition, changes in diaphragm end-expiratory thickness were observed over the first week of ventilation in 56% of patients. About 80% of these patients showed a decrease in thickness of >10%, which was associated with increased risk of delayed extubation.

Causes and mechanisms

In this section we summarise three mechanisms by which invasive ventilation contributes to the development of diaphragm weakness. Figure 1 provides a schematic overview of these mechanisms.

Disuse atrophy There is strong evidence that disuse of the diaphragm due to ventilator overassist is the critical contributor to diaphragm weakness. This has been demonstrated both *in vivo* and *in vitro*. Diaphragm inactivity is associated with activation of proteolytic pathways, which results in myofibrillar atrophy and contractile force reduction. Studies in animals and brain-dead patients suggest an important role for oxidative stress and mitochondrial dysfunction in the development of diaphragm weakness. However, recent studies investigating diaphragm biopsies from ICU patients showed significant diaphragm fibre atrophy and weakness in the absence of mitochondrial dysfunction and oxidative stress. Further research is required to understand the cellular mechanisms causing

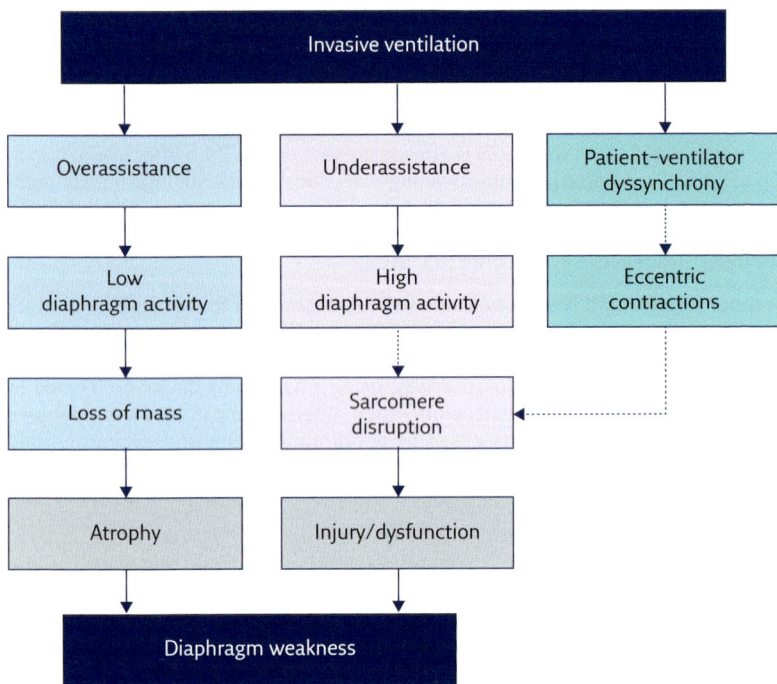

Figure 1. Schematic illustration of invasive ventilation-related mechanisms involved in the development of diaphragm weakness. Dashed lines represent uncertain causation.

disuse atrophy. Importantly, ultrasound studies indicate that diaphragm atrophy occurs rapidly (<4 days) and that the change in diaphragm thickness (*i.e.* rate and magnitude) is correlated with the extent to which respiratory effort is suppressed by the ventilator.

Excessive loading It has been demonstrated that, in nonventilated patients, excessive inspiratory loading can result in diaphragm muscle injury and prolonged loss of force production. Whether inadequate ventilator support also results in diaphragm injury in critically ill patients is less clear. However, strong breathing efforts are common in patients on partially supported modes. In addition, histological patterns in the diaphragm muscle of these patients are consistent with load-induced injury. In addition to high breathing effort, patient–ventilator dyssynchrony, especially eccentric (lengthening) contractions, may promote load-induced diaphragm injury. Whether eccentric contractions are sufficiently severe and frequent to contribute to diaphragm weakness in ICU patients is as yet unknown. Nevertheless, this emphasises the importance of good patient–ventilator synchrony during invasive ventilation, which is another rationale for monitoring patient effort. The concept of load-induced diaphragm injury may explain recent ultrasound findings in which an increase in diaphragm thickness of >10% during the course of invasive ventilation was associated with high levels of patient inspiratory effort and decreased likelihood of extubation. This increase in thickness possibly reflects muscle inflammation and oedema.

Longitudinal atrophy Diaphragm muscle loss affecting the length of muscle fibres was recently described as an effect of excessive PEEP. An increase in PEEP applied during invasive ventilation results in a larger end-expiratory lung volume and, consequently, shorter diaphragm length at the zone of apposition. Experimental work showed that PEEP results in loss of sarcomeres, resulting in a decreased optimal length for force generation. If similar effects occur in the human diaphragm, an acute reduction in PEEP (*i.e.* during a spontaneous breathing trial) would result in an overstretched diaphragm above its adapted optimal length and, consequently, result in diaphragm dysfunction. The clinical relevance of this hypothesis remains to be investigated.

Other risk factors In critically ill patients, it is likely that multiple factors play a role in the development or aggravation of diaphragm weakness. Next to the mechanisms related to invasive ventilation, the diaphragm can be involved in shock-related organ failure present at the time of ICU admission. For instance, animal studies have demonstrated that cardiogenic shock is associated with contractile impairment and fatigue of the respiratory muscles, resulting from increase in diaphragm work and reduction in diaphragm oxygen delivery. In addition, sepsis could impair diaphragm force through activation of inflammation in the muscle. There is some evidence that medication such as sedatives, neuromuscular blockers and corticosteroids affect the severity of diaphragm weakness, but this is beyond the scope of this chapter.

Diaphragm-protective ventilation

Considering the potentially detrimental effects of controlled invasive ventilation on the diaphragm, there is a strong rationale for applying partially assisted ventilator modes when feasible and safe. Maintaining spontaneous breathing under invasive ventilation should minimise disuse atrophy, and avoiding excessive spontaneous inspiratory efforts potentially limits the development of load-induced diaphragm injury. In clinical practice, we should aim to titrate inspiratory support and sedation to maintain levels of inspiratory effort that are considered physiological (figure 2).

Further research is needed to define the optimal level of inspiratory effort in critically ill patients. This probably depends on the underlying condition, the maximal strength of the diaphragm and respiratory rate. Until further data are available, it seems reasonable from a physiological perspective to maintain a breathing

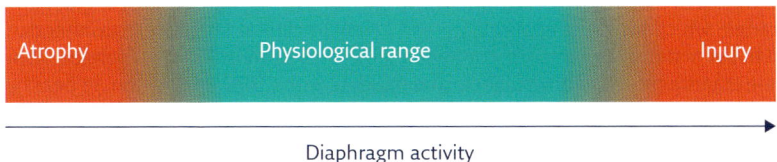

Diaphragm activity

Figure 2. Concept of diaphragm-protective ventilation, aiming to keep diaphragm activity within physiological range and preventing muscle atrophy and injury.

effort similar to that of healthy subjects at rest. A study in patients weaning from invasive ventilation showed that patients who were successfully weaned from the ventilator exhibited inspiratory effort within this physiological range (approximately 4–8 cmH$_2$O). In addition, using ultrasound, patients with a TF$_{di}$ of 15–30% during the first 72 h of invasive ventilation had the shortest duration of ventilation.

A diaphragm-protective ventilation strategy enables a new opportunity to minimise, prevent or recover from the effects of invasive ventilation on the diaphragm. To apply such a strategy, bedside monitoring of breathing effort is required.

Monitoring techniques for the diaphragm

Today, the state-of-the-art method for monitoring respiratory muscle effort is assessment of changes in pleural pressure using an oesophageal balloon catheter. This enables direct and continuous measurement of inspiratory effort. However, this technique requires expertise in positioning of the catheter and interpretation of waveforms. Recommended reading regarding this monitoring technique is provided in the reading list at the end of this chapter.

With the introduction of neurally adjusted ventilator assist (NAVA), a mode for partially assisted ventilation that synchronises ventilation to diaphragm electrical activity (EA$_{di}$), continuous monitoring of crural EA$_{di}$ has become available for ICU patients. EA$_{di}$ is measured using a dedicated nasogastric feeding tube with embedded electrodes at the level of the diaphragm. The EA$_{di}$ curve can be displayed during any mode of ventilation and is a valuable tool for detecting diaphragm inactivity, ventilator overassistance and patient–ventilator asynchronies.

Ultrasound is a noninvasive and feasible bedside technique for assessment of diaphragm excursions, thickness and thickening. For more detailed information on diaphragm ultrasound, see the chapter "Monitoring respiratory muscles: respiratory muscle ultrasound".

Prevention and therapeutic strategies

Few studies have evaluated strategies to improve respiratory muscle function in patients with critical-illness-associated diaphragm weakness. This section will summarise the role of pharmacological interventions and training of inspiratory muscles.

Today, no drug is approved to improve respiratory muscle function. There has been interest in improving contractile efficiency of muscle fibres by using phosphodiesterase-4 inhibitors or the calcium sensitiser levosimendan. In a retrospective cohort study, improvement in diaphragm movement was found in 21 out of 40 patients with ventilator-induced diaphragm dysfunction after receiving a low dose of theophylline. However, theophylline has a narrow non-toxic therapeutic range, which limits its applicability and safety in clinical practice. Levosimendan has been shown to enhance contractile efficiency of muscle fibres isolated from the diaphragm of healthy subjects and patients with COPD. In addition, in healthy volunteers it was demonstrated that levosimendan improved neuromuscular efficiency of the diaphragm and reversed fatigue. The effect of this drug on the diaphragm function of ICU patients remains to be investigated.

Inspiratory muscle training (IMT) is safe and feasible in ICU patients. A typical hand-held inspiratory threshold device that can be used for IMT is shown in

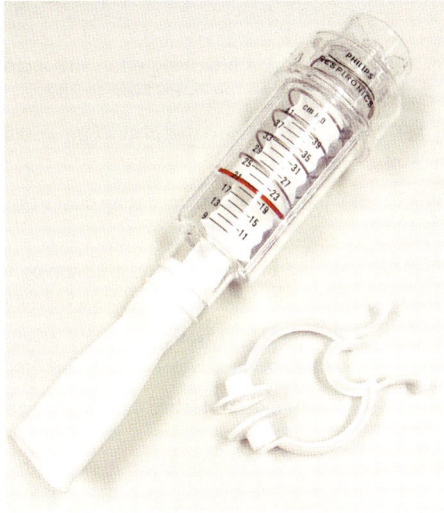

Figure 3. A threshold IMT device. The threshold can be increased by adjusting the spring length.

figure 3. Patients should be sufficiently alert to cooperate with the training method. When performing IMT, the patient is disconnected from the ventilator and the device is connected to the tracheostomy tube or endotracheal tube with the cuff inflated. Different loading protocols have been applied. We use the protocol applied by Martin *et al.* (2011): four sets of 6–10 loaded breaths. Loading is set such that subjects can consistently open the valve during inspiration and loading is gradually increased daily as tolerated. This strategy has been shown to improve P_{Imax} and to reduce the duration of ventilator weaning. Optimal training protocols should be further developed and the impact of IMT on clinical outcomes requires future studies. Other strategies that are currently being investigated are phrenic nerve pacing for the prevention of disuse and restoring diaphragm function. Phrenic nerve pacing has been applied in experimental and human studies, using a transvenous phrenic nerve pacing system designed to be applied percutaneously in the left subclavian vein. Whether there is a potential role of phrenic nerve pacing in difficult-to-wean ICU patients will be determined in the near future.

Summary

Invasive ventilation may have detrimental effects on the respiratory muscles. A diaphragm-protective ventilation strategy therefore has great potential for improving patient outcomes. Clinicians should consider monitoring respiratory muscle effort during the course of invasive ventilation. The right balance between lung-protective ventilation, adequate gas exchange, patient comfort and maintaining inspiratory effort may be challenging to achieve. Further studies are needed to determine the optimal level for inspiratory effort and the effects of a diaphragm-protective ventilation strategy on patient outcomes.

Further reading

- de Vries H, *et al.* (2018). Assessing breathing effort in mechanical ventilation: physiology and clinical implications. *Ann Transl Med*; 6: 387.

- Dres M, *et al.* (2017). Critical illness-associated diaphragm weakness. *Intensive Care Med*; 43: 1441–1452.

- Heunks LM, *et al.* (2015). Monitoring and preventing diaphragm injury. *Curr Opin Crit Care*; 21: 34–41.

- Martin AD, *et al.* (2011). Inspiratory muscle strength training improves weaning outcome in failure to wean patients: a randomized trial. *Crit Care*; 15: R84.

- Mauri T, *et al.* (2016). Esophageal and transpulmonary pressure in the clinical setting: meaning, usefulness and perspectives. *Intensive Care Med*; 42: 1360–1373.

- Schepens T, *et al.* (2019). Diaphragm-protective mechanical ventilation. *Curr Opin Crit Care*; 25: 77–85.

Artificial airways

Christian S. Bruells and Tim Frenzel

Artificial airways have been or have to be established during an ICU stay for a variety of reasons. They can be subdivided into supraglottic devices and transglottic, intratracheally placed tubes. The latter are the most common in ICU. However, supraglottic airways have their role, besides during routine anaesthesia in the operating room, mainly in emergency situations and in the management of a difficult airway. Airway devices placed in the trachea with an inflated cuff are defined as being a "secured airway", which describes the fact that risk of macro-aspiration is reduced. In this chapter we describe different devices with techniques and hints for their correct and safe placement.

Different tubes/types/locations

A secured airway can be established transorally, transtracheally (or *via* the cricothyroid ligament in an emergency) or *via* the nostrils during a planned fibreoptic intubation in the expected difficult airway. The classic tube is the Mallinckrodt tube, which is available in different sizes. Usually tube sizes of 7.0 or 7.5 mm inner diameter are used for women and 8.0 or 8.5 mm inner diameter are used for men, depending on body size. Tubes are basically plastic tubes with a balloon around the distal edge (cuff), that can be inflated *via* a small tube (cuff-line) after insertion in the trachea sealing it against leakage (from the lung) and aspiration (form the pharyngeal side). The plastic material has a certain stiffness and is bent slightly following the anatomical structure between orifice and glottis. However, if a steeper angle is needed, a guidewire can be used (discussed later in this chapter).

Key points

- Artificial airways in the ICU usually describe endotracheal devices, *i.e.* an endotracheal tube or a tracheal cannula.

- Intubation in the ICU deserves careful preparation.

- Supraglottic airway devices may help to bridge a difficult-to-intubate situation.

- Videolaryngoscopy is a promising device to insert the endotracheal tube in difficult anatomical situations; the fibreoptic placement cannot be replaced completely.

Tracheal cannulas are shorter and a variety of brands exist with different advantages and disadvantages. Often, when tracheal cannula placement is planned as a temporary measure (for a period of ICU stay), flexible cannulas with shorter and larger dimensions (outer dimensions 9–11 mm) are used. In continuously tracheostomised patients (*i.e.* cerebral pathology, swallowing disorder and after surgery) stiff cannulas with different inlay management are inserted, but should be limited to units with long-term ventilation focus (specialised weaning wards). The cuffs have larger volumes resulting in lower tissue pressures that limit trauma and possibly long periods of tracheal stenosis.

Nasal tubes are mainly used during fibreoptic intubation, *e.g.* in an expected difficult airway. They are longer and smaller in diameter, in order to pass the nasal structures. Due to their higher resistance (Hagen–Poiseuille equation), they are not the tube of choice for longer ventilation or even spontaneous breathing efforts and are only a bridging method, most often for a planned tracheostomy in an ICU setting.

Mask ventilation

Before endotracheal placement of the tube, every operator should be capable of handling a ventilation mask connected to a handbag. This is of crucial importance for upholding oxygenation and as a backup if the airway cannot be secured with endotracheal intubation for example. An unskilled ICU practitioner must be trained in the handling of a mask. First, the mask is placed on the bridge of the nose and then placed completely on the face. One hand forms a "C" and presses the mask onto the face. Then, the third and fourth fingers lift the chin and pull the head backwards to open up the pharyngeal space by moving the tongue, while the other hand presses the bag gently to deliver a sufficient minute volume (*i.e.* 12–14 compressions per minute with fitting V_T). The bag usually has a volume of around 1.5 L, so you must not empty it completely (about one-third is enough). Ventilation can be improved by inserting a small tube, called the "Guedel tube", which helps to open up the pharyngeal space and move the tongue ventrally. In most cases, using a Guedel tube with skilled mask ventilation allows oxygenation until an artificial airway can be established (figure 1). If you consider using a PEEP valve with the bag you can expect to have a considerable amount of atelectatic lung areas after anaesthesia induction, especially in obese patients.

Guidewires

Guidewires/stylets can help to insert the tube when the hyomental distance is small, resulting in a "curve" the tube has to follow when inserted. The tube can be pre-formed as a "hockey" stick and inserted into the trachea. It is important that the stylet does not stick out at the distal end of the tube and it is retracted during the passage into the trachea to prevent perforation. For example, if the pars membranacea of the trachea is perforated by the stylet, a mediastinal emphysema results and the patient's life is at stake. Lubricating the stylet before inserting it into the tube (silicon spray, *etc.*) helps to retract it (otherwise plastic on plastic does not glide smoothly).

The intubation procedure

Preparation Before intubation is started the preparation of the procedure and patient-related risks is crucial; some basic questions should be answered, even in emergency situations:

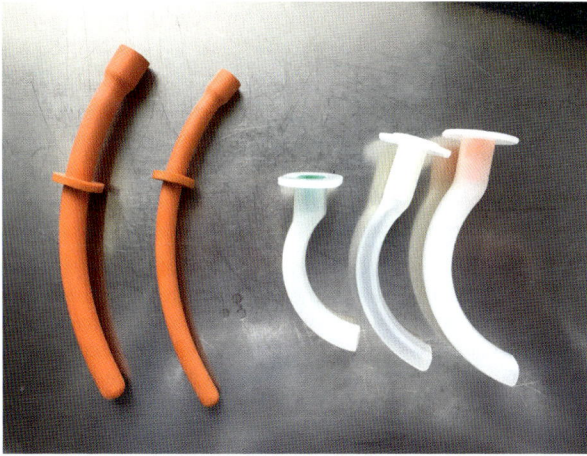

Figure 1. Wendel and Guedel tubes of different sizes. The Wendel tubes, shown on the left, can be used after extubation and in an awake patient. Guedel tubes of different sizes are shown on the right. Please be aware that insertion of a Guedel tube may evoke vagal reflexes with vomiting.

- Is there increased risk of aspiration?
- Is there intra-abdominal pathology?
- When was the last meal?
- Is there increased gastric pressure?
- Is there gastric sphincter pathology?
- Is there heartburn?
- Is there trauma?

If there is any doubt, precautions against aspiration must be taken. You must not underestimate the risk of aspiration. That implicates the intubation risk of aspiration which implies performing the intubation using a "rapid sequence induction" protocol possibly avoiding mask ventilation after anaesthesia induction and the use of a rapid acting muscle relaxant (succinylcholine or rocuronium in high dose). The head of the bed should be elevated to 30°; placement of a nasogastric tube should be considered to reduce the amount of gastric content and relieve gastric pressure (consider use of abdominal sonography to assess gastric filling). If a nasogastric tube is in place, suctioning should be continued using a second suctioning device.

Risks Intubation in the ICU is seldom a planned procedure in a healthy person, unlike in the operating room. The main risks of emergency intubations are:

- Unforeseen difficult airway
- Cannot intubate, cannot ventilate situation
- Failed intubation
- Hypoxia
- Aspiration

- Damage to teeth
- Damage to laryngeal structures
- Airway obstruction
- Haemodynamic instability (before the start of the procedure or caused by induction of anaesthesia)

Most of these risks are life threatening within a very short time. Table 1 gives an overview about the preparative steps prior to intubation.

Intubation using a Macintosh blade

Positioning Ideally, the patient is placed in a position called the "Jackson position", *i.e.* the head is lifted upwards towards the trunk, which allows a better view of the vocal cords. This is more difficult in an ICU bed than in the operating room but with the help of small pillows this can be established. Be aware that the trunk/neck and head should be in line, and your position should be as ideal as possible, which is behind the patient. Try to improve the space around the bed so that the team can work adequately.

Direct laryngoscopy The "classic" approach to inserting a tracheal tube is direct laryngoscopy. It consists of a handle to which blades of different sizes and shapes can be attached (figure 2a). A regular sized adult patient can usually be intubated using a size 3 Macintosh blade. The basic mechanism is lifting the mandible and head so that a direct view of the glottis is established.

Table 1. An overview of measures to be prepared prior to an intubation procedure

Airway	Ventilator prepared
	Handbag with 30 L·min^{-1} oxygen flow and reservoir, fitting facemask
	Two laryngoscopes and two different blade sizes, function tested
	Two different tube sizes
	Intubation stylet/bougie
	Cuff-blocker syringe 20 mL or manometer
	Capnography working
	Supraglottic airway reachable
Drugs	Well working *i.v.* for drug administration
	Hypnotic
	Opioid
	Muscle relaxant
	Catecholamines 100 and 10 µg·mL^{-1}
	Pressurised infusion bag (fluid challenge)
Suction	Running, tested
	Large suctioning tube
NIV	Pre-intubation with F_{IO_2} of 1.0 for 5 min, if possible (pre-oxygenation)
Team	Crew resource management principles
	• Who is who?
	• Who does what?
	• What if?
	• May we need help?
	• How long would it take to arrive?

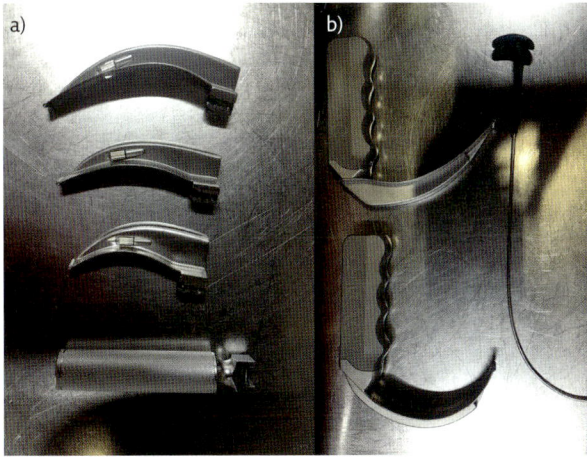

Figure 2. a) Three different sizes of a Macintosh blade (5, 4 and 3) with the handle. b) Two different spatulas of a videolaryngoscope (C-MAC; Karl-Storz, Tuttlingen, Germany). Note the different angle of the regular blade (top) and the hyperangulated shape (bottom). For the latter a special shaped stylet has to be used (right-hand side).

Insert the blade on the right and move towards the left when in the mouth taking the tongue out of the picture. The tip of the blade is placed above the epiglottis (so the epiglottis is not loaded on the spatula) and the whole device is pulled footwards, not kinked. Kinking puts pressure on the front teeth with the danger of breaking them and worsens the axis of sight making it more difficult to gain a direct view of the vocal cords. The resulting bleeding can make it impossible to intubate because reflection of light by the inner pharyngeal wall is disrupted in a bleeding situation. One predefined member of the team can perform a so-called "BURP" manoeuvre which is the acronym for "backwards-upwards-rightwards-pressure" to improve sight and facilitate placement of the tube. The tube is inserted until the first black line has passed the vocal cords and the cuff is inflated. Ventilation should start as soon as one member of the team can auscultate the stomach (failed intubation) and as a second step the lungs (lung ventilated? both sides ventilated?). Correct positioning of the tube is confirmed using waveform capnography. The hand of the intubating person keeps the tube in place until it is fixed on the patient's face. This has been demonstrated by Kabrhel *et al.* (2007).

Videolaryngoscopy

This technique has become more available and popular in recent years. Primarily constructed for training reasons its use has become routine in many operating rooms and ICUs. Videolaryngoscopes use a camera at the tip of the blade, for example, that is inserted in the mouth (indirect laryngoscopy). A main advantage is that all staff members involved in the procedure have a direct view of the larynx and can help to either identify the correct structures or apply manoeuvres (BURP, *etc.*) to ease intubation. Two different blade variations exist: either regular Macintosh blades with a camera and light at its tip, and hyperangulated versions (designed for difficult intubations) that allow a view of the larynx when the larynx is located ventrally and the intubating person has to "look around the corner".

There are a number of advantages and disadvantages of indirect laryngoscopy compared to direct laryngoscopy.

1) Advantages

- Eye and airway don't need to be in line
- Better view with limited mouth opening or mobility (c-spine precautions)
- Others can see and help
- Higher success rate, especially in difficult situations
- Education

2) Disadvantages

- Variable learning curves
- Fogging or secretions may obscure view
- Potential for equipment failure
- More expensive

Device selection Several companies provide videolaryngoscopes: C-MAC (Karl-Storz, Tuttlingen, Germany), Glidescope (Verathon, Bothell, WA, USA), AWS (Pentax, Tokyo, Japan), and King vision (Ambu, Ballerup, Denmark). For further examples see figure 2b.

Handling In general a four-step approach is used (mouth – screen – mouth – screen):

- Mouth: look in the mouth as you insert the videolaryngoscope (to avoid oropharyngeal trauma).
- Screen: look at the screen to visualise the epiglottis followed by the glottis itself, use minimal force to protract the mandible.
- Mouth: look in the mouth as you insert the endotracheal tube into the mouth (to avoid oropharyngeal trauma).
- Screen: look at the screen as you slowly pass the tube through the larynx.

With hyperangulated devices like the Glidescope or the D-blade of the C-MAC device tilt it downwards a little to bring the line of view and the axis of the airway more in line making driving the tip of the tube into the larynx easier. With these hyperangulated blades come preformed stylets that contain a handle with which the tube can be rotated and led into position. When the tip of the tube has passed the cords retract the stylet and pass the tube deeper. Conversely to pulling footwards with the regular blades, the hyperangulated blades must be pulled towards the ceiling.

Awake fibreoptic intubation

This procedure is used especially in cases with difficult airways in compliant patients. Besides this an experienced operator is necessary. In most settings in the ICU this is not the case. An advantage of this technique is that the patient would secure their own airway until the endotracheal tube is in place. Local anaesthetics (spray-as-you-go and/or transtracheal injection) and, for example, ketamine, remifentanil and/or dexmedetomidine can be used to facilitate patient compliance during the procedure while staying awake. Xylomethazoline should be administered to both nostrils to reduce the risk of bleeding. The bronchoscope is preloaded with a tube and inserted through the nostrils or orally, the connector of the tube to the machine is removed and kept in a place where it is available directly after intubation. There are two different ways to handle the procedure. The tube can be prepositioned in the epipharynx (such as a Wendel tube, *i.e.* small tubing used to keep the airway open and positioned through the nose) and the bronchoscope passed through it. Another way is the complete fibreoptic passage first; when the bronchoscope has safely reached the trachea, the tube is slid down the bronchoscope passing the nose, pharynx and glottis. Use 5–10 mL of lidocaine 1% to anesthetise the glottis and trachea before passing it. Bleeding may occur in several cases and can aggravate the intubation procedure or even make it impossible for the untrained and trained.

When the bronchoscope has passed through the glottis and the tube has been advanced in the trachea (correct position confirmed *via* bronchoscope) anaesthesia is induced with a hypnotic most often combined with an opioid.

It must be emphasised, that although pulmonologists are more familiar with a bronchoscope than a Macintosh device, fibreoptic intubation is the most skilful procedure of all procedures described. This has been demonstrated by Heidegger (2011).

Supraglottic devices

In the ICU setting, supraglottic airway devices are part of emergency airway management when placement of an endotracheal tube cannot be performed. Two different types exist and consist of laryngeal masks and (rarely) laryngeal tubes (figure 3). Both devices do not protect the lungs from macro-aspiration and their ability to apply high pressures in a situation of reduced compliance of the respiratory

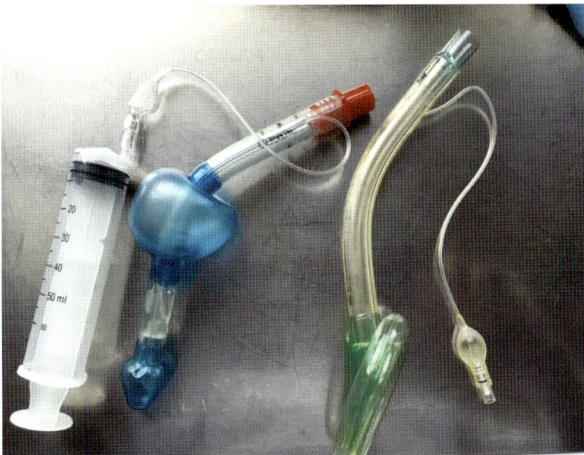

Figure 3. Laryngeal tube with insufflation syringe for cuff (left) and laryngeal mask (right).

system is limited: peak pressures must remain <20 cmH$_2$O to avoid gastric inflation. The masks are inserted with a prefilled cuff pointing in the direction of the hard palate. The mask is then guided into the pharynx; the tongue must remain in its position. These devices are only a bridging method in the ICU but may allow oxygenation until other devices (videolaryngoscope or fibreoptic bronchoscope) are in place. Specialised laryngeal masks allow the (fibreoptically guided) insertion of a small flexible tube. This has been demonstrated by Lighthall *et al.* (2013).

Emergency cricothyroidotomy

Indication is a "can't intubate, can't ventilate" scenario. With an extended neck in the supine position the thyroid cartilage is stabilised and a 4-cm vertical incision with a scalpel blade is made over the cricothyroid membrane. After identification of the cricothyroid membrane it is incised horizontally and a bougie ("stylet") is passed. An endotracheal tube (internal diameter 6 mm) is then passed *via* the bougie and the cuff is inflated. Correct placement is confirmed using waveform capnography. In most cases a cricothyroidotomy is converted within a short time to a surgical tracheostomy in the operating theatre.

It is of importance to have a plan and the skills to manage a "can't intubate, can't ventilate" scenario. Regular simulation training in this technique and setting, using the coniotomy kits in the ICU, can be an important part of the strategy.

Percutaneous dilatational tracheotomy

Tracheotomy is a subglottical airway inserted directly into the trachea.

Examples of indications can be upper airway obstruction, the inability to protect and clear the airway (inadequate coughing), long-term ventilation and to facilitate weaning from prolonged invasive ventilation. Advantages include the reduced need for sedation, possibly communication (phonation), training of swallowing, decreased work of breathing and patients might be transferred to wards. Timing has to be on an individual basis (advantages and disadvantages of an early percutaneous dilatational tracheotomy strategy). Examples of relative contraindications are no informed consent, bleeding disorders, infection, mass (*e.g.* big thyroid) or history of radiation therapy at site of placement, difficult anatomy (short neck, distortion, *etc.*), emergency setting, difficult intubation or patient still on high respiratory support (PEEP >10 cmH$_2$O, F_{IO_2} >0.5). Ultrasound can help identify the anatomy and possible crossing vessels before or during the procedure. In the case of difficult anatomy or difficult intubation a surgical approach might be a preferable option compared to the described dilatational technique.

The patient is put under general anaesthesia and positioned supine with the head in hyperextension (hint: put a towel in between the shoulders). The setting is comparable to intubation (ready for re-intubation, *etc.*) (see above). The patient should be fasted to reduce risk of aspiration during this elective procedure. The team consists of an airway manager and a surgeon in addition to assistance. Capnography is used during whole procedure. The procedure is sterile. The most commonly used Ciaglia technique is described below.

- Ventilate patient with F_{IO_2} 1.0, pressure control (set minute volume low alarm off or as low as possible regarding leakage during procedure).
- Bronchial and pharyngeal toilet.

- Cuff is deflated and airway manager retracts endotracheal tube under (video-) laryngoscopic view until the cuff is situated between or right above the vocal cords. As an alternative a laryngeal mask can be considered as an airway.
- Bronchoscope is inserted through endotracheal tube (or laryngeal mask).
- Surgeon uses local anaesthetic (possibly with adrenaline) at site of incision.
- Incision about 2.5 cm in between first and second tracheal ring (if not well palpable, use the line from half-way thyroid jugulum).
- Needle puncture in between first and second ring (air aspiration), position and depth checked *via* bronchoscope (cave: perforation of posterior wall).
- Guidewire is placed through the needle and graduated dilatation takes place (Ciaglia).
- Tracheotomy cannula is placed and position is checked with bronchoscope.
- Never inflate cuff of tracheal cannula while still ventilating patient *via* endotracheal tube due to risk of tracheal perforation.
- If accidental decannulation takes place in first 1–3 days use oral intubation rather than attempting to put the cannula back (risk of malpositioning).

Short-term complications can include equipment failure, malposition, damage to local structures, emphysema, pneumothorax or mediastinum possibly leading to death. Delayed complications can include infection, accidental decannulation, ulceration of local tissue and obstruction of cannula. Late complications such as bleeding due to tracheal granulomata or tracheal stenosis or malacia can occur.

Summary

Establishing an artificial airway in the ICU is a common procedure. The handling of the devices needs skilful operators and knowledge of the anatomical structures and pitfalls. Artificial airways in ICU are most often tracheal tube and tracheal cannula, the placements of which are most likely to be done by every ICU physician. Nevertheless, the handling of emergency settings, supralaryngeal airways, mask ventilation, *etc.* is crucial for the patients being treated.

Further reading

- Apfelbaum JL, *et al.* (2013). Practice guidelines for management of the difficult airway: an updated report by the American Society of Anesthesiologists Task Force on Management of the Difficult Airway. *Anesthesiology*; 118: 251–270.

- Ciaglia P, *et al.* (1985). Elective percutaneous dilatational tracheostomy. A new simple bedside procedure; preliminary report. *Chest*; 87: 715–719.

- De Jong A, *et al.* (2014). Video laryngoscopy *versus* direct laryngoscopy for orotracheal intubation in the intensive care unit: a systematic review and meta-analysis. *Intensive Care Med*; 40: 629–639.

- Frerk C, *et al.* (2015). Difficult Airway Society 2015 guidelines for management of unanticipated difficult intubation in adults. *Br J Anaesth*; 115: 827–848.

- Heidegger T (2011). Fiberoptic intubation. *N Engl J Med*; 364: e42.

- Hosokawa K, *et al.* (2015). Timing of tracheotomy in ICU patients: a systemic controlled review of randomized controlled trials. *Crit Care*; 19: 424.

- Kabrhel C, *et al.* (2007). Orotracheal intubation. *N Engl J Med*; 356: e15.

- Lafferty BD, *et al.* (2015). Videolaryngoscopy as a new standard of care. *Br J Anaesth*; 115: 136–137.

- Lighthall G, *et al.* (2013). Laryngeal mask airway in medical emergencies. *N Engl J Med*; 369: e26.

- Ortega R, *et al.* (2007). Positive-pressure ventilation with a face mask and a bag-valve device. *N Engl J Med*; 357: e4.

- Ortega R, *et al.* (2012). Monitoring ventilation with capnography. *N Engl J Med*; 367: e27.

- Paolini JB, *et al.* (2013). Review article: video-laryngoscopy: another tool for difficult intubation or a new paradigm in airway management? *Can J Anaesth*; 60: 184–191.

Controlled modes

Jakob Wittenstein, Robert Huhle and Marcelo Gama de Abreu

Invasive ventilation is often unavoidable in the critical phase of illness and represents an important lifesaving measure. Nonetheless, further damage to the lung can occur during ventilation. VILI can increase mortality and must be avoided.

Following the principle of *primum non nocere*, a strictly evidence-based patient-centred choice of ventilation settings is recommended. These settings constitute the so-called "lung-protective ventilation". The main components of lung-protective ventilation are V_T, low P_{plat} and ΔP, and adequate levels of PEEP. Respiratory rate (RR) and respiratory gas flow should also be taken into account. Taken together, these variables will determine the amount of energy that is stored and also dissipated in the lungs due to cyclical deformation, possibly triggering pro-inflammatory and pro-fibrotic responses, and even breaking the alveolar–capillary barrier if the plastic characteristics of the parenchyma are exceeded. Usually, lung protection is more easily accomplished during controlled invasive ventilation, *i.e.* without spontaneous breathing activity. Although this can be accomplished with all modes, the particularities of each mode can be used to optimise the ventilatory approach.

In this chapter, basic concepts of controlled invasive ventilation are revised, modes are briefly explained, and state-of-the-art information on the practice of lung-protective ventilation settings revised.

Key points

- Controlled invasive ventilation modes are among the oldest and most frequently used modes of invasive ventilation in clinical practice.

- Lung-protective ventilation strategies can be accomplished with both volume-controlled ventilation (VCV) and pressure-controlled ventilation (PCV).

- Lung recruitment manoeuvres are better conducted under PCV.

- Titration of PEEP is more easily conducted under VCV.

Controlled invasive ventilation modes

Modern intensive care and anaesthesia ventilators offer several different ventilation modes. Regarding lung protection in patients without lung injury, superiority of one specific mode over the others has not been demonstrated. Table 1 depicts some of the most frequently used modes for controlled invasive ventilation.

Conventional controlled invasive ventilation modes The most commonly used modes of controlled invasive ventilation are pressure- and volume-controlled ventilation (PCV and VCV, respectively), where VCV corresponds to the default mode in most ventilators.

Figure 1a shows typical tracings of tracheal pressure, ventilator system airway pressure, flow and volume during VCV. VCV is a time cycled and volume-targeted invasive ventilation mode. In VCV, V_T, RR and I:E ratio represent the basic settings, whereas a constant inspiratory flow is adjusted by the ventilator itself to deliver the desired settings. Also, an inspiratory pause can be set, which will lead to a relatively short period of zero flow at the end of inspiration. In some ventilators, this pressure may also be determined by means of an inspiratory hold manoeuvre. The inspiratory pause can be useful to allow equilibration of airway pressure across different lung units, and also to assess the so-called airway P_{plat}, which is more closely related to the pressure in the alveoli than the peak airway pressure. This mode allows for better control of the end-expiratory partial carbon dioxide pressure.

PCV is a time cycled and pressure-limited invasive ventilation mode (figure 1b). In PCV the main setting is the inspiratory pressure, and the ventilator adjusts flow during inspiration in order to achieve an approximately constant airway pressure, resulting in a decelerating flow pattern.

VCV has also been implemented in combination with an automatic flow adjustment, where the lowest possible inspiratory pressure is achieved. This adjustment results in a decelerating flow pattern that resembles PCV. This mode has been termed pressure–regulated VCV, which is similar to PC-VG.

In most ICU ventilators, and some modern anaesthesia devices, VCV and PCV may allow triggering by the patient's inspiratory effort. Usually, the inspiratory trigger is based on inspiratory flow or pressure, or both. When the patient triggers a spontaneous breath, the ventilator delivers a cycle, with similar characteristics as the respective controlled breaths. Usually, they are referred to as assisted/controlled VCV and PCV, but their description is beyond the scope of this chapter. Furthermore, it should be kept in mind that under assisted/controlled ventilation, V_T is not under control, and so-called pendelluft (shift of gas among different lung regions despite no delivery of flow by the ventilator) may occur.

Further time cycled, pressure-controlled modes APRV is a time cycled ventilation mode that applies two levels of airway pressure. The higher continuous airway pressure is usually maintained for longer periods of time (usually >2 s), and released in intervals until a lower pressure is reached (for example PEEP, but also zero) for short periods of time (usually <1 s, typically 0.5 s). These settings are intended to result in an inverse I:E ratio, but physiological ratios are also possible. As a result of inverse I:E ratio, so-called auto- or intrinsic-PEEP may occur due to limitation of the time for expiration. An important difference from conventional PCV is the fact that nonassisted spontaneous breathing activity is possible at any time, both

Table 1. Common modes used for controlled invasive ventilation

Mode	Comment	Possible indications
VCV	VCV is targeted at volume and cycled by time; available in most mechanical ventilators in ICU and operating room.	Control of V_T in protective invasive ventilation; control of $P_{a}CO_2$; decremental PEEP trials.
PCV	PCV is targeted at pressure and cycled by time.	Control of plateau and peak airway pressure; offers a decelerating inspiratory flow pattern that might theoretically homogenise air mixture across lung regions; allows better control of ΔP in protective invasive ventilation; recruitment manoeuvres more easily performed.
VCV with AutoFlow	Adjusts the flow to achieve the desired tidal volume. Also known as pressure control with volume guarantee (PC-VG).	Volume guarantee at lowest possible airway pressure and with decelerating inspiratory flow pattern.
Airway pressure release ventilation (APRV)	APRV is a time cycled ventilation with a higher and lower continuous airway pressure. Typically, inspiratory times are much higher than expiratory times, resulting in an inverse inspiratory to expiratory (I:E) ratio of up to 10:1. Nonassisted spontaneous breathing activity is possible at any time under a bias flow.	Increase of mean airway pressure; smooth transition from controlled to spontaneous breathing.
Biphasic airway pressure ventilation/bi-level positive airway pressure	Airway pressure is changed between two levels, but can sense and respond to inspiratory efforts to trigger inspiration. It can be combined with pressure support at the lower airway pressure level, and also at the higher airway pressure level in some ventilators, which is known as bi-level positive airway pressure ventilation.	Transition from controlled to assisted spontaneous breathing.
High frequency jet ventilation (HFJV)	HFJV uses respiratory rates above the physiological value (100–150 breaths per min) and working pressures at the ventilator higher than usual (1.5–2.5 bar).	Airway surgery; diagnostic procedures of the upper airways; one-lung ventilation; transtracheal ventilation in emergency airway situations.
High frequency oscillatory ventilation (HFOV)	HFOV uses respiratory rates even higher than HFJV (600–900 breaths per min); promotes active expiration.	Recruitment of lungs and ventilation under higher mean airway pressure; lung surgery requiring a quiet lung; surgery or diagnostic procedures of the airways; CT-guided procedures where movement artefacts should be reduced.

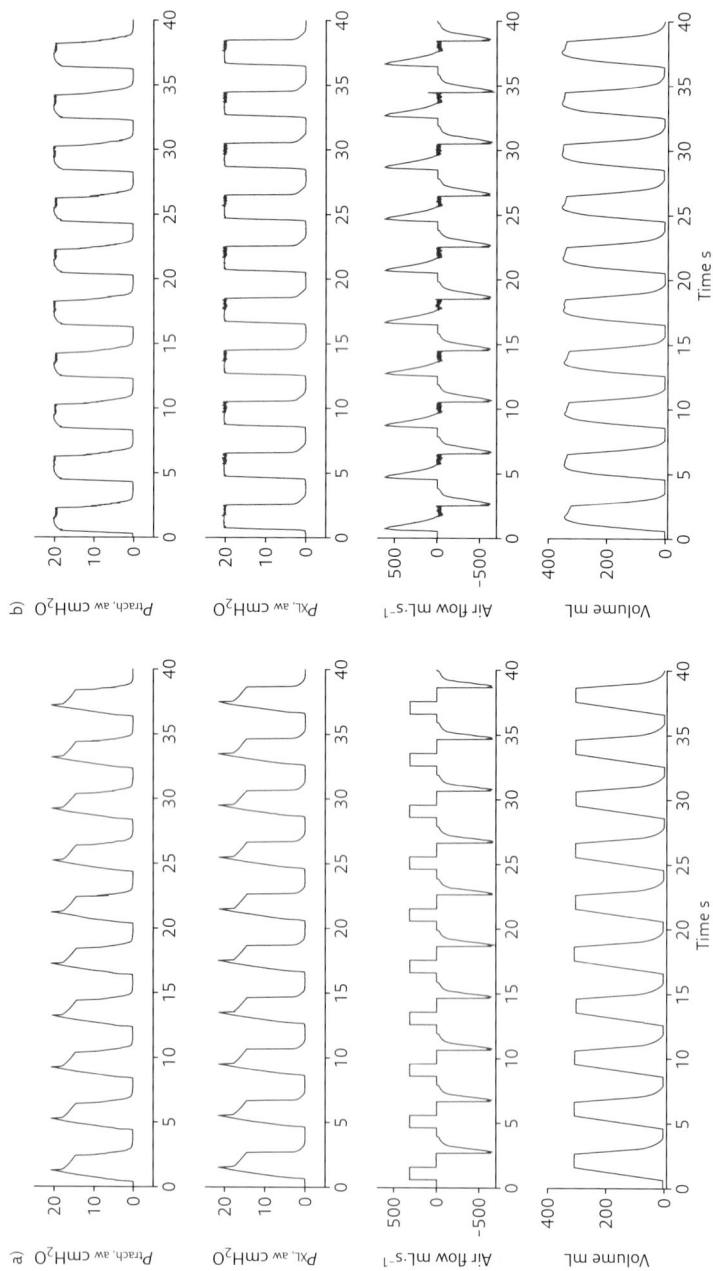

Figure 1. Tracing of tracheal airway pressure (P$_{trach, aw}$), airway pressure in the ventilator (P$_{XL, aw}$), air flow and volume in the respiratory system (volume) during a) VCV and b) PCV at the bench. Note the differences in the time patterns between these modes.

at the higher and the lower airway pressures. For controlled invasive ventilation, APRV has similar indications to PCV, while permitting a smooth transition from controlled to assisted spontaneous breathing.

Biphasic airway pressure ventilation resembles APRV in some respects. However, biphasic airway pressure ventilation can be used with time windows that are modulated by inspiratory and expiratory efforts. Also, it allows pressure-supported breaths at the lower airway pressure level and, in certain devices, also at the higher airway pressure, so-called bi-level positive airway pressure mode. Thus, unlike in APRV, asynchrony between patient inspiratory or expiratory effort and ventilator may occur.

In most ventilators, in controlled ventilation modes an inspiratory trigger based on inspiratory flow or pressure can be set. When the patient triggers a spontaneous breath, the ventilator delivers a cycle, similar to the mandatory breaths. The combination of controlled ventilation allowing for extra spontaneous breaths is referred to as assisted/controlled ventilation.

Nonconventional controlled invasive ventilation modes Nonconventional modes of controlled invasive ventilation are usually reserved for severe impairment of lung function and selected indications during surgery, for example, to facilitate the surgical approach of the airways, emergency situations and diagnostic procedures. They include the so-called high frequency ventilation modes, especially HFJV and HFOV.

Unlike conventional ventilation, HFJV can be accomplished using a conventional endotracheal tube, or a small bore cannula placed above and below the glottis through a transtracheal or a transglottic approach. Jet ventilators may differ importantly from conventional ventilators, since they need to apply pressures in the range of 1.5–2.5 bar, with an above physiological RR of 100–150 breaths per min. These settings result in airway pressures lower than those obtained with conventional controlled invasive ventilation, and in $V\text{T}$ as low as 1–3 mL·kg^{-1}. Due to possible air entrainment, inspiratory oxygen fractions during HFJV are higher than usual (50–100%), but the effective oxygen fraction in the trachea is usually lower.

In HFOV a diaphragm or piston pump is used to obtain sinusoidal oscillations in airway pressure. Described as early as 1972, this mode uses RR of 5–15 Hz. The mean airway pressure is determined by the so-called inspiratory bias flow and a gas outflow valve. The pressure differences at the ventilator are situated in the range of 60–90 cmH$_2$O. Despite this high value, the ΔP in HFOV is high, the downstream pressure in the airways is obviously much lower, and the resulting $V\text{T}$ is only a fraction of that obtained with conventional invasive ventilation, being situated in the range of 1–3 mL·kg^{-1}. The major factors that determine the $V\text{T}$ during HFOV are the diameter and length of the endotracheal tube, ΔP itself, inspiratory time, the impedance of the respiratory system and the oscillation frequency, whereby higher frequencies result in lower $V\text{T}$.

The combination of ultra-low $V\text{T}$ with an increased mean airway pressure makes this mode attractive for protective lung ventilation. However, there is no evidence it is superior to conventional controlled invasive ventilation.

Protective controlled invasive ventilation settings

Whether under VCV, PCV or any other mode of controlled invasive ventilation, ventilation should be conducted to protect the lungs from excessive stress, while providing adequate gas exchange. Since no mode has been shown to be superior in terms of impact on lung injury, the recommendations given here apply to all modes.

The role of V_T Despite several clinical studies showing potential benefits of low V_T, high V_T is still common during surgery and in the ICU, even in patients with ARDS. In ARDS a V_T ≤6mL per kg predicted body weight (PBW) reduced mortality, whereas in surgical patients two-lung ventilation with a V_T of 6–8 mL per kg PBW reduced the rate of postoperative pulmonary complications. Therefore, a low protective V_T should be used in all patients under controlled invasive ventilation, whereby the calculation of V_T should be based on ideal weight or PBW, and not on actual body weight. This ensures that both obese and cachectic patients are ventilated with an adequate V_T. The following equations can be used to calculate the ideal body weight in kg:

$$PBW \text{ in males} = 50 + 0.91 \times (\text{height in cm} - 152.4)$$

$$PBW \text{ in females} = 45.5 + 0.91 \times (\text{height in cm} - 152.4)$$

When using time cycled modes, for example PCV, electronic warning and reporting systems and staff training can help to improve compliance with a protective ventilation regime with reduced V_T. If hypercapnia develops, it can usually be well tolerated. However, it should be borne in mind that hypercapnia can increase pulmonary hypertension and thus aggravate right ventricular dysfunction. Further consequences may be myocardial depression and reduced renal blood flow. Finally, hypercapnia should be avoided if intracerebral pressure is already elevated.

The role of plateau and inspiratory peak pressures The inspiratory P_{plat} results from the interaction between V_T, PEEP and the mechanical properties of the respiratory system. This value should be approximately the same under VCV and PCV. The ARDS Network showed that a P_{plat} ≤30 cmH$_2$O was associated with reduced mortality when compared to values as high as 50 cmH$_2$O.

In patients without injured lungs, P_{plat} is usually <15 cmH$_2$O, even when a V_T as high as 10 mL per kg PBW is used. When the P_{plat} exceeds 15–20 cmH$_2$O, a reduction of V_T to <6 mL per kg PBW should considered. However, absolute values may differ in patients with increased intra-abdominal pressure or stiff chest, since P_{plat} is only a surrogate for the transpulmonary pressure.

The inspiratory peak pressure also depends on V_T, PEEP and the mechanical properties of the respiratory system. However, it is strongly influenced by the gas flow and, consequently, the resistive component of the respiratory circuit and system. In this regard, VCV and PCV differ importantly. At similar V_T and PEEP, the constant inspiratory flow of VCV, especially if combined with an inspiratory pause, will lead to higher peak pressures as compared with PCV. This difference is not easily predictable in clinical routine, but must be considered when adjusting protective controlled invasive ventilation. Ideally, peak and plateau pressure should be monitored by end-inspiratory occlusions.

The role of ΔP The interest in ΔP, which represents the relationship between V_T and compliance of the respiratory system, and can be calculated from the difference between plateau and end-expiratory pressure, has increased in recent years. Given that the protective range of V_T may vary according to the lung volume available for ventilation ("baby lung" concept), assessment of ΔP can contribute to a more individual titration of controlled invasive ventilation. Accordingly, ΔP serves as an indicator of the functional lung volume. In patients with ARDS, ΔP >14 cmH$_2$O was associated with mortality (Amato *et al.*, 2015), while in surgical patients an increase in ΔP as a response to PEEP adjustments was associated with higher rates of pulmonary complications (Neto *et al.*, 2016). Nonetheless, it must be kept in mind that the influence of the thoracic wall is not mirrored by ΔP, and that its prognostic value is limited when spontaneous breathing is present.

The role of PEEP During VCV and PCV, PEEP is achieved by closure of the expiratory valve in the ventilator; whereas in APRV, PEEP represents a continuous positive pressure with a bias flow that is able to react to inspiratory effort demands. Intended to stabilise lung units at expiration, improve oxygenation and minimise cyclic opening and closing of alveoli, PEEP represents one of the most controversial aspects of protective controlled invasive ventilation. Higher PEEP values have been recommended in severe ARDS, but this has been challenged recently. Excessively high PEEP values lead to atrophy of longitudinal muscle fibres of the diaphragm. Also, inappropriate PEEP settings, especially in presence of expiratory flow limitation, may lead to trapping of air at end-expiration, resulting in airway pressures higher than those set in the mechanical ventilator (auto-PEEP), to redistribution of air within lung units with different time constants (pendelluft), and impairment of haemodynamics. Individual titration of PEEP has been claimed to mitigate these adverse effects. Although many techniques have been proposed for PEEP titration, perhaps the most widely used one is the evaluation of the elastance or compliance of the respiratory system during a stepwise decrease of PEEP following lung recruitment, a so-called decremental PEEP trial (figure 2). This titration is better accomplished during VCV than PCV, since VCV allows the direct measurement of the elastance at constant V_T. However, it must be kept in mind that titration of PEEP using a decremental trial is controversial, and has been associated with higher mortality in patients with ARDS.

The role of lung recruitment manoeuvres Recruitment manoeuvres aim at increasing the number of lung units available for ventilation, and require that regional opening pressures be exceeded for sufficient time. Their use is controversial both in the ICU and during surgery. Current evidence supports that they should be used only as a rescue during hypoxaemia, and carried out in a standardised manner. Also, they should preferably be conducted during tidal ventilation, *i.e.* without stopping the ventilator. For this purpose, PCV is superior to VCV. PCV allows the PEEP to be gradually increased until the desired opening pressure is exceeded, while keeping ΔP constant (figure 2). Importantly, V_T will decrease during this procedure, possibly reducing the chance of trauma of the lung parenchyma.

Summary

Controlled invasive ventilation modes, specifically VCV and PCV, are among the oldest and most frequently used modes of invasive ventilation in clinical practice. Accordingly, every physician should be able to use them, whether working in the ICU, operating room, emergency room or any other specialty. Controlled invasive ventilation modes have served as basis for the development of several other modes, including those that allow synchronisation with the patient's respiratory effort and even nonassisted spontaneous breathing. Although the flow and pressure *versus* time profiles from VCV and PCV differ importantly, the clinical outcome associated

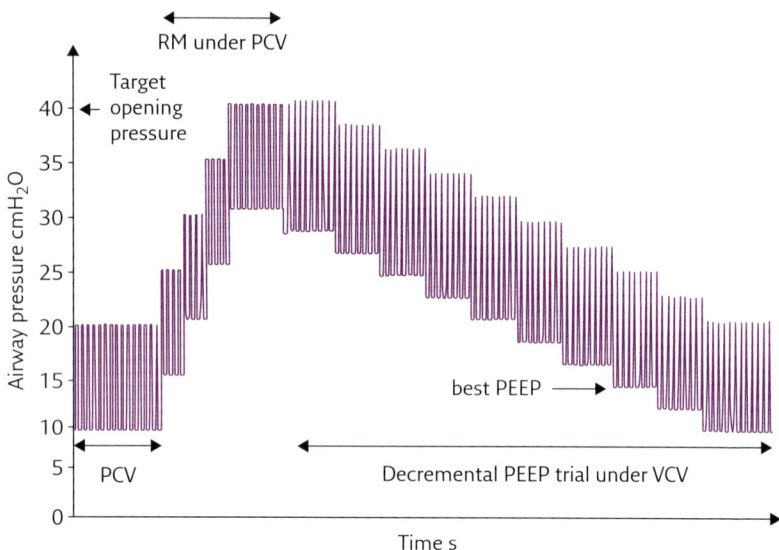

Figure 2. Recordings of airway pressure and time during a typical lung recruitment manoeuvre (RM) under PCV, followed by a decremental PEEP trial under VCV. The RM is performed with a stepwise increase of PEEP and fixed ΔP until exceeding the target opening pressure. The decremental PEEP trial aims to determine the PEEP that leads to the highest compliance of the respiratory system (best PEEP). Values must be individualised and the RM conducted only if there are no contraindications.

with their use does not differ significantly. Accordingly, settings of variables for lung protection, especially V_T, RR and PEEP, can be accomplished with both modes. However, they differ in terms of their ability to deliver recruitment manoeuvres and in facilitating the evaluation of PEEP able to stabilise lungs. While PCV offers the advantage of a constant ΔP during a stepwise increase of PEEP, VCV allows direct assessment of elastance during a decremental PEEP trial. The appropriate use and ability to choose the controlled invasive ventilation mode that best fits to a specific situation or task demands training and knowledge of the underlying functioning principles.

Further reading

- The Acute Respiratory Distress Syndrome Network (2000). Ventilation with lower tidal volumes as compared with traditional tidal volumes for acute lung injury and the acute respiratory distress syndrome. *N Engl J Med*; 342: 1301–1308.

- Amato MB, *et al.* (2015). Driving pressure and survival in the acute respiratory distress syndrome. *N Engl J Med*; 372: 747–755.

- Bellani G, *et al.* (2016). Epidemiology, patterns of care, and mortality for patients with acute respiratory distress syndrome in intensive care units in 50 countries. *JAMA*; 315: 788–800.

- Briel M, *et al.* (2010). Higher *vs* lower positive end-expiratory pressure in patients with acute lung injury and acute respiratory distress syndrome: systematic review and meta-analysis. *JAMA*; 303: 865–873.

- Buczkowski PW, *et al.* (2007). Air entrainment during high-frequency jet ventilation in a model of upper tracheal stenosis. *Br J Anaesth*; 99: 891–897.

- Chatburn RL, *et al.* (2014). A taxonomy for mechanical ventilation: 10 fundamental maxims. *Respir Care*; 59: 1747–1763.

- Cools F, *et al.* (2009). Elective high frequency oscillatory ventilation *versus* conventional ventilation for acute pulmonary dysfunction in preterm infants. *Cochrane Database Syst Rev*; 3: CD000104.

- Esteban A, *et al.* (2013). Evolution of mortality over time in patients receiving mechanical ventilation. *Am J Respir Crit Care Med*; 188: 220–230.

- Fritzsche K, *et al.* (2010). Anasthesiologische Besonderheiten bei der laryngotrachealen Chirurgie. Hochfrequenzjetventilation als spezielle Beatmungsstrategie wahrend der Narkose.Anesthetic management in laryngotracheal surgery [High-frequency jet ventilation as strategy for ventilation during general anesthesia]. *Anaesthesist*; 59: 1051–1061.

- Gattinoni L, *et al.* (2005). The concept of "baby lung". *Intensive Care Med*; 31: 776–784.

- Gavriely N, *et al.* (1985). Pressure-flow relationships of endotracheal tubes during high-frequency ventilation. *J Appl Physiol*; 59: 3–11.

- Güldner A, *et al.* (2015). Intraoperative protective mechanical ventilation for prevention of postoperative pulmonary complications: a comprehensive review of the role of tidal volume, positive end-expiratory pressure, and lung recruitment maneuvers. *Anesthesiology*; 123: 692–713.

- Hemmes SN, *et al.* (2013). Intraoperative ventilatory strategies to prevent postoperative pulmonary complications: a meta-analysis. *Curr Opin Anaesthesiol*; 26: 126–133.

- Henderson-Smart DJ, *et al.* (2009). High frequency oscillatory ventilation *versus* conventional ventilation for infants with severe pulmonary dysfunction born at or near term. *Cochrane Database Syst Rev*; 3: CD002974.

- Krishnan JA, *et al.* (2000). High-frequency ventilation for acute lung injury and ARDS. *Chest*; 118: 795–807.

- LAS VEGAS Investigators (2017). Epidemiology, practice of ventilation and outcome for patients at increased risk of postoperative pulmonary complications: LAS VEGAS - an observational study in 29 countries. *Eur J Anaesthesiol*; 34: 492–507.

- Lunkenheimer PP, *et al.* (1972). Application of transtracheal pressure oscillations as a modification of "diffusing respiration". *Br J Anaesth*; 44: 627.

- Marchak BE, *et al.* (1981). Treatment of RDS by high-frequency oscillatory ventilation: a preliminary report. *J Pediatr*; 99: 287–292.

- Neto AS, *et al.* (2016). Association between driving pressure and development of postoperative pulmonary complications in patients undergoing mechanical ventilation for general anaesthesia: a meta-analysis of individual patient data. *Lancet Respir Med*; 4: 272–280.

- The PROVEnet Investigators (2014). Higher *versus* lower positive end-expiratory pressure during general anaesthesia for open abdominal surgery – the PROVHILO trial. *Lancet*; 384: 495-503.

- Putensen C, *et al.* (2009). Meta-analysis: ventilation strategies and outcomes of the acute respiratory distress syndrome and acute lung injury. *Ann Intern Med*; 151: 566-576.

- Writing Group for the PReVENT Investigators, *et al.* (2018). Effect of a low *vs* intermediate tidal volume strategy on ventilator-free days in intensive care unit patients without ARDS: a randomized clinical trial. *JAMA*; 320: 1872-1880.

Partially supported modes

Christian Putensen and Stefan Muenster

Partial ventilatory support is commonly used not only to separate patients from invasive ventilation, but also to provide stable ventilatory assistance of a desired degree. Because excessive workload may lead to muscle fatigue, sufficient ventilatory support has to be provided to maintain the work of breathing at a tolerable level. However, increasing the level of ventilatory support beyond an adequate level of spontaneous work of breathing and alveolar ventilation has not been demonstrated to be advantageous for the patient. Therefore, full ventilatory support should be seen as an extreme level of ventilatory support.

Conventional partially supported ventilator modes (table 1) either provide ventilatory assistance to every inspiratory effort and modulate the V_T of the patient (*e.g.* pressure support ventilation (PSV)), or modulate minute ventilation by periodically adding mechanical insufflations to unsupported spontaneous

Key points

- The potential benefits of preserved spontaneous breathing during invasive ventilation are an increased aeration of nonventilated lung regions close to the diaphragm, less need for sedation, improved cardiac filling and better matching of pulmonary ventilation and perfusion, and thus, oxygenation.

- Disadvantages of spontaneous breathing during invasive ventilation include the possibility that high spontaneous breathing effort in patients with respiratory failure may cause a high transpulmonary pressure (P_L), which has the potential to aggravate VILI. In addition, high spontaneous breathing efforts may result in uncontrolled high and injurious V_T.

- Airway pressure release ventilation (APRV)/biphasic positive airway pressure allows unrestricted spontaneous breathing in any phase of the ventilator cycle and has been associated with lower inflation pressure, better oxygenation, less sedative use and less pneumonia when compared with other modes of invasive ventilation in patients with ARDS.

Table 1. Ventilator modes for partially supported ventilation

PSV	Assisted spontaneous breathing (every spontaneous breathing effort made by the patient will be supported with a preset inspiratory pressure)
Assist-control ventilation	The ventilator will deliver a fixed V_T when a breathing effort made by the patient is detected
APRV and biphasic positive airway pressure	Ventilation by time-cycled switching between two pressure levels in a CPAP circuit Unrestricted and unassisted breathing are permitted in any phase of the mechanical ventilator cycle
Synchronised intermittent mandatory ventilation (SIMV)	In SIMV the ventilator attempts to deliver the mandatory breaths in synchrony with the patient's own inspiratory efforts

breathing (*e.g.* intermittent mandatory ventilation). In contrast, ventilatory support techniques such as biphasic positive airway pressure, which is equivalent to APRV, allow unrestricted spontaneous breathing in any phase of the mechanical cycle.

Advantages and disadvantages of spontaneous breathing during invasive ventilation

To understand the advantages and disadvantages of preserved spontaneous breathing (unassisted breathing) during invasive ventilation, it is helpful to first gain some insight into the basic physiology of spontaneous breathing in a nonventilated person. In a nonventilated person, the posterior muscular sections of the diaphragm show greater movement than the anterior tendon plate. Consequently, the decrease in intrapleural pressure and the increase in P_L is higher in the dependent lung regions close to the diaphragm when compared with nondependent lung regions. This increase in P_L accounts for the recruitment of non-aerated lung regions close to the diaphragm in nonventilated individuals.

This effect can also be partially observed in invasively ventilated patients where the mode of the ventilator allows spontaneous breathing (*e.g.* APRV or biphasic positive airway pressure). In spontaneously breathing patients with concomitant invasive ventilation, radiographic imaging using CT demonstrated that spontaneous breathing distributes most of the V_T to the dependent lung regions close to the diaphragm, thereby reducing the cyclic alveolar collapse. Thus, the dependent lung regions tend to be better aerated during spontaneous breathing in ventilated patients compared with controlled ventilation, especially when they are in a supine position. Therefore, ventilation–perfusion matching improves in ventilated patients during partial ventilator support (assisted breathing) when compared with controlled invasive ventilation (the absence of spontaneous breathing). Moreover, improved oxygenation and decarboxylation of the blood has been reported in several studies when spontaneous breathing is preserved during invasive ventilation. Spontaneous breathing in ventilated patients leads to a periodic reduction in the intrathoracic pressure, which supports venous return and ventricular filling. Consequently, cardiac output and oxygen transport capacity increase in patients with normal cardiac function. However, in ventilated patients with congestive heart failure increased venous return due to spontaneous breathing may worsen cardiac function. Restricted use of neuromuscular blocking agents (NMBAs) in ventilated patients allows for concomitant spontaneous breathing and lower levels of sedation (*e.g.* Richmond Agitation–Sedation Scale (RASS) of –2 to –3); and subsequently, less use of vasopressors, which is associated with better survival. Even short periods of invasive ventilation (<3 days) with complete diaphragm inactivity have been shown to cause diaphragm muscle atrophy and dysfunction, and were associated with prolonged weaning from invasive ventilation.

Although the physiology suggests that spontaneous breathing during invasive ventilation may be beneficial, some disadvantages have been linked with spontaneous breathing in ventilated patients. Even moderate increases in P_L have been linked to the release of inflammatory markers and translocation of microorganisms, which may contribute to pulmonary and extrapulmonary organ dysfunction and an increase in mortality in patients with ARDS. Thus, an increase in P_L caused by spontaneous breathing during ventilation may induce VILI. Some authors report that high spontaneous breathing efforts in ventilated patients with respiratory failure cause high P_L, which has the potential to aggravate VILI. In addition, spontaneous breathing in ventilated patients may result in uncontrolled high and injurious V_T. Although a regional increase in P_L with spontaneous breathing in ventilated patients has been shown to promote recruitment and reduce cyclic alveolar collapse, its role in VILI in the dependent lung regions is not yet fully understood.

Interaction between spontaneous breathing and invasive ventilation

Modulation of V_T through mechanical support of each breath – assisted invasive ventilation Every spontaneous breathing attempt at inspiration should be followed by mechanical support provided by the ventilator. Although the spontaneous breath is supported in different ways in different ventilation modes, an increase in the patient's respiratory rate, caused by increased ventilatory demand, will always result in more mechanical support. By contrast, a reduction in respiratory rate will lead to a reduction in mechanical ventilatory support, which in the case of apnoea will be nil.

Modulation of minute volume (through the intermittent application of mechanical V_T in addition to non-assisted spontaneous breathing) – partial ventilator support In these modes, the mechanical ventilatory support is constant and does not depend on the inspiratory efforts of the patient. Increased ventilatory demand does not result in any change in the level of mechanical support. However, by regulating the mechanical ventilatory rate, infinitely variable support of spontaneous breathing from 0% to 100% is possible. In the event of apnoea, the set minute volume will be applied.

Controlled invasive ventilation *versus* partial ventilator support in allowing concomitant spontaneous breathing in patients with severe ARDS

The ARDS et Curarisation Systematique (ACURASYS) RCT using lung-protective controlled invasive ventilation and deep sedation (Ramsay Score of 6, which corresponds to a RASS of –4 to –5) demonstrated that early and short-term (48 h) infusion of the NMBA cisatracurium besilate improved 90-day survival rate and time-off the ventilator in severe ARDS (defined as a P_{aO_2}/F_{IO_2} ratio <150 mmHg (20.0 kPa)).

Based on this trial, early and short-term use of NMBAs has been recommended as the standard of care to achieve better synchronisation with the ventilator, decrease VILI and improve oxygenation in severe ARDS. However, controlled invasive ventilation with deep sedation and use of NMBAs precludes clinical monitoring of neurological signs, and has been associated with an increased risk of:

- critical illness polyneuropathy and myopathy
- delirium
- post-traumatic stress disorder

when compared with patients managed with partial ventilatory support and lighter and shorter sedation. Furthermore, an analysis of the ACURASYS trial demonstrated that the study was underpowered for its primary outcome, which is reflected by the lack of a statistically significant difference shown for 90-day crude mortality and the confidence intervals.

In many ICUs intensivists aim to minimise the use of sedatives and to wake-up patients early. Implementation of spontaneous awakening and spontaneous breathing trials, thereby reducing the amount and duration of sedation and days on invasive ventilation, is associated with less time in the ICU and in the hospital, and improved ICU, in-hospital and 1-year survival. Recently, the Reevaluation of Systemic Early Neuromuscular Blockade (ROSE) trial was conducted to assess the efficacy and safety of early NMBA use during deep sedation (RASS of −4 to −5) in patients with moderate-to-severe ARDS. The control group did not receive NMBA during a lighter sedation regimen (RASS of −2 to −3). The investigators found no significant difference in 90-day mortality between patients who received an early and continuous NMBA infusion and those who were treated with a usual-care approach with lighter sedation targets. However, the ROSE trial did not intend to investigate preserved early spontaneous breathing during assist-control ventilation.

Although the use of deep sedation with NMBAs during controlled invasive ventilation has been a recommended standard of care, this concept needs to be re-evaluated in the light of the recently published ROSE trial to balance the risks and benefits of the two approaches to invasive ventilation in the early phase of moderate-to-severe ARDS.

Traditionally, controlled invasive ventilation is provided *via* an artificial airway to completely unload a patient's work of breathing and ensure adequate gas exchange during the acute phase of respiratory insufficiency, until the underlying respiratory function has resolved. Recent research suggests that even in patients with moderate-to-severe ARDS partial ventilator support may be safely administered (provided that the respiratory drive is not too high and can be controlled by the ventilator). Although introduced as weaning techniques, modes providing assisted or partial support of spontaneous breathing are increasingly used to provide primary mechanical ventilatory support in critically ill patients.

Pressure support ventilation

PSV provides a preset pressure during inspiration to support spontaneous breathing by the patient. PSV eases the patient's ability to overcome the resistance of the endotracheal tube and is useful during weaning because it decreases the work of breathing. PSV requires the patient to trigger every single breath. Typically, the ventilator detects spontaneous breathing by the patient through a generated inspiratory gas flow or a lower airway pressure. When this occurs, the ventilator will generate an inspiratory gas flow to deliver a preset inspiratory pressure (pressure support). Thus, each spontaneous breath is delivered as a spontaneous assisted breath. Inspiration is terminated when the inspiratory gas flow reaches a predefined threshold, typically 10–25% of the peak flow rate or a fixed flow (usually 5 $L \cdot min^{-1}$), although higher values may be used in patients with obstructive airway disease. V_T depends on spontaneous breathing by the patient, respiratory system mechanics, and the level of pressure support. In contrast to assist-control ventilation, V_T is determined partially by the patient's muscular effort and partially by the ventilator.

In PSV mode, most ventilators allow modulation of the following parameters:

- trigger sensitivity
- inspiratory rise time (IRT)
- level of pressure support
- the cycling-off criteria

Triggering of inspiration is initiated by patient effort and is detected by a pressure or flow sensor. Some ventilators allow clinicians to adjust the trigger sensitivity to receive an optimal triggering signal from the patient. Once inspiration has been initiated, the ventilator delivers a high inspiratory flow, which rapidly decreases throughout the rest of inspiration (figure 1). The IRT determines the time to reach the selected airway pressure. A short IRT results in a high peak inspiratory flow and a short time to reach that peak. However, this may be disadvantageous in some cases, for example patients with restrictive lung disease. Here, a prolonged IRT leads to a longer inspiratory flow phase, and therefore, helps patients with a restrictive lung disease to generate a sufficient V_T. The optimal IRT must be evaluated for each patient together with clinical parameters such as V_T, *etc*. The level of pressure support depends on the patient. The level of support should generate a V_T of 4–6 mL·kg^{-1} bodyweight. However, increasing the level of pressure support reduces the work of breathing, and pressure support levels of ≥10 cmH$_2$O may result in a total loss of work of breathing. Most ventilators allow the cycling-off criteria to be modulated: the termination of inspiration can be varied by altering the predefined threshold for the inspiratory gas flow rate. For example, an increase in the threshold to 30% of the inspiratory peak flow rate results in starting the expiration earlier and thereby reduces the inspiratory time.

The benefits of PSV are variable V_T, inspiratory times and respiratory rates, which contribute to increased patient comfort. Moreover, spontaneous breathing during PSV may potentially avoid muscle atrophy of the diaphragm during invasive ventilation. However, asynchrony between the patient and the ventilator may still be present as the ventilator may not detect every patient breath, especially in the presence of auto-PEEP. This phenomenon may lead to an increased work of breathing and results in patient discomfort. PSV is entirely dependent on the spontaneous breathing effort of the patient. In the absence of spontaneous inspiratory efforts, PSV will not provide any ventilator support and will switch to a "backup" mode, which is usually assist-control ventilation. Despite limited pressure support levels, PSV often results in a large V_T (mainly caused by a high respiratory drive) that is not compatible with a lung-protective ventilation strategy to avoid VILI.

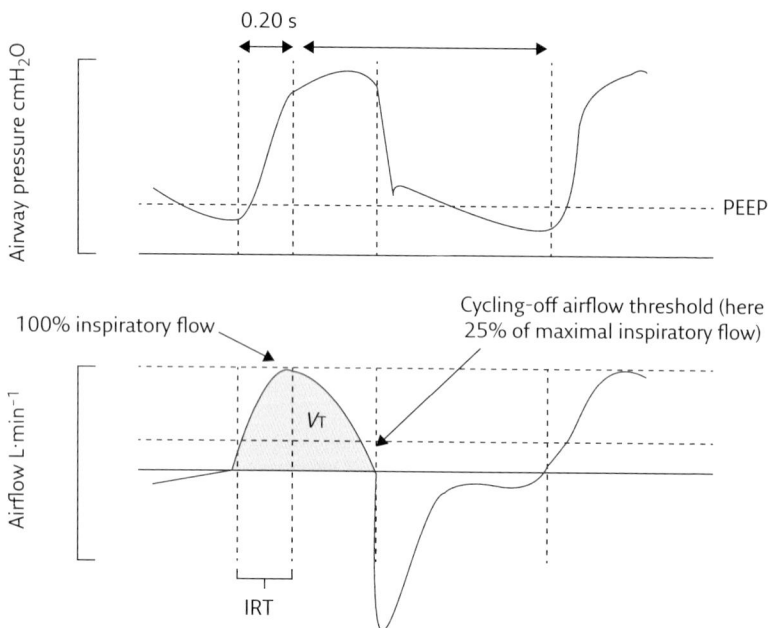

Figure 1. *In PSV, the delivered VT is calculated by integrating the area under the flow curve (purple shaded area). The IRT defines how fast the maximal airflow (100%) is achieved. Thereafter, the inspiratory airflow continuously decreases because, once the pressure target is reached, maintaining this level requires progressively less air to flow into the lungs. As soon as the cycling-off airflow threshold (i.e. a preset percentage of maximal air flow) is reached, the ventilator ceases to deliver inspiratory flow and the expiratory valve is opened to allow passive exhalation.*

Sufficiently powered prospective clinical trials comparing PSV *versus* controlled invasive ventilation during acute respiratory failure or moderate-to-severe ARDS, and focusing on outcomes such as mortality, length of ICU stay or quality of life, are lacking. One clinical trial showed improved patient comfort with PSV when compared with assist-control ventilation in patients with acute respiratory failure. Observational studies comparing PSV with assist-control ventilation in ARDS patients did not observe a difference in oxygenation, but carbon dioxide elimination was slightly improved. The results of clinical trials in patients with mild-to-moderate ARDS suggested poor oxygenation, cardiac index, and ventilation-perfusion matching with PSV when compared with APRV.

Assist-control ventilation

Assist-control ventilation is either a volume- or pressure-controlled time-cycled mode of ventilation. In general, five parameters can be modified by the user in the volume-controlled mode:

- *V*T
- respiratory rate

- PEEP
- inspiratory gas flow
- trigger sensitivity

Thus, the ventilator will deliver a fixed V_T when a patient breath is detected. The preset V_T is constant and peak or plateau pressures may increase when lung compliance decreases. Thus, assist-control ventilation is almost a controlled invasive ventilation mode, despite the fact that the delivery of V_T is synchronised with the spontaneous breathing of the patient and thus represents an assisted breathing option.

Advantages of assist-control ventilation include:

- support of spontaneous breathing by the ventilator,
- a low work of breathing, and
- easy carbon dioxide removal, as ventilation is still controlled mainly by the operator rather than the patient.

Disadvantages of assist-control ventilation include the following:

- As assist-control ventilation is volume-controlled and time cycled, asynchrony and stacked breaths are a concern as a fixed V_T will be delivered regardless of the patient's demand.
- Hyperventilation, and subsequently respiratory alkalosis, can occur as the patient is only able to initiate breaths.
- Tachypnoea can be an issue as the time for exhalation can be too short to complete expiration; this can lead to breath stacking or auto-PEEP, which may decrease patient comfort.

Although assist-control ventilation has been widely used by intensivists, no clinical trials have been reported that compare controlled invasive ventilation *versus* assist-control ventilation.

APRV and biphasic positive airway pressure

APRV is frequently called biphasic positive airway pressure or bilevel positive airway pressure (bi-level) by investigators and ventilator manufactures. APRV/biphasic positive airway pressure ventilates using time-cycled switches between two pressure levels in a high flow or demand valve CPAP circuit. Therefore, unrestricted and unassisted breathing are permitted in any phase of the mechanical ventilator cycle (figure 2). The degree of ventilator support with APRV/biphasic positive airway pressure is determined by the duration of the two CPAP levels and the mechanically delivered V_T, which mainly depends on respiratory compliance and the difference between the two CPAP levels. By design, changes in ventilatory demand do not alter the level of mechanical support. When spontaneous breathing is absent, APRV/biphasic positive airway pressure does not differ from conventional pressure-controlled, time-cycled invasive ventilation.

Based on the initial description, APRV keeps the duration of the low CPAP level (release time) at 1.5 s or less. Expiratory lung collapse is prevented during APRV by creating intrinsic PEEP during the short expiration (pressure release), while in the traditional description of biphasic positive airway pressure "PEEP" is directly set with the lower CPAP level. When biphasic positive airway pressure is used,

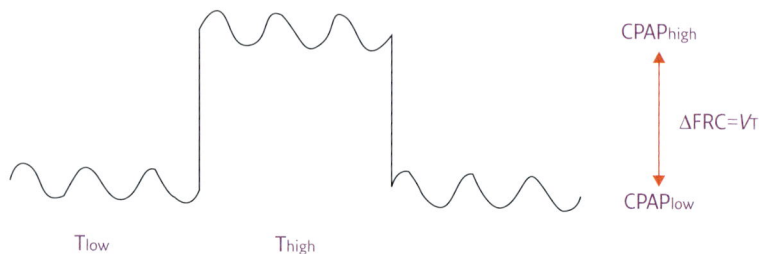

Determinants of V_T:
ΔP_{aw}
Compliance
Resistance

Figure 2. APRV/biphasic positive airway pressure. Unrestricted and unassisted spontaneous breathing is allowed in any phase (CPAPhigh and CPAPlow) of the ventilator cycle. Tlow: time during the expiration phase; Thigh: time during the inspiration phase; FRC: functional residual capacity; Paw: airway pressure.

expiratory time is usually set to avoid an end-expiratory gas flow or auto-PEEP/intrinsic PEEP. To allow spontaneous breathing on the high CPAP level, inspiratory time during APRV/biphasic positive airway pressure must not be decreased to <1.0 s. An inspiratory time of ≥2.0 s is recommended.

Clinical trials that compared APRV/biphasic positive airway pressure with assist-control ventilation did not reveal any differences in mortality, length of ICU stay, level of sedation, and days on invasive ventilation. APRV/biphasic positive airway pressure has been associated with lower inflation pressure, better oxygenation, less sedative usage and less pneumonia when compared with other modes of invasive ventilation in patients with mild-to-moderate ARDS. In the absence of protocolised sedation and preserved spontaneous breathing strategies, a case-matched analysis could not demonstrate an advantage of APRV/biphasic positive airway pressure on outcomes in a mixed population of critically ill patients. By contrast, preserving early spontaneous breathing with APRV/biphasic positive airway pressure in patients with mild-to-moderate ARDS was associated with a shorter duration of ventilator support and length of ICU stay in a small RCT. Recently, another RCT demonstrated less time on invasive ventilation and in the ICU with early spontaneous breathing during APRV when compared with assist-control ventilation in moderate-to-severe ARDS.

Synchronised intermittent mandatory ventilation

In synchronised intermittent mandatory ventilation (SIMV) the ventilator attempts to deliver the mandatory breaths in synchrony with the patient's own inspiratory efforts. SIMV allows spontaneous breathing between a preset number of patient-triggered (synchronised) and ventilator-delivered mandatory breaths. If the patient makes an inspiratory effort during a window of time determined by the intermittent mandatory ventilation rate, the ventilator delivers a mandatory breath in response to the patient's inspiratory effort. However, if no inspiratory effort is detected by the ventilator, a time-triggered breath will be delivered. The mechanically delivered breaths (assisted breathing) can be either volume or pressure controlled.

When volume-controlled SIMV is used, the V_T will be controlled by the ventilator setting and therefore supports protective ventilation strategies. However, spontaneous breathing may lead to breath stacking, which is mainly due to a double trigger that causes a second inspiratory breath without an expiration cycle. Consequently, the V_T may be doubled. There is increasing evidence that the use of pressure-controlled rather than volume-controlled ventilation may diminish this problem.

In general, SIMV may aggravate hyperventilation with the risk of developing a respiratory alkalosis, and it may cause an excessive work of breathing during spontaneous breathing. Debate exists as to whether interaction between the patient and the ventilator may contribute to VILI. Moreover, SIMV does not allow unrestricted spontaneous breathing. RCTs have demonstrated less weaning success with SIMV when compared with PSV.

Further reading

- Hering R, *et al.* (2002). Effects of spontaneous breathing during airway pressure release ventilation on renal perfusion and function in patients with acute lung injury. *Intensive Care Med*; 28: 1426–1433.

- Kaplan LJ, *et al.* (2001). Airway pressure release ventilation increases cardiac performance in patients with acute lung injury/adult respiratory distress syndrome. *Crit Care*; 5: 221–226.

- National Heart, Lung, and Blood Institute PETAL Clinical Trials Network, *et al.* (2019). Early neuromuscular blockade in the acute respiratory distress syndrome. *N Engl J Med*; 380: 1997–2008.

- Papazian L, *et al.* (2010). Neuromuscular blockers in early acute respiratory distress syndrome. *N Engl J Med*; 363: 1107–1116.

- Putensen C, *et al.* (1999). Spontaneous breathing during ventilatory support improves ventilation-perfusion distributions in patients with acute respiratory distress syndrome. *Am J Respir Crit Care Med*; 159: 1241–1248.

- Putensen C, *et al.* (2001). Long-term effects of spontaneous breathing during ventilatory support in patients with acute lung injury. *Am J Respir Crit Care Med*; 164: 43–49.

- Putensen C, *et al.* (2006). The impact of spontaneous breathing during mechanical ventilation. *Curr Opin Crit Care*; 12: 13–18.

- Yoshida T, *et al.* (2013). Spontaneous effort causes occult pendelluft during mechanical ventilation. *Am J Respir Crit Care Med*; 188: 1420–1427.

- Yoshida T, *et al.* (2017). Volume-controlled ventilation does not prevent injurious inflation during spontaneous effort. *Am J Respir Crit Care Med*; 196: 590–601.

- Zhou Y, *et al.* (2017). Early application of airway pressure release ventilation may reduce the duration of MV in acute respiratory distress syndrome. *Intensive Care Med*; 43: 1648–1659.

Proportional modes

Michela Rauseo and Lise Piquilloud

Key points

- If the integrity of the pathway from respiratory centres to respiratory muscles is intact and if neuromuscular transmission is not impaired, electrical diaphragmatic activity (EA_{di}) is a surrogate of neural respiratory drive.

- EA_{di} can be recorded at the bedside using a nasogastric tube equipped with electrodes.

- EA_{di} can be used to pilot the ventilator: to initiate and terminate pressurisation in synchrony with the patient's breath; and to deliver assistance in proportion to the patient's inspiratory demand.

- Neurally adjusted ventilator assist (NAVA) improves patient–ventilator synchrony compared to conventional modes of assisted ventilation and can limit lung overdistension.

- Multicentre studies assessing the use of NAVA in patients prone to benefitting from the technique (*e.g.* patients with poor patient–ventilator synchrony or patients at risk of difficult weaning) are lacking.

- Assistance can be delivered in proportion to the patient's inspiratory effort using proportional assist ventilation (PAV).

- PAV+ automatically measures resistance and elastance through short end-inspiratory occlusions.

- PAV+ improves patient–ventilator synchrony compared to standard modes of assisted ventilation and prevents overassist.

- Multicentre studies assessing the use of PAV+ in large ICU patient populations are lacking.

Definition of proportional modes

Proportional modes of assisted ventilation are designed to deliver, on a breath-by-breath basis, ventilator assistance in proportion to the patient's demand. Two different systems of proportional ventilation are available.

- Neurally adjusted ventilator assist (NAVA) delivers assistance in proportion to crural diaphragmatic electrical activity (EA_{di}). If the pathway from the respiratory centres to the respiratory muscles is intact and if neuromuscular transmission is not impaired, EA_{di} is a reliable surrogate of the brain stem respiratory centre activity (or respiratory drive).
- Proportional assist ventilation (PAV) delivers assistance in proportion to the inspiratory airflow and volume generated by the patient's inspiratory effort. This results in delivering, at any time during inspiration, airway pressure in proportion to the muscular pressure generated by the inspiratory muscles (P_{mus}).

Proportional ventilation is fundamentally different from conventional assisted ventilation, during which a set amount of assistance (selected by the clinician) is delivered independently of the patient's demand.

Neurally adjusted ventilator assist

Working principle of NAVA Breathing is an autonomic action initiated and terminated in the brainstem respiratory centres where electrical outputs are generated by networks of neurons. These electrical outputs (respiratory drive) are transmitted through the respiratory motor neurons to the diaphragm and the other respiratory muscles. In response, muscle fibre depolarisation and contraction occur. This generates negative pressure in the pleural space and alveoli, and allows flow of ambient air into the alveoli.

At the diaphragm level, muscle fibre depolarisation is reflected by crural EA_{di}, which is well correlated to the global electrical activity of the diaphragm. If the pathway from the respiratory centres to the respiratory muscles is intact and if the neuromuscular transmission is not impaired, EA_{di} is a reliable surrogate of respiratory drive. EA_{di} can be recorded at the bedside through the oesophageal wall using a specialised nasogastric tube equipped with electrodes (EA_{di} catheter). This catheter is similar in size and function to a conventional nasogastric tube. Correct positioning of the catheter is checked using the transoesophageal electrocardiographic signal also recorded by the electrodes as a guide. Practically, the operator can check correct positioning on the ventilator screen based on a simple algorithm.

After signal filtering by the ventilator software (*e.g.* to suppress ECG) and if the pathway from respiratory centres to respiratory muscles is intact, the EA_{di} signal can be used to pilot the ventilator in order to deliver assistance in synchrony with and in proportion to the patient's inspiratory drive. In practical terms, during NAVA, the ventilator pressurisation is initiated as soon as the EA_{di} signal increases over a threshold value set by the clinician (neural inspiratory trigger). The pressure delivered throughout the breath is instantaneously proportional to the EA_{di} amplitude. Ventilator-delivered pressurisation thus parallels the morphology of EA_{di} during inspiration. The proportionality factor between EA_{di} amplitude (measured in μV) and the amount of assistance delivered by the ventilator (in cmH_2O) is called the NAVA level. It must be set by the clinician. Expiratory cycling occurs when EA_{di} decreases to 70% of its maximum inspiratory value. This setting cannot be modified by the clinician. The working principle of NAVA is illustrated in figure 1. For safety reasons, in cases of poor EAdi signal quality, the system uses a conventional pneumatic trigger as a backup triggering system. Neural and pneumatic triggers can be used alternatively on a "first come, first served" basis, meaning that if a pneumatic triggering signal is detected earlier than an increase in EAdi, the ventilator will be triggered by the pneumatic signal. Depending on the subsequent detection of the EAdi signal, pressurisation is delivered either in proportion to EAdi or as a pressure-regulated cycle. Depending on the software version, the system uses either pressure support ventilation (PSV) (older versions) or pressure-controlled ventilation (more recent versions) as backup ventilation. If apnoea occurs, the apnoea ventilation is automatically activated as in other spontaneous modes.

How to use NAVA in practice The use of NAVA requires the insertion of a dedicated EAdi catheter and its positioning using the ventilator's dedicated software. Concerning the ventilator settings, F_{IO_2} and PEEP are set as usual. The neural inspiratory trigger default value of 0.5 µV is adequate in most cases. It can be increased if signal artefacts lead to inadequate ventilator pressurisations. Different approaches have been described for NAVA level setting but no definitive recommendations are available. Theoretically, the NAVA level to select should be the level associated with adequate diaphragm discharge. Practically, the NAVA level can be set using the previsualisation system implemented in the ventilator software in order to obtain a maximal inspiratory pressure during NAVA equal to the inspiratory pressure used during PSV. Alternatively, a NAVA level titration procedure has been proposed to determine the NAVA level threshold associated with the absence of further significant increases in airway pressure and V_T ("adequate" NAVA level). This titration procedure is, however, time consuming and not easy to perform at the bedside. To adapt NAVA level during the weaning phase, it has also been suggested to measure the EAdi maximal peak value during a period of minimal ventilator assistance and then to titrate the gain in order to reduce the EAdi peak to 60% of this maximal value.

A practical solution to setting NAVA level is sequentially using the previsualisation system implemented in the ventilator software and the minimal ventilator assistance technique previously described to adapt NAVA level as soon as a transient reduction of the amount of assistance is feasible and safe. Another pragmatic solution is to use the ventilator's built-in module to set the initial NAVA level and then titrating the NAVA level to find the minimal level associated with the absence of respiratory distress.

Regardless of the strategy used to set NAVA level, as soon as the NAVA level is modified, the amount of pressure delivered by the ventilator changes. This influences V_T and respiratory profile, and is responsible for nearly immediate feedback from chemo- and mechanoreceptors to the brainstem respiratory centres. This feedback influences the output delivered by the respiratory centres. With NAVA, the amount of assistance delivered is always related to the patient's demand. This is one of the main advantages of the proportional modes but, compared to conventional modes of assisted ventilation, limits the ability to impose a fixed amount of assistance.

Use of NAVA and limitations of its use NAVA is safe, and can be used both for invasive ventilation and NIV. The only formal contraindication to NAVA use is a contraindication to inserting a nasogastric tube.

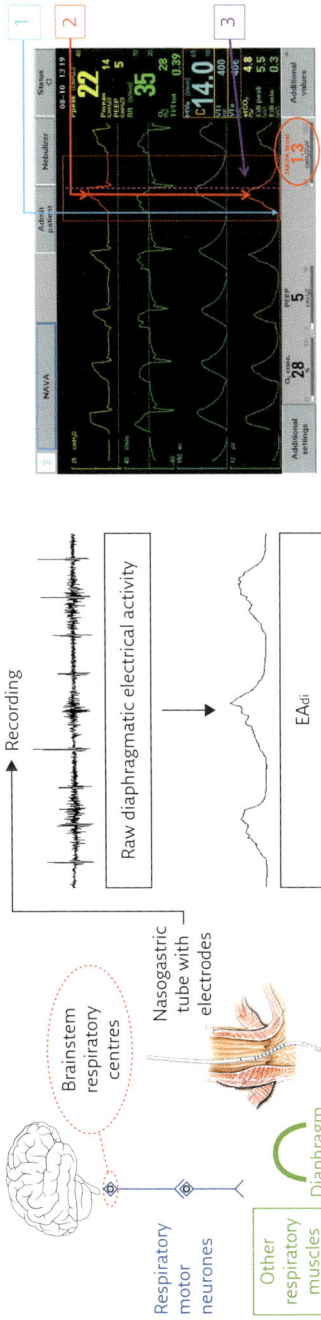

Figure 1. *Illustration of the working principle of NAVA. In the NAVA system, the EAdi signal is used 1) to trigger the ventilator, 2) to deliver proportional assistance and 3) to cycle off the ventilator. Paw (in cmH$_2$O) is calculated as EAdi (in µV) × NAVA level (in cmH$_2$O·µV^{-1}) + PEEP (in cmH$_2$O).*

Obtaining a reliable EAdi signal requires the absence of impairment of the neural transmission pathway from the brainstem respiratory centres to the diaphragm, including the integrity of the phrenic nerves and neuromuscular junctions. Practically, EAdi cannot, for example, be obtained in presence of proximal cervical spine cord injury, bilateral phrenic lesions or severe myasthenia gravis. Obtaining a reliable EAdi signal can also sometimes be difficult in the presence of hiatal hernia or unilateral phrenic paralysis. Except in these very specific situations, NAVA can be used as soon as spontaneous respiratory activity is present. A reduction in sedation is, however, sometimes required to obtain an EAdi signal of sufficient amplitude to have a good signal to noise ratio. NAVA ventilation can be difficult to use when the patient's respiratory drive is clearly abnormal. This can be the case with cerebral lesions or when respiratory drive is markedly increased, for example, due to severe systemic inflammation.

Advantages of using NAVA Diaphragm fibre depolarisation and associated EAdi increase (neural trigger) occur earlier than airflow and airway pressure variations commonly used to trigger a ventilator (pneumatic trigger). The trigger delay between breath initiation in the brainstem respiratory centres and the start of ventilator pressurisation is thus reduced with NAVA compared to conventional modes of assisted ventilation. In contrast to the pneumatic trigger, the neural trigger is not perturbed by the presence of dynamic air trapping or leaks. This suggests a particular advantage of using NAVA in obstructive patients and during NIV. During NAVA, the transition from inspiration to expiration occurs when EAdi decreases to 70% of the peak value observed during the same breath. This has been shown to improve patient–ventilator synchrony compared to conventional modes of assisted ventilation. Fewer asynchrony events per minute and/or lower asynchrony index have been observed under NAVA compared to PSV. This has been observed both during invasive ventilation and NIV.

As an increase in NAVA level results in a decrease in EAdi amplitude, the V_T increase is limited when NAVA level is increased. NAVA thus limits the risk of lung overdistension compared to PSV. Overdistension can, however, still occur in some patients when high NAVA levels (>2 $cmH_2O \cdot \mu V^{-1}$) are selected. Compared to PSV, NAVA improves diaphragm contractility efficiency. This suggests a potential advantage of using NAVA in patients at risk of difficult weaning. This, however, has not been formally assessed in a large cohort of patients. Compared to conventional modes of assisted ventilation, NAVA also allows more physiological respiratory variability, and could improve ventilation distribution within the lungs and sleep quality.

A first multicentre randomised study comparing NAVA and PSV in a general population of invasively ventilated patients confirmed that NAVA was safe to use over a prolonged period of time and improved patient–ventilator synchrony. The use of NAVA was, however, not associated with improved outcome in terms of ventilation or ICU stay duration, or mortality. In this randomised study, EAdi signal was available both for patients ventilated with NAVA and PSV. This could have influenced the PSV settings. In addition, the general population of patients included in the study was not expected to obtain great benefits from NAVA. It cannot thus be excluded, based on this study, that specific patient groups, for example, patients with poor patient–ventilator interaction or at risk of difficult weaning, could benefit from NAVA.

In conclusion, concerning the advantages of using NAVA, studies on clinically relevant outcomes in patients prone to benefit from the NAVA technology are still lacking.

NAVA for monitoring If the pathway from the respiratory centres to the respiratory muscles is intact and if neuromuscular transmission is not impaired, EA$_{di}$ is a surrogate of patient's respiratory drive. EA$_{di}$ can be used to monitor patient–ventilator asynchronies at the bedside. Using EA$_{di}$ to detect patient–ventilator asynchronies is much more sensitive than using flow and airway pressure–time curves only. EA$_{di}$ can also be used to optimise the ventilator settings during PSV. The use of EA$_{di}$ for this purpose allows a reduction of the ventilator response time. EA$_{di}$ amplitude variations can be used to assess variations in inspiratory effort intensity. Finally, neuroventilatory efficiency measured as V_T/EA$_{di}$ is a recently described parameter to assess the ability of the diaphragm to convert neuromuscular activity into tidal ventilation or, in other words, to assess diaphragm strength.

Proportional assist ventilation

Working principle of PAV PAV is a proportional mode of assisted ventilation in which the ventilator generates pressure throughout inspiration in proportion to the inspiratory airflow and volume generated by the patient's inspiratory effort. This results in delivering, at any time during inspiration, airway pressure (P_{aw}) in proportion to P_{mus}. The pressure delivered by the ventilator (P_{aw}) is not square shaped but follows the P_{mus} profile, resulting in a progressive increase from the start of inspiration with gradual pressurisation. Maximal assistance is reached only at the end of inspiration. Therefore, during PAV, P_{aw} is not a set value as it is during PSV.

According to the motion equation of the respiratory system, the total pressure that must be applied to insufflate the lungs (P_{tot}) is equal to the sum of the resistive pressure ($P_{resistive}$=flow×resistance), the elastic retraction pressure ($P_{elastic}$=volume above end-expiratory lung volume at PEEP×elastance) and the pressure at baseline (P_0), immediately before inspiration.

The equation of motion can be written as:

$$P_{tot} = P_{resistive} + P_{elastic} + P_0 = (flow \times resistance) + (volume \times elastance) + P_0 \quad (1)$$

During assisted ventilation, P_{tot} is the sum of P_{aw} and P_{mus}. This corresponds to the following equation:

$$P_{tot} = P_{aw} + P_{mus} \quad (2)$$

In this situation, the equation of motion of the respiratory system can be written as:

$$P_{tot} = P_{aw} + P_{mus} = (flow \times resistance) + (volume \times elastance) + P_0 \quad (3)$$

During PAV, the amplitude of the assistance delivered is determined by proportionality factors (gains) selected by the clinician. In the original PAV system, the user had to select independently a percentage of assistance for the $P_{resistive}$ component and a percentage of assistance for the $P_{elastic}$ component. Practically, the clinician had to select two factors called flow assist (FA) and volume assist (VA). FA is expressed as a fraction of resistance. It reflects the assistance delivered by the

Equation of motion of the respiratory system in an actively breathing patient (assisted ventilation):

$$P_{tot} = P_{aw} + P_{mus} = \underbrace{(flow \times R)}_{P_{resistive}} + \underbrace{(volume \times E)}_{P_{elastic}} + P_0$$

PAV+ general principle:

- Automated short end-inspiratory occlusion → determination of R and E
- Continuous measurement of flow and volume (flow transducer)
- P_0 = set PEEP
- P_{aw} = gain % $\times P_{tot}$
- $P_{aw} = P_{mus} \times \dfrac{gain \%}{100 - gain \%}$

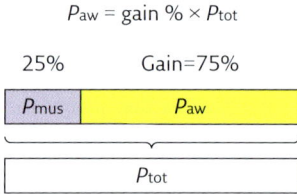

$$P_{aw} = gain \% \times P_{tot}$$

25%   Gain=75%

P_{mus}	P_{aw}

P_{tot}

Figure 2. Summary of the working principle of PAV+. R: resistance; E: elastance.

ventilator per unit of measured flow. In other words, FA is the assist pressure per unit flow (in $cmH_2O \cdot L^{-1} \cdot s$). VA is expressed as a fraction of elastance. It reflects the assistance delivered per unit of measured volume. In other words, VA is the assist pressure per unit volume (in $cmH_2O \cdot L^{-1}$).

We can thus write that during PAV:

$$P_{aw} = (FA \times flow) + (VA \times volume) \tag{4}$$

Selecting FA and VA requires an estimation of the respiratory mechanics (resistance and elastance) at the start and on an intermittent basis during PAV ventilation.

In practical terms, estimating resistance and compliance is difficult, and often not reliable in spontaneously breathing patients. In addition, independently selecting FA and VA is not easy. For these reasons, a simplified system called proportional assist ventilation with load adjustable gain factor (PAV+) has been developed. PAV+ offers two improvements. First, the system automatically performs brief (300 ms) pauses at the end of inspiration every 8–15 breaths to measure resistance and elastance. Second, with PAV+, only a single level of FA and VA, called the PAV+ gain, must be selected by the clinician. Only PAV+ can be used in critically ill patients. Figure 2 summarises the working principle of PAV+.

With the PAV+ system, the ventilator automatically performs short end-inspiratory occlusions to iteratively determine resistance and elastance. Flow and volume are measured by the ventilator flow sensor throughout the breath. Flow is obtained by direct measurement and volume is computed by integration of the flow signal. Based on the intermittent measurement of resistance and elastance, and on the instantaneous measurement of flow and volume, instantaneous $P_{resistive}$ and $P_{elastic}$ can be measured. If P_0 is considered equal to the set PEEP, based on equation 3, P_{tot} can be measured on a continuous basis and it is possible to deliver an amount of assistance corresponding to a given proportion of P_{tot}. This proportion is determined by the proportionality factor (or gain) set by the clinician.

The relationship between P_{tot} and delivered P_{aw} is illustrated by the following equation:

$$P_{aw} = \text{gain } (\%) \times P_{tot} \tag{5}$$

By combining the equations 2 and 5, we can write:

$$P_{aw} = P_{mus}\left(\frac{\text{gain }\%}{100 - \text{gain }\%}\right) \tag{6}$$

The amount of assistance delivered is thus proportional to P_{mus}.

As an example, if the gain is set to 75%, P_{aw} is, at any time, three times higher than P_{mus}, meaning that, in this situation, the ventilator is responsible for 75% of the total "work" whereas the patient performs 25% of the work. If the patient's demand increases, P_{mus} and P_{tot} immediately increase. In response, the PAV+ system increases the amount of assistance delivered by the ventilator in order to maintain the same P_{aw}/P_{mus} ratio. Oppositely, when the patient's demand decreases, the amount of assistance delivered by the ventilator decreases.

How to use PAV+ in practice Ventilating a patient with PAV+ requires a dedicated ventilator but no special equipment. The clinician must set the pneumatic trigger, PEEP and F_{IO_2} as for conventional modes of assisted ventilation. The transition from inspiration to expiration (expiratory valve opening) occurs when inspiratory flow decreases to a pre-set level. The by default value of 3 L·min^{-1} is usually adequate.

To use PAV+, the clinician must select the gain, *i.e.* the proportion of P_{tot} that has to be delivered by the ventilator. The gain can be selected between 0% (absence of ventilator assistance) and 85% (nearly the full assistance delivered by the ventilator). How to set the gain during PAV+ is still matter of debate. Carteaux *et al.* (2013) proposed an algorithm that allows setting the gain in PAV+ in order to target a reasonable range of patient's inspiratory effort, defined as a respiratory muscle pressure–time product (PTP$_{mus}$) between 50 and 150 cmH$_2$O·s·min^{-1}. Practically, as PTP$_{mus}$ cannot be measured at the bedside as a standard of care, a surrogate of PTP$_{mus}$ is used. This surrogate is the peak muscle pressure ($P_{mus_{peak}}$), which represents the maximum pressure swing generated by the inspiratory muscle contraction during inspiration. $P_{mus_{peak}}$ is defined as follows:

$$P_{mus_{peak}} = \left(P_{aw_{peak}} - PEEP\right)\left(\frac{100 - \text{gain }\%}{\text{gain }\%}\right) \tag{7}$$

Setting the gain at the bedside according to this method requires using a grid specifying the $Pmus_{peak}$ corresponding to ΔPaw (Paw_{peak} – PEEP) displayed on the ventilator screen and to the set gain. The aim is to adapt the gain in order to target a $Pmus_{peak}$ between 5 and 10 cmH$_2$O. This approach has been demonstrated to be feasible in clinical practice.

Use of PAV and PAV+, and limitations of use The original PAV system can be used both during invasive ventilation and NIV. As it requires a clinical estimation of resistance and elastance, and does not take into account changes in respiratory mechanics over time, it can, however, be of limited reliability. It cannot be used in acutely ill patients. The PAV+ system takes into account actual respiratory mechanisms and their variations over time. It is easy to use at the bedside in invasively ventilated patients but cannot be used for NIV as the measurement of resistance and elastance with short end-inspiratory occlusions cannot be performed in presence of leaks. It is important to note that the PAV+ system considers set PEEP to assess $Ptot$ and does not take into account intrinsic PEEP. In presence of significant intrinsic PEEP, this could lead to delivery of low assistance levels.

Advantages of using PAV+ PAV+ can be used in critically ill, invasively ventilated patients. Patients in the early weaning phase are more prone to remain under assisted ventilation when PAV+ is used compared to PSV. Compared to PSV, sleep can be of improved quality (increase in deep sleep and rapid eye movement sleep periods, and fewer sleep disruptions) when PAV+ is used. However, controversial results have been published on this topic.

Clinical studies have compared PAV+ to PSV on physiological outcomes. Compared to PSV, PAV+ increases respiratory variability and improves patient–ventilator synchrony. As during PAV+, the ventilator is triggered by a pneumatic signal (same triggering system as for PSV), PAV+ is not expected to have a major impact on reducing trigger delays compared to PSV. It could nevertheless indirectly reduce trigger delays in presence of air trapping. Indeed, compared to PSV, PAV+ reduces lung overdistension and could thus facilitate ventilator triggering when air trapping is present. As PAV+ allows expression of feedback mechanisms, it reduces the risk of overassist and of potentially related diaphragmatic atrophy. This is a major advantage compared to traditional modes of assisted ventilation, as with these modes, overassist is nearly the rule.

Recent systematic reviews and meta-analyses found discordant results concerning the potential advantages of using PAV+ compared to conventional modes of assisted ventilation. As PAV+ has demonstrated clear positive physiological effects, prospective randomised studies assessing the effect of PAV+ on clinically relevant outcomes must be performed.

PAV+ for monitoring With the PAV+ system, it is possible to monitor respiratory mechanics, as resistance and compliance are measured by the system on a semi-continuous basis. The PAV+ systems also allows estimation of $Pmus$ on a continuous basis. $Pmus$ values could be used to titrate the amount of assistance delivered with conventional modes of assisted ventilation, in order to target a physiological value with the aim of avoiding both under- and overassist.

Summary

Proportional modes deliver assistance in proportion to patients' inspiratory demand. Two different systems are available. NAVA delivers assistance in proportion to EAdi, usually a surrogate of neural respiratory drive. PAV delivers assistance in proportion to the inspiratory airflow and volume generated by the patient's inspiratory effort. This results in delivering, at any time during inspiration, P_{aw} in proportion to P_{mus}. Both systems are safe to use at the bedside. Proportional modes improve patient–ventilator asynchrony and restore respiratory variability. They can limit the risk of lung overdistension and of overassist. Their potential to improve patients' outcomes in terms of mechanical ventilation, ICU or hospital stay duration, or in terms of mortality remain to be demonstrated in prospective studies.

Further reading

- Alexopoulou C, et al. (2013). Patient–ventilator synchrony and sleep quality with proportional assist and pressure support ventilation. *Intensive Care Med*; 39: 1040–1047.

- Barwing J, et al. (2009). Evaluation of the catheter positioning for neurally adjusted ventilatory assist. *Intensive Care Med*; 35: 1809–1814.

- Beloncle F, et al. (2016). Accuracy of delivered airway pressure and work of breathing estimation during proportional assist ventilation: a bench study. *Ann Intensive Care*; 6: 30.

- Beloncle F, et al. (2017). A diaphragmatic electrical activity-based optimization strategy during pressure support ventilation improves synchronization but does not impact work of breathing. *Crit Care*; 21: 21.

- Blankman P, et al. (2013). Ventilation distribution measured with EIT at varying levels of pressure support and neurally adjusted ventilatory assist in patients with ALI. *Intensive Care Med*; 39: 1057–1062.

- Bosma K, et al. (2007). Patient–ventilator interaction and sleep in mechanically ventilated patients: pressure support *versus* proportional assist ventilation. *Crit Care Med*; 35: 1048–1054.

- Bosma KJ, et al. (2016). A pilot randomized trial comparing weaning from mechanical ventilation on pressure support *versus* proportional assist ventilation. *Crit Care Med*; 44: 1098–1108.

- Brander L, et al. (2009). Titration and implementation of neurally adjusted ventilatory assist in critically ill patients. *Chest*; 135: 695–703.

- Carteaux G, et al. (2013). Bedside adjustment of proportional assist ventilation to target a predefined range of respiratory effort. *Crit Care Med*; 41: 2125–2132.

- Carteaux G, et al. (2016). Comparison between neurally adjusted ventilatory assist and pressure support ventilation levels in terms of respiratory effort. *Crit Care Med*; 44: 503–511.

- Colombo D, et al. (2011). Efficacy of ventilator waveforms observation in detecting patient–ventilator asynchrony. *Crit Care Med*; 39: 2452–2457.

- Costa R, *et al.* (2011). A physiologic comparison of proportional assist ventilation with load-adjustable gain factors (PAV+) *versus* pressure support ventilation (PSV). *Intensive Care Med*; 37: 1494–1500.

- Delisle S, *et al.* (2011). Sleep quality in mechanically ventilated patients: comparison between NAVA and PSV modes. *Ann Intensive Care*; 1: 42.

- Demoule A, *et al.* (2016). Neurally adjusted ventilatory assist as an alternative to pressure support ventilation in adults: a French multicentre randomized trial. *Intensive Care Med*; 42: 1723–1732.

- Di Mussi R, *et al.* (2016). Impact of prolonged assisted ventilation on diaphragmatic efficiency: NAVA *versus* PSV. *Crit Care*; 20: 1.

- Doorduin J, *et al.* (2014). Automated patient–ventilator interaction analysis during neurally adjusted non-invasive ventilation and pressure support ventilation in chronic obstructive pulmonary disease. *Crit Care*; 18: 550.

- Doorduin J, *et al.* (2015). Assisted ventilation in patients with acute respiratory distress syndrome: lung-distending pressure and patient-ventilator interaction. *Anesthesiology*; 123: 181–190.

- Eldridge FL (1975). Relationship between respiratory nerve and muscle activity and muscle force output. *J Appl Physiol*; 39: 567–574.

- Kacmarek RM (2011). Proportional assist ventilation and neurally adjusted ventilatory assist. *Respir Care*; 56: 140–148.

- Kataoka J, *et al.* (2018). Proportional modes *versus* pressure support ventilation: a systematic review and meta-analysis. *Ann Intensive Care*; 8: 123.

- Lourenco RV, *et al.* (1966). Nervous output from the respiratory center during obstructed breathing. *J Appl Physiol*; 21: 527–533.

- Mauri T, *et al.* (2016). Esophageal and transpulmonary pressure in the clinical setting: meaning, usefulness and perspectives. *Intensive Care Med*; 42: 1360–1373.

- Moorhead KT, *et al.* (2013). NAVA enhances tidal volume and diaphragmatic electro-myographic activity matching: a Range 90 analysis of supply and demand. *J Clin Monitoring Computing*; 27: 61–70.

- Oyer LM, *et al.* (1989). Patterns of neural and muscular electrical activity in costal and crural portions of the diaphragm. *J Appl Physiol*; 66: 2092–2100.

- Patroniti N, *et al.* (2012). Respiratory pattern during neurally adjusted ventilatory assist in acute respiratory failure patients. *Intensive Care Med*; 38: 230–239.

- Piquilloud L, *et al.* (2011). Neurally adjusted ventilatory assist improves patient-ventilator interaction. *Intensive Care Med*; 37: 263–271.

- Piquilloud L, *et al.* (2012). Neurally adjusted ventilatory assist (NAVA) improves patient-ventilator interaction during non-invasive ventilation delivered by face mask. *Intensive Care Med*; 38: 1624–1631.

- Rozé H, *et al.* (2011). Daily titration of neurally adjusted ventilatory assist using the diaphragm electrical activity. *Intensive Care Med*; 37: 1087-1094.

- Ruiz-Ferron F, *et al.* (2009). [Respiratory work and pattern with different proportional assist ventilation levels]. *Medicina Intensiva*; 33: 269-275.

- Schmidt M, *et al.* (2015). Neurally adjusted ventilatory assist and proportional assist ventilation both improve patient-ventilator interaction. *Crit Care*; 19: 56.

- Sinderby C, *et al.* (1998). Voluntary activation of the human diaphragm in health and disease. *J Appl Physiol*; 85: 2146-2158.

- Sinderby C, *et al.* (1999). Neural control of mechanical ventilation in respiratory failure. *Nat Med*; 5: 1433-1436.

- Sun Q, *et al.* (2017). Effects of neurally adjusted ventilatory assist on air distribution and dead space in patients with acute exacerbation of chronic obstructive pulmonary disease. *Crit Care*; 21: 126.

- Terzi N, *et al.* (2012). Clinical review: update on neurally adjusted ventilatory assist – report of a round-table conference. *Crit Care*; 16: 225.

- Tirupakuzhi Vijayaraghavan BK, *et al.* (2018). Evidence supporting clinical use of proportional assist ventilation: a systematic review and meta-analysis of clinical trials. *J Intensive Care Med*: 885066618769021.

- Xirouchaki N, *et al.* (2008). Proportional assist ventilation with load-adjustable gain factors in critically ill patients: comparison with pressure support. *Intensive Care Med*; 34: 2026-2034.

- Younes M, *et al.* (2001). A method for measuring passive elastance during proportional assist ventilation. *Am J Respir Crit Care Med*; 164: 50-60.

- Younes M, *et al.* (2001). A method for noninvasive determination of inspiratory resistance during proportional assist ventilation. *Am J Respir Crit Care Med*; 163: 829-839.

- Younes M (1992). Proportional assist ventilation, a new approach to ventilatory support. Theory. *Am Rev Respir Dis*; 145: 114-120.

Automated modes

Jean-Michel Arnal and Cenk Kirakli

Closed-loop ventilation modes automatically adapt certain ventilator settings to keep the patient's physiological variables within the target ranges set by the clinician. The clinician determines the target, the strategy and the safety limits, and the ventilator then adjusts the settings within these boundaries. The main advantages are:

- Continuous adaptation of ventilation to the patient's condition
- Application of lung-protective ventilation in all patients
- The ability to switch from controlled to spontaneous breaths automatically
- The gradual decrease in pressure support during weaning
- The smaller number of manual adjustments needed

ASV is a closed-loop control system for ventilation settings, first launched in 1998 and modified in 2016 (ASV 1.1). Further development of ASV led to INTELLiVENT-ASV, which was launched in 2010 and offers fully closed-loop control of both oxygenation and ventilation settings.

Adaptive support ventilation

ASV is a closed-loop ventilation mode that combines adaptive pressure-controlled ventilation for passive patients with adaptive pressure support ventilation if the patient is triggering. The aim of this mode is to optimise the patient's work of breathing, minimise the mechanical power delivered by the ventilator, improve patient safety and comfort, and decrease the workload for ICU staff.

Key points

- Adaptive support ventilation (ASV) is a closed-loop ventilation mode suitable for both passive and spontaneously breathing patients.

- ASV determines the combination of V_T and respiratory rate according to the target minute volume set by the clinician and the patient's respiratory mechanics.

- INTELLiVENT-ASV represents fully closed-loop control of ventilation and oxygenation settings.

- INTELLiVENT-ASV adjusts all settings to reach the targets set by the clinician.

How does it work? The user sets patient's sex and height and the target minute ventilation ($V'E$) in %. The ventilator calculates the patient's ideal body weight (IBW), target $V'E$ in L·min⁻¹ and the anatomical dead space volume (VD) based on the IBW (100% $V'E$=100 mL·kg⁻¹ IBW and VD=2.2×IBW). Subsequently, the ventilator measures the patient's respiratory mechanics, namely the expiratory time constant (RCexp). RCexp is the product of airway resistance multiplied by compliance. RCexp for a normal lung patient is in the range 0.5–0.7 s. RCexp shorter than 0.5 s is measured in the case of decreased compliance, such as ARDS or chest wall stiffness. By contrast, RCexp longer than 0.7 s occurs in the case of increased resistance, such as COPD or asthma. The ASV algorithm enters the target $V'E$, RCexp and VD values into the Otis and Mead equations, to calculate the combination of respiratory rate (RR) and VT associated with the lowest force and work of breathing (WOB) (figure 1). In passive patients, ASV delivers pressure-controlled breaths, adjusting inspiratory pressure and RR to reach the optimal combination of VT and RR. In spontaneously breathing patients, ASV delivers pressure-supported breaths, adjusting the pressure support to reach the optimal VT. When the patient recovers, pressure support decreases automatically in preparation for weaning. In spontaneously breathing patients, ASV has no control over the patient's RR. RCexp is measured breath-by-breath. If a restrictive or obstructive pathology develops during ventilation, this enables ASV to adapt by decreasing VT and increasing RR in the first case, and increasing VT and decreasing RR in the latter. In ASV mode, PEEP and FIO_2 are set manually.

Initial settings, adjustments and monitoring Table 1 outlines the initial settings, adjustments and monitoring for ASV in passive and spontaneously breathing patients, as well as the settings for use during weaning.

ASV for weaning In spontaneously breathing patients, ASV automatically decreases pressure support when the patient's efforts become stronger.

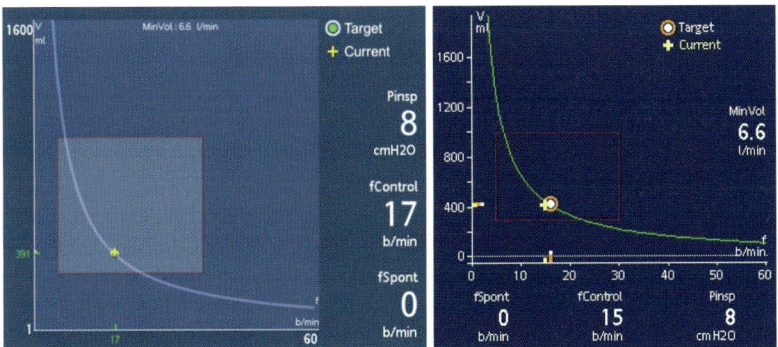

Figure 1. The ASV graph displays the multiple combinations of VT and RR possible to reach the target $V'E$ (MinVol in the software) set by the clinician. The circle represents the target combination of VT and RR determined by the ASV algorithm, while the yellow cross indicates the patient's actual combination of VT and RR. The red square represents the safety limits.

Table 1. Initial settings, adjustments and monitoring of ASV for passive and spontaneously breathing patients, and for use during weaning

	Passive patients	Spontaneously breathing patients	Weaning
Initial settings			
V'_E%	100%	100%	25%
PEEP and F_{IO_2}	Manually according to P_{aO_2} or S_{pO_2}		
Inspiratory trigger	Not active	2 L·min⁻¹ (titrated individually for each patient)	
Pressure rise time	Not active	50 ms (titrated according to patient–ventilator synchronisation)	
Expiratory trigger	Not active	25% (titrated according to patient–ventilator synchronisation)	
Pressure limit	30 cmH₂O (may be increased to 35 cmH₂O in severe COPD)		
Adjustments			
V'_E%	±10% according to P_{aCO_2}	±20% according to the patient's effort and RR	No change
PEEP and F_{IO_2}	According to P_{aO_2} or S_{pO_2}		
Monitoring			
Respiratory mechanics	RCexp, compliance, resistance	RCexp	RCexp
Lung protection	V_T/IBW, P_{plat}, total PEEP, ΔP	V_T/IBW	
Ventilation support		Pressure support and RR	Pressure support and RR
Blood gas	P_{aO_2}, P_{aCO_2} and pH		

When the actual pressure support is below 12 cmH₂O, a weaning trial can be performed by decreasing the target V'_E to 25%. This setting decreases pressure support to 5–6 cmH₂O during the trial, with the possibility of increasing pressure support again if the patient's efforts are very weak. If the patient tolerates these settings for 30 min and the pressure support remains low, extubation can be considered.

Evidence The evidence shows that ASV can select different combinations of V_T and RR for normal-lung, COPD and ARDS patients, as well as decrease WOB and improve patient–ventilator synchrony, with the need for fewer manual adjustments and fewer arterial blood gas analyses when compared with conventional modes. Several RCTs show that ASV shortens weaning duration in different patient groups (post-surgical, medical and COPD).

INTELLiVENT-ASV

INTELLiVENT-ASV is a fully closed-loop ventilation mode based on ASV, which manages both the ventilation and oxygenation settings automatically using the data supplied by an end-tidal carbon dioxide tension (P_{ETCO_2}) and S_{pO_2} sensor.

The goal is to reach the ventilation and oxygenation targets set by the clinician, using the same functions and safety features of the ASV mode.

How does it work? The user sets patient's sex and height, and the patient's condition (choosing between normal lungs, ARDS, chronic hypercapnia and brain injury). By selecting the patient's condition, the algorithm proposes different default P_{ETCO_2} and S_{pO_2} target ranges. In passive patients, the ventilation controller adjusts the target V'_E according to the measured P_{ETCO_2} and target P_{ETCO_2} set by the clinician (figure 2). In spontaneously breathing patients, the ventilation controller adjusts the target V'_E to keep the patient's RR in an acceptable range. For any given target V'_E, the ASV controller determines the optimal combination of V_T and RR and delivers either an

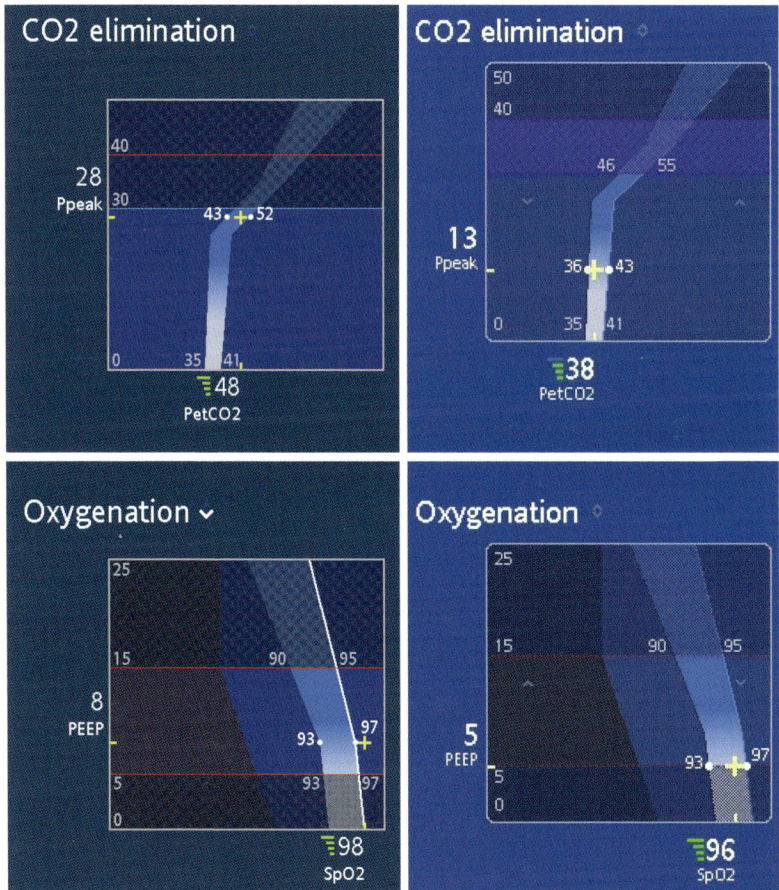

Figure 2. The ventilation map (top panel) displays the P_{ETCO_2} target ranges set by the user and the actual P_{ETCO_2} with a quality index (green bars); the oxygenation map (bottom panel) displays the S_{pO_2} target ranges set by the user and the actual S_{pO_2} with a quality index (green bars).

adaptive pressure-controlled breath in passive patients, or an adaptive pressure-supported breath in spontaneously breathing patients.

The oxygenation controller adjusts F_{IO_2} and PEEP to keep the patient's S_{pO_2} within the target S_{pO_2} range set by the clinician (figure 2). A PEEP/F_{IO_2} table derived from the ARDSnet publications is used to determine the combination of PEEP and F_{IO_2}.

Initial settings, adjustments and monitoring Table 2 outlines the initial settings, adjustments and monitoring for INTELLiVENT-ASV in passive and spontaneously breathing patients (see also the video in the online supplementary material, available at: https://books.ersjournals.com/).

INTELLiVENT-ASV for weaning INTELLiVENT-ASV has an automatic weaning protocol that can be customised by the clinician. When activated, the ventilator starts by gradually decreasing pressure support if the patient's RR remains

Table 2. Initial settings, adjustments and monitoring of INTELLiVENT-ASV for passive and spontaneously breathing patients

	Passive patients	Spontaneously breathing patients
Initial settings		
P_{ETCO_2} target	According to lung condition	Maximum P_{ETCO_2} according to lung condition
Pressure limit	30 cmH$_2$O (may be increased to 35 cmH$_2$O in severe COPD)	
S_{pO_2} target	According to lung condition	
Minimum PEEP	5 cmH$_2$O or higher	5 cmH$_2$O
Maximum PEEP	According to lung condition	
Minimum F_{IO_2}	21% to 30%	
Inspiratory trigger	Not active	2 L·min^{-1} (titrated individually for each patient)
Pressure rise time	Not active	50 ms (titrated according to patient–ventilator synchronisation)
Expiratory trigger	Not active	25% (titrated according to patient–ventilator synchronisation)
Adjustments		
P_{ETCO_2} target	According to change in lung condition and P_{aCO_2}–P_{ETCO_2} gradient	No change
S_{pO_2} target	According to change in lung condition	
Monitoring		
Respiratory mechanics	RCexp, compliance, resistance	RCexp
Lung protection	V_T/IBW, P_{plat}, total PEEP, ΔP	V_T/IBW
Ventilation support	Pressure support and RR	
Blood gas	P_{aO_2}, P_{aCO_2} and pH	

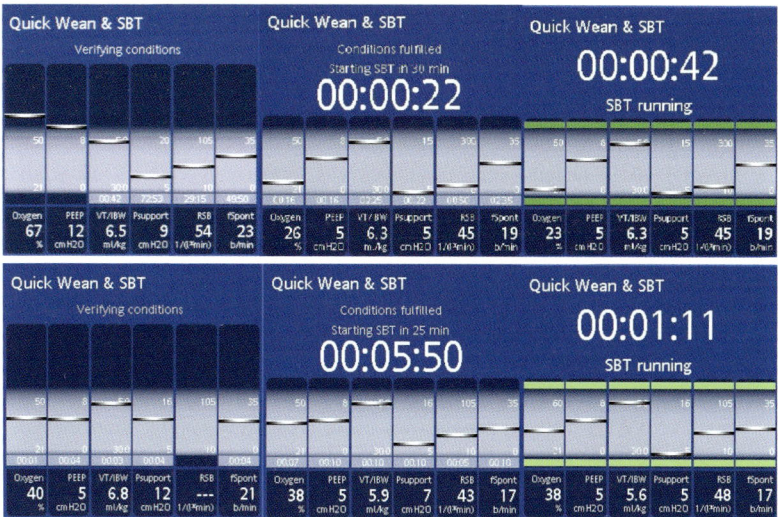

Figure 3. The three steps of the automatic weaning protocol (from left to right): screening of the readiness to wean criteria, observation phase, and weaning trial.

within the target range and screening the readiness to wean criteria set by the clinician: PEEP, FIO_2, pressure support, RR, VT–RR combination and percentage of spontaneous breaths. When all the criteria have been met, an observation period starts during which pressure support continues to decrease gradually. The duration of the observation period is determined by the clinician. At the end of this period, a weaning trial starts automatically using the PEEP, $V'E$ % and duration set by the clinician (figure 3). During the weaning trial, the FIO_2 controller continues to run so that FIO_2 is adjusted according to SpO_2, and all the readiness to wean criteria are monitored continuously. If some parameters move out of their respective target ranges set by the clinician, the weaning trial aborts automatically and a failure message is displayed. However, if all the parameters remain within their target ranges for the duration of the weaning trial, the trial is completed and a message is displayed that extubation should be considered. A dedicated window displays the progress of the weaning protocol and the parameters causing failure, if applicable.

Evidence Results in passive and spontaneously breathing patients both in the ICU and after cardiac surgery have shown INTELLiVENT-ASV to be safe, as well as having a high degree of both feasibility and usability. Preliminary outcome studies in the ICU comparing INTELLiVENT-ASV with conventional modes reported similar outcomes for both, with a dramatic decrease in the number of manual ventilator settings. Evidence obtained from paediatric ICUs remains scarce.

Summary

ASV and INTELLiVENT-ASV continuously adapt the ventilator settings according to the patient's condition, in order to apply the strategy set by the clinician. They result in improved safety for the patients and the constant delivery of lung-protective ventilation. Monitoring of the dynamic changes of ventilator settings and the patient's physiological variables provides clinicians with useful information, which allows them to adjust the strategy and start weaning at the earliest possible opportunity.

Further reading

- Arnal JM (2015). Adaptive support ventilation. *In:* Rimensberger P, ed. Pediatric and Neonatal Mechanical Ventilation: from Basics to Bedside. Berlin, Springer.

- Arnal JM, *et al.* (2008). Automatic selection of breathing pattern using adaptive support ventilation. *Intensive Care Med*; 34: 75–81.

- Arnal JM, *et al.* (2012). Safety and efficacy of a fully closed-loop control ventilation (IntelliVent-ASV) in sedated ICU patients with acute respiratory failure: a prospective randomized crossover study. *Intensive Care Med*; 38: 781–787.

- Arnal JM, *et al.* (2013). Feasibility study on full closed-loop control ventilation (IntelliVent-ASV) in ICU patients with acute respiratory failure: a prospective observational comparative study. *Crit Care*; 17: R196.

- Arnal JM, *et al.* (2018). Closed loop ventilation mode in intensive care unit: a randomized controlled clinical trial comparing the numbers of manual ventilator setting changes. *Minerva Anestesiol*; 84: 58–67.

- Arnal JM, *et al.* (2018). Parameters for simulation of adult subjects during mechanical ventilation. *Respir Care*; 63: 158–168.

- Belliato M (2016). Automated weaning from mechanical ventilation. *World J Respirol*; 6: 49–53.

- Bialais E, *et al.* (2016). Closed-loop ventilation mode (IntelliVent-ASV) in intensive care unit: a randomized trial. *Minerva Anestesiol*; 82: 657–668.

- Clavieras N, *et al.* (2013). Prospective randomized crossover study of a new closed-loop control system *versus* pressure support during weaning from mechanical ventilation. *Anesthesiology*; 119: 631–641.

- Fot EV, *et al.* (2017). Automated weaning from mechanical ventilation after off-pump coronary artery bypass grafting. *Front Med (Lausanne)*; 4: 31.

- Gruber PC, *et al.* (2008). Randomized controlled trial comparing adaptive-support ventilation with pressure-regulated volume-controlled ventilation with automode in weaning patients after cardiac surgery. *Anesthesiology*; 109: 81–87.

- Kirakli C, *et al.* (2015). A randomized controlled trial comparing the ventilation duration between adaptive support ventilation and pressure assist/control ventilation in medical patients in the ICU. *Chest*; 147: 1503–1509.

- Kirakli C, *et al.* (2011). Adaptive support ventilation for faster weaning in COPD: a randomised controlled trial. *Eur Respir J*; 38: 774–780.

- Lellouche F, *et al.* (2013). Evaluation of fully automated ventilation: a randomized controlled study in post-cardiac surgery patients. *Intensive Care Med*; 39: 463–471.

- Rose L, *et al.* (2015). Automated versus non-automated weaning for reducing the duration of mechanical ventilation for critically ill adults and children: a Cochrane systematic review and meta-analysis. *Crit Care*; 19: 48.

Invasive ventilation in ARDS

Irene Telias, Lieuwe D. Bos and Eddy Fan

Invasive ventilation is the cornerstone of supportive care in patients with ARDS and a source of harm. Physiological evidence on principles to guide ventilation strategies is extensive. However, RCTs are scarce and interpretation of their results challenging. Therefore, understanding the principles allows us to adapt available evidence to specific patients and guide invasive ventilation when there is no evidence in the trials.

Pathophysiology of ARDS, risks and aims of invasive ventilation

Inflammation leads to increased permeability of the alveolo-capillary membrane, extravascular lung water and collapse of the dependent lung (figure 1). The remaining aerated lung available for gas exchange in the non-dependent areas is small (*i.e.* the baby lung) resulting in lower functional residual capacity (or end-expiratory lung volume (EELV)). These changes result in alterations to:

- Respiratory mechanics: decreased respiratory system compliance (C_{rs}) proportional to the size of the baby lung.
- Gas exchange: impaired oxygenation and carbon dioxide clearance due to ventilation/perfusion mismatch including shunt (lack of ventilation with

Key points

- ARDS is characterised by inflammatory pulmonary oedema resulting in altered mechanics, oxygenation and systemic inflammation.

- Recognising ARDS is the first step to setting the ventilator appropriately.

- All patients should receive controlled invasive ventilation with low V_T (6–8 mL·kg^{-1} predicted body weight) limiting P_{plat} to <30 cmH$_2$O (2.9 kPa) during the early phase.

- Patients with moderate and severe ARDS should be considered for a higher PEEP strategy, prone position and transferred to an ECMO referral centre if lack of improvement.

- Uncertainties include the best technique to set PEEP and managing invasive ventilation during spontaneous breathing.

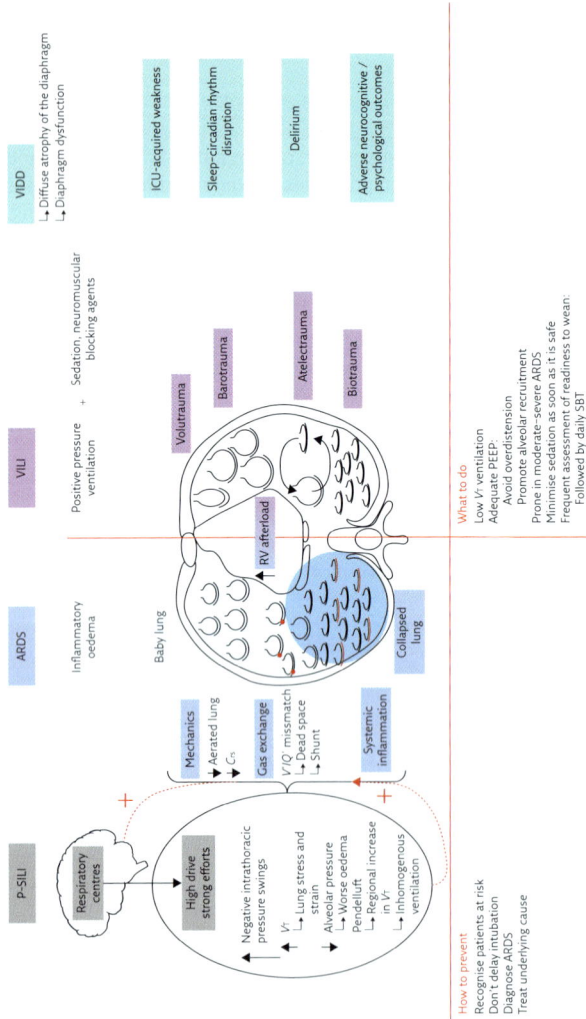

Figure 1. Pathophysiology of ARDS, risks of invasive ventilation and strategies to minimise harm. In the centre of the figure, pathophysiology of ARDS is contrasted to pathophysiological mechanisms of VILI. To the left, mechanisms that lead to patient self-inflicted lung injury (P-SILI) are highlighted; these occur more prominently in patients with moderate–severe ARDS before, but also during, invasive ventilation. On the right, other adverse consequences of invasive ventilation and critical illness that need to be considered when setting the ventilator and adjusting sedation and use of other adjunctive therapies like neuro-muscular blocking agents are shown. For simplicity, the consequences of ARDS and invasive ventilation on other organs (worsening multiorgan failure) are not displayed, but are inherent to the concepts of systemic inflammation and biotrauma. Strategies to prevent worsening and to minimise harm are also listed. VIDD: ventilator-induced diaphragm dysfunction; C_{rs}: respiratory system compliance; SBT: spontaneous breathing trials; V'/Q': ventilation/perfusion ratio.

preserved perfusion in collapsed areas) and dead space (microcirculatory occlusion in ventilated areas).
- Other organs: increased right ventricular afterload and failure, due to increased pulmonary vascular resistance; multiorgan failure, due to systemic inflammation arising from the lung.

Respiratory drive during early ARDS is often high, and strong breathing efforts in moderate and severe ARDS can worsen injury through various mechanisms; so-called patient self-inflicted lung injury.

Invasive ventilation can also worsen lung injury and promote multiorgan failure (*i.e.* VILI) by:

- Excessive stress and strain due to increased volume and pressure applied to the baby lung (volutrauma and barotrauma). Overdistension of aerated lung promoting collapse of pulmonary vessels, increasing dead-space and right ventricular afterload.
- Repeated opening and closing of alveolar units and small airways (atelectrauma).
- Release of inflammatory mediators with further damage to the lung and distant organs (biotrauma).

During controlled ventilation, respiratory muscles are at risk of ventilator-induced diaphragm dysfunction due to disuse atrophy resulting in dysfunction.

Therefore, ventilator strategies in ARDS should aim at maintaining adequate gas exchange while decreasing the risk of VILI and ventilator-induced diaphragm dysfunction by:

- Promoting lung recruitment by increasing EELV (*i.e.* increasing the size of the baby lung) and improving gas exchange.
- Limiting excessive stress, strain and cyclic opening and closure of alveolar units.
- Allowing for spontaneous breathing as soon as it is safe.

How to set the ventilator in patients with early phase ARDS

Aim for low V_T *ventilation and limit inspiratory pressures to avoid excessive stress and strain* During the initial phase, a controlled mode of ventilation should be used and V_T should be set according to predicted body weight (PBW) based on height and sex, proportional to the size of the normal lung. The clinical evidence supports the use of low V_T ventilation (LTVV) (6–8 mL·kg^{-1} PBW) and limitation of P_{plat} to <30 cmH$_2$O (2.9 kPa). From a practical standpoint, starting with 6 mL·kg^{-1} of PBW is reasonable. LTVV can result in hypercapnia, acidosis, high respiratory drive and need for deep sedation. If respiratory drive is high with flow starvation or double cycling, increasing to 8 mL·kg^{-1} PBW is safe if no further worsening is seen.

Setting PEEP in patients with ARDS Higher PEEP in ARDS can: 1) promote recruitment of collapsed alveolar units (increasing the size of the baby lung/ EELV); 2) avoid cyclic alveolar (and possibly small airways) opening and closure; and 3) result in overdistension of aerated lung. The relative weight of each consequence depends on the lung's recruitability. Data suggest that using higher PEEP is beneficial in moderate-to-severe ARDS; however, the risk of overdistension in some patients within this group might also be higher and RCTs compared the use of higher *versus* lower PEEP regardless of patient's physiological response to PEEP.

Practically speaking, initial PEEP can be set using any of the methods from the RCTs: high PEEP–F_{IO_2} table (ALVEOLI and LOV studies), or the highest PEEP that results in P_{plat} from 28 cmH$_2$O (2.7 kPa) to 30 cmH$_2$O (2.9 kPa) (ExPRESS study). Increasing PEEP usually leads to an increase in P_{plat} (especially if no recruitment occurs), which should be monitored carefully.

Based on extensive physiological evidence, monitoring the response to an increase in PEEP should be done to estimate recruitability and risk of overdistension (figure 2). Different bedside methods have been proposed, none of which have been tested in an RCT:

- Oxygenation response to PEEP (considering the interaction with haemodynamics)
- Improvement of C_{rs} (considering the risk of measuring tidal recruitment)
- Single breath de-recruitment manoeuvre
- Use of various parameters derived from electrical impedance tomography, amongst others

We suggest judging the overall clinical response to PEEP and carrying out at least one of the listed measures of recruitability to decide if higher PEEP is beneficial or risky to the specific patient. The combination of more than one might be informative, for example higher PEEP resulting in better compliance but worsening oxygenation might imply recruitability but suggest possible interaction with haemodynamics (*e.g.* intracardiac shunt or lower cardiac output).

Adjuvant therapies for moderate and severe ARDS Patients with moderate-to-severe ARDS (with a P_{aO_2}/F_{IO_2} <150 mmHg (20 kPa)) should be considered early for prone positioning lasting >12 h. Prone positioning allows for a homogeneous distribution of ventilation related to a decrease in chest wall compliance and change in the location of the aerated and non-aerated lung regions improving ventilation/perfusion match. It can promote alveolar recruitment and less injurious ventilation with improvement in oxygenation and mortality. The main adverse effects from prone positioning include tube obstruction and pressure ulcers.

Patients with severe ARDS that do not respond to these measures should be considered for transfer to a referral centre that can provide ECMO relatively early in the course of the disease. Veno-venous ECMO is the most frequently used configuration in this setting and results in improved gas exchange while allowing lung rest with extremely low V_T and inspiratory pressures, thus further mitigating VILI.

High-frequency oscillatory ventilation (HFOV), despite having the theoretical advantage of minimising VILI by delivering relatively high mean airway pressure with very small V_T (at high frequency), should not be routinely used. A large RCT demonstrated higher mortality with HFOV compared to LTVV with higher PEEP. However, it can be considered as a rescue therapy in patients with refractory hypoxaemia not eligible for ECMO.

Later in the course of ARDS There are no RCTs that have evaluated spontaneous breathing during invasive ventilation in patients with ARDS. However, there is enough evidence to suggest that as the patient improves, sedation should be minimised and, when the patient meets readiness to wean criteria (improvement in oxygenation and reasonable haemodynamic stability), daily spontaneous breathing trials should be performed and patients should be extubated as soon as possible.

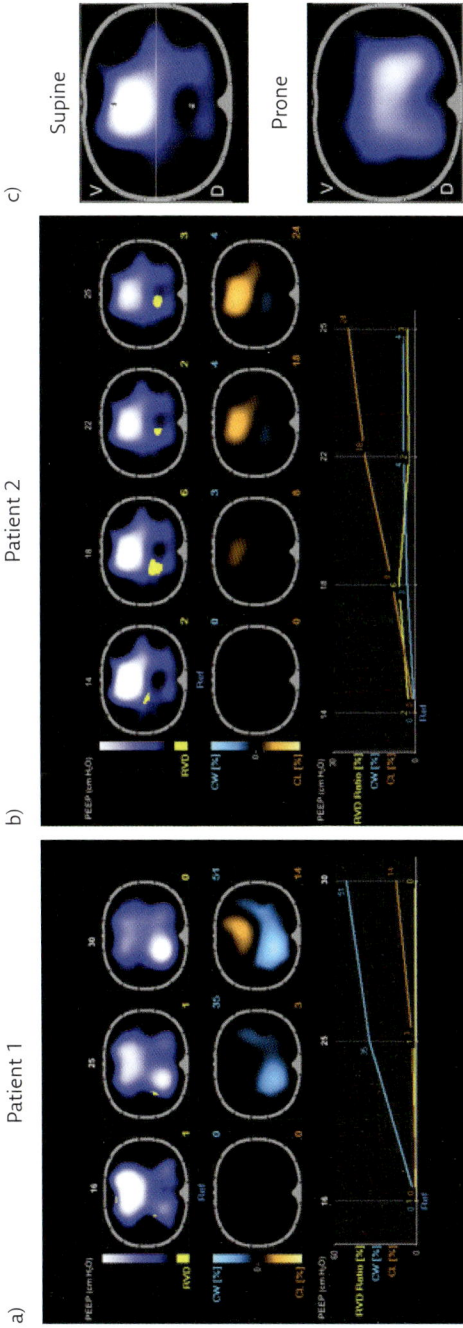

Figure 2. Heterogeneity in the response to high PEEP and difference with prone position. Electrical impedance tomography (EIT) measures change in lung impedance (global and regional) as a surrogate of change in aeration. a, b) Two patients with moderate ARDS undergoing PEEP titration using EIT to monitor their response in the supine position. The upper panel shows the distribution of aeration at each PEEP level (white meaning higher aeration and blue meaning less aeration). The middle panel shows the regional change in compliance estimated using this method as PEEP increases compared to the reference (low PEEP). Areas in blue represent areas with increased compliance and orange refers to areas with a loss in compliance with respect to the reference. The lower panel shows global increase in compliance (blue) and decrease in compliance (orange) over time. Patient 1 shows an increase in compliance at high PEEP together with a more homogeneous distribution of aeration (potential for recruitment with PEEP). At the highest PEEP level there is coexistence of areas of increased and decreased compliance (possible overdistension with PEEP). Patient 2 shows negligible increase in compliance and mostly a decrease in compliance together with a heterogeneous distribution of aeration. c) The same patient shows a more homogeneous distribution of aeration when in the prone position. RVD: regional ventilation delay; CW: compliance win; CL: compliance loss; V: ventral; D: dorsal. Images provided courtesy of Thomas Piraino (St. Michael's Hospital, Toronto, ON, Canada).

Current considerations during invasive ventilation in patients with ARDS

During controlled invasive ventilation The use of neuromuscular blocking agents during the first 48 h of invasive ventilation in ARDS patients with P_{aO_2}/F_{IO_2} <150 mmHg (20 kPa) improved mortality in the ACURASYS trial. Potential mechanisms may include the prevention of reverse triggering (present during deep sedation and controlled ventilation) and inhibiting activity of the expiratory muscles. There are ongoing concerns related to the risk of ICU-acquired weakness and the concomitant need for heavy sedation. Therefore, a larger confirmatory trial was conducted by the PETAL Network. It was stopped early and will help inform whether neuromuscular blocking agents should be routinely used.

Clinicians should be cautious about using aggressive recruitment manoeuvres in patients with moderate and severe ARDS. These consist in applying high pressure to open alveolar units during a short time. The ART trial showed increased mortality when combining them with high PEEP compared to low PEEP–F_{IO_2} table in moderate and severe ARDS.

The use of driving pressure ($\triangle P = P_{plat} - PEEP$) to titrate ventilation is supported by a strong physiological rationale. However, no prospective RCT tested an intervention based on this rationale that doesn't consider possible tidal recruitment. $\triangle P$ represents the distending pressure of the respiratory system and is a possible surrogate of stress and strain to the baby lung that is highly associated with mortality. C_{rs} is directly proportional to the size of the baby lung and inversely proportional to the $\triangle P$. Therefore, adjusting V_T to target a safe $\triangle P$ might normalise V_T to the size of the baby lung ($\triangle P = V_T / C_{rs}$).

Using transpulmonary pressure measured with oesophageal pressure to set PEEP considers the difference in mechanics of the lung and chest wall. Transpulmonary pressure represents the distending pressure of the lung. Some patients have an increased contribution of the chest wall to airway pressure due to oedema, obesity or intra-abdominal hypertension. Setting PEEP to achieve transpulmonary pressure >0 at end-expiration might avoid lung collapse and cyclic opening and closing of alveolar units. A recent RCT proved no benefit of titrating PEEP using a simplistic approach based on this rationale compared to a high PEEP–F_{IO_2} table. No harm was found; therefore, other approaches to calculate transpulmonary pressure and personalise PEEP titration accordingly may be considered and could be tested in future studies.

The use of ultraprotective ventilation (V_T <6 mL·kg^{-1} PBW) with low-flow extracorporeal carbon dioxide removal is a possible alternative to decrease VILI in moderate and severe ARDS. A pilot trial proved its feasibility; however, balance between efficacy and safety need to be tested in a larger RCT.

During spontaneous breathing Around 30% of patients with ARDS are ventilated in a spontaneous mode; however, evidence on how to manage the ventilator under this circumstance is scarce.

There is agreement that strong spontaneous breathing efforts are harmful early in patients with moderate/severe ARDS. On the contrary, moderate efforts in less severe patients might be beneficial by preventing atelectasis, improving haemodynamics, avoiding atrophy and requiring less sedation. However, there is no evidence on whether controlled ventilation should be completely avoided in mild ARDS and whether any degree of spontaneous breathing should be allowed early in moderate ARDS.

When transitioning to a spontaneous mode in the recovery phase, persistent altered mechanics and oxygenation, high drive, strong efforts and dyssynchronies are frequent. Based on large cohort and physiological studies, an intermediate range of inspiratory effort might be warranted. To achieve this, noninvasive measures of drive and effort, such as airway occlusion pressure or diaphragm ultrasound, might be used in all patients. Those patients at higher risk of injury (*e.g.* strong efforts, severe injury, systemic inflammation, haemodynamic instability or worsening with spontaneous breathing), may require invasive measures such as oesophageal pressure. However, no prospective study tested an intervention to control effort and, if applied, it should not delay extubation if the patient's overall clinical condition is improving. Patient–ventilator dyssynchronies were associated with poor outcome. However, it is uncertain if implementing an intervention to avoid dyssynchronies is beneficial. Nevertheless, not all dyssynchronies are equal: monitoring them, and understanding its mechanism provides useful information regarding the patient's overall condition.

Summary

Managing invasive ventilation during ARDS is challenging, can lead to harm and is associated with many unanswered questions. However, there is enough evidence to support the need for early recognition of the syndrome, use of LTVV, limit inspiratory pressure and use of adequate PEEP in the initial phase, as well as prone position in more severe patients. Understanding physiological principles and clinical evidence helps adjust best practices to specific patients.

Further reading

- Amato MB, *et al.* (2015). Driving pressure and survival in the acute respiratory distress syndrome. *N Engl J Med*; 372: 747–755.

- Bellani G, *et al.* (2016). Epidemiology, patterns of care, and mortality for patients with acute respiratory distress syndrome in intensive care units in 50 countries. *JAMA*; 315: 788–800.

- Brochard L, *et al.* (2017). Mechanical ventilation to minimize progression of lung injury in acute respiratory failure. *Am J Respir Crit Care Med*; 195: 438–442.

- Fan E, *et al.* (2017). An Official American Thoracic Society/European Society of Intensive Care Medicine/Society of Critical Care Medicine Clinical Practice Guideline: mechanical ventilation in adult patients with acute respiratory distress syndrome. *Am J Respir Crit Care*; 195: 1253–1263.

- Gattinoni L, *et al.* (2016). The "baby lung" became an adult. *Intensive Care Med*; 42: 663–673.

- Goligher EC, *et al.* (2016). Clinical challenges in mechanical ventilation. *Lancet*; 387: 1856–1866.

- Pham T, *et al.* (2017). Mechanical ventilation: state of the art. *Mayo Clin Proc*; 92: 1382–1400.

- Ranieri VM, *et al.* (2012). Acute respiratory distress syndrome: the Berlin definition. *JAMA*; 307: 2526–2533.

Invasive ventilation in obstructive airway disease

Louis-Marie Galerneau, Claude Guérin and Nicolas Terzi

Patients with obstructive airway diseases (COPD or asthma) receive invasive ventilation in the ICU when acute respiratory failure is severe and/or NIV (the standard of care in COPD patients) is contraindicated or has failed. As RCTs on invasive ventilation are lacking, ventilator management relies on pathophysiological considerations, of which acute dynamic pulmonary hyperinflation (DPH) and increased work of breathing (WOB) are cardinal features. As for any patient receiving invasive ventilation in the ICU, the primary goal is to protect the lung from a further injury.

Once intubated the patient is commonly sedated and paralysed. Initial ventilator settings should include low V_T, low respiratory rate, short inspiratory time (t_I) and long expiratory time (t_E).

In this chapter we will provide a brief reminder of the pathophysiological basis, and then discuss passive and active invasive ventilation and the settings and monitoring in each. This chapter does not discuss nebulisation of medications like bronchodilators and administration of steroids. However, it is stressed that these should not be withheld. Also, we stress that it is important to titrate morphine wisely in these patients.

Pathophysiological basis

DPH, defined as higher end-expiratory lung volume than expected (gas trapping), results from an imbalance between lung expiratory time constant (the product of compliance and resistance) and expiratory time set out by the caregiver.

Key points

- NIV is the standard of care in the management of patients with obstructive airway disease in acute respiratory failure.

- Invasive ventilation in this setting is therefore performed in selected and severe patients or in those contraindicated for NIV.

- Invasive ventilation in patients with obstructive airway disease is not fed by evidence-based medicine recommendations but based on pathophysiological principles with the primary aim of not worsening dynamic pulmonary hyperinflation.

The time constant is the time required to exhale 63% of V_T according to a single compartment lung model (figure 1). Resting lung volume (functional residual capacity) is reached after 3–4 time constants. Due to acute airflow obstruction, airflow resistance increases and so does the time constant. Typical inspiratory and expiratory resistance in COPD patients under invasive ventilation is 22 cmH$_2$O·s·L^{-1} and 18 cmH$_2$O·s·L^{-1}, respectively, *versus* 13 cmH$_2$O·s·L^{-1} and 12 cmH$_2$O·s·L^{-1}, respectively, in ICU patients with normal lung. The time constant may also increase if an emphysema component is present. However, in COPD patients in the ICU a typical compliance value of 59 mL·cmH$_2$O^{-1} has been found, which is close to that in normal subjects. Therefore, the time constant is 1.1 s on average in COPD *versus* 0.6 s in normal subjects. In patients with acute severe airway obstruction due to asthma, respiratory resistance is much higher, up to 50–70 cmH$_2$O·s·L^{-1} (figure 1).

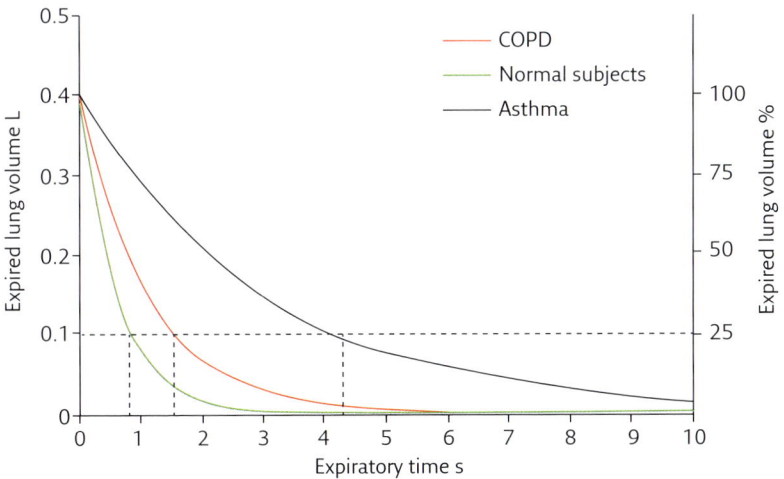

Respiratory rate breaths·min^{-1}		18	10	6
	Total breath duration s	3.33	6.00	10.00
tI/tE 0.50	tI s	1.66	3.00	5.00
	tE s	1.66	3.00	5.00
tI/tE 0.25	tI s	0.83	1.50	2.50
	tE s	2.50	4.50	7.50

Figure 1. Exponential decay of lung volume during expiration according to the single compartment lung model in COPD, a normal subject and asthma. In a single time constant the lung deflates by 63% (horizontal broken line), which markedly differs across conditions (vertical broken lines). The constant of the lung volume decay is the ratio of tE to time constant. Therefore, the ventilator settings should be adjusted to match both times. The table displays the resulting tE from manipulation of respiratory rate at different tI/tE ratios. In patients with severe asthma even the highest tE may not allow resting lung volume recovery.

Furthermore, with DPH right ventricle afterload increases and, hence, the risk of acute cor pulmonale. The primary goal of invasive ventilation is therefore to make every effort to not worsen and even to reduce DPH.

Passive invasive ventilation

Settings Lowering V_T to 6–8 mL·kg^{-1} predicted body weight contributes to this task in association with limiting P_{plat} <30 cmH$_2$O. Because DPH is a time-dependent phenomenon its reduction will better benefit from an increase in t_E. Lowering respiratory rate is the most powerful adjustment to make at the ventilator to increase t_E at the same t_I/t_E ratio and inspiratory flow (figure 1).

Lowering both V_T and respiratory rate could promote hypercapnia because minute ventilation goes down. To help minimise this, instrumental dead space should be minimised by using a heated humidifier and connecting the ventilator circuit Y-piece directly at the endotracheal tube. However, some degree of hypercapnia and respiratory acidosis can be tolerated. Indeed, the concept of permissive hypercapnia stemmed from pioneering studies done more than 30 years ago in patients with acute severe asthma receiving invasive ventilation. Slowing the rate of P_{aCO_2} decrease is extremely important to maintain stable haemodynamics and avoid rebound alkalosis, which can be associated with hypokalaemia/hypophosphataemia and concurrent cardiac arrhythmias.

Whether the volume-controlled or pressure-controlled mode should be used is not evidence based. Given that respiratory mechanics can vary dramatically over a short period of time in these patients and that the primary goal is to control the lung volume, there is a strong rationale for using the volume-controlled mode. It is worth emphasising that in pressure-controlled mode the set pressure reflects P_{plat} only if end-inspiratory flow is nil. Due to high inspiratory resistance this is commonly not the case, and hence end-inspiratory occlusion must be carried out. Furthermore, inspiratory resistance cannot be computed because the inspiratory flow is not constant.

The systematic use of PEEP is not justified, even if it is a field of debate, and PEEP can be set to 0 if DPH is dramatic. The rationale for using PEEP would be to prevent atelectrauma in some lung regions, even though there is an overall lung hyperinflation. However, the distribution of intrinsic PEEP (PEEPi), the pressure counterpart of DPH, is heterogeneous and hence there is a risk with PEEP of worsening DPH regionally. If used PEEP should be set to 85% PEEPi because the haemodynamic consequence is minimised. However, depending on the prevalence of the distribution of low expiratory time constants, and hence regional DPH, impairment of haemodynamics can occur at lower values of PEEP/PEEPi ratio. In selected COPD patients it has been shown that end-expiratory lung volume can be reduced by PEEP. PEEP would then reopen small airways and favour exhalation in these regions. It is highly likely that this effect would come from a large prevalence of expiratory flow limitation and small airways collapse. If used, PEEP should be titrated in 1 cmH$_2$O steps as long as the closely monitored P_{plat} and PEEPtotal (=PEEP+PEEPi) does not increase.

Monitoring Respiratory monitoring of DPH is of paramount importance. Static PEEPi is measured by performing end-expiratory interruption of flow (figure 2) and

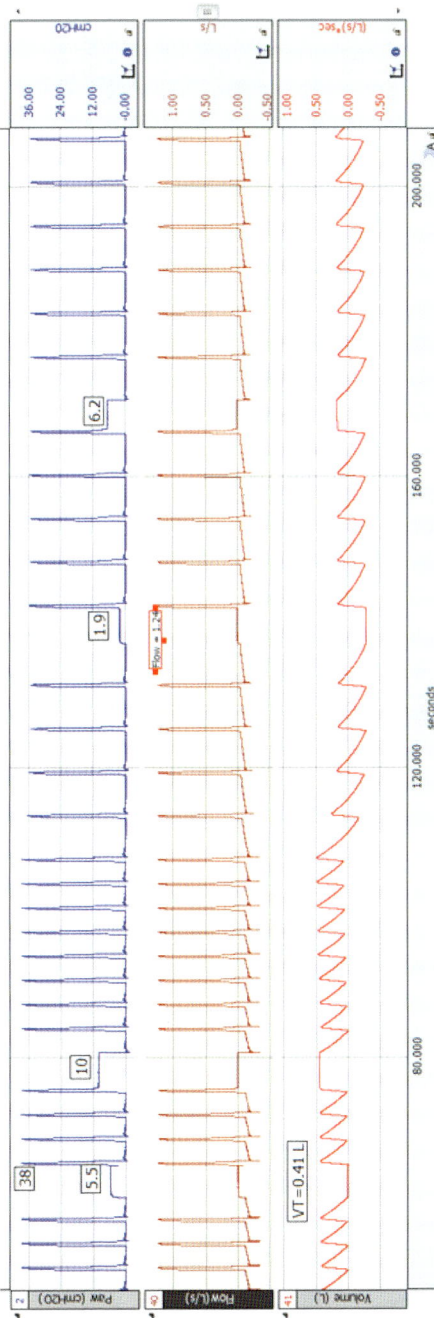

Figure 2. From top to bottom, traces of airway pressure (Paw), flow and volume against time in a COPD patient under invasive ventilation at constant flow inflation. After three breaths the airways are occluded and total end-expiratory pressure is measured (5.5 cmH₂O). After three further breaths the airways are occluded again at the end of inspiration to measure the Pplat (10 cmH₂O). From the ninth breath after baseline ventilation resumption the respiratory rate is lowered. That allows the end-expiratory lung volume to decrease and total end-expiratory pressure to go down to 1.9 cmH₂O. Elastance of the respiratory system is 11 cmH₂O·L⁻¹ (compliance 91 mL·cmH₂O⁻¹). Total inspiratory resistance of the respiratory system is 26.5 cmH₂O·s·L⁻¹.

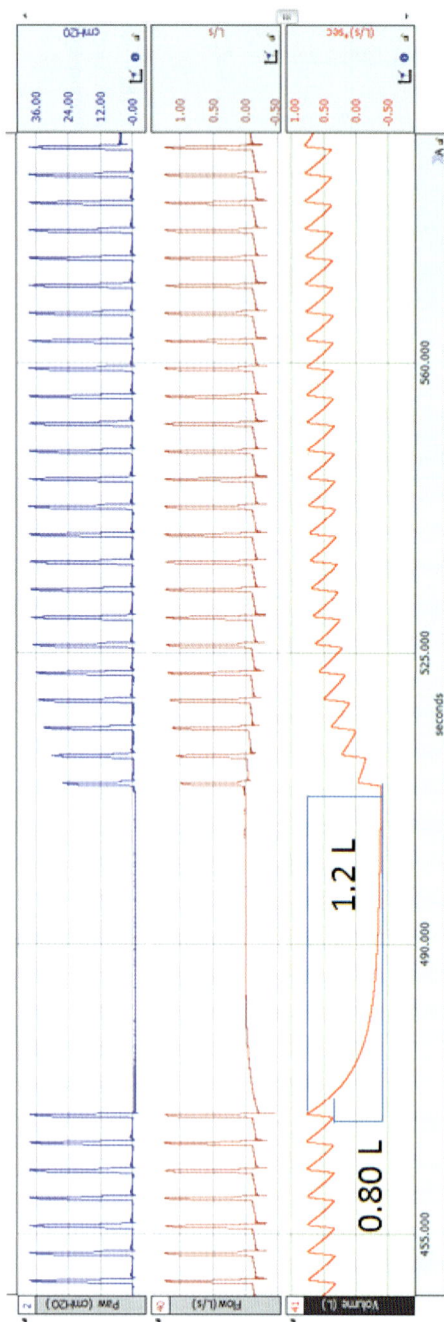

Figure 3. Measurement of DPH. After the seventh baseline breath, the respiratory rate is suddenly decreased to 1 breath·min[-1] (alternately the patient can be disconnected from the ventilator and left freely exhaling to the atmosphere) until zero flow is reached. The change in end-expiratory lung volume is 0.80 L, which is the amount of air trapping. Once the baseline ventilation is restored the process of DPH happens again. It took almost nine breaths to reach the new equilibrium, i.e. where it was before the manoeuvre. The total end-inspiratory lung volume is equal to the dynamic pulmonary inflation plus VT (almost 1.2 L).

recorded at the time of the plateau. P_{plat} is measured by performing end-inspiratory occlusion (figure 2). DPH can be measured by allowing the patient to exhale to the atmosphere until the flow becomes nil (figure 3).

Pressure support ventilation

Settings Once paralysis and sedation are stopped patients are moved to pressure support ventilation (PSV). WOB is now shared with the respiratory muscles and protecting the respiratory muscles from myotrauma becomes a key objective, together with lung protection. The issues are still DPH and the PEEPi the respiratory muscles have to overcome before mechanical assistance can happen, but patient comfort and prevention of patient–ventilator asynchrony must also be considered. Although PSV has been proven valuable in several acute clinical conditions, predefined airway pressure that remains unchanged from breath to breath is unlikely to provide optimal assistance all the time especially in obstructive patients. Indeed, assisted modes generally aim at synchronising the ventilator insufflation to the patient's effort, both to optimise comfort and to minimise WOB. V_T should be lowered by reducing the level of pressure support, targeting a window of 25–35 breaths·min^{-1} total respiratory rate (including inefficient efforts) without dyspnoea. Lowering V_T and DPH can also be done by reducing tI, and hence increasing tE. This is achieved not only by lowering PSV but also by setting the expiratory trigger closer to the maximal inspiratory flow rate. Inspiratory triggering should be as sensitive as possible to minimise the inspiratory effort without auto-triggering. PEEP is useful in favouring the efficiency of inspiratory muscles contraction. Setting PEEP is not easy, because measurement of PEEPi requires invasive assessment of oesophageal pressure. PEEP should be used at a low level and titrated according to the rate inefficient efforts and comfort.

The price to pay for this strategy is a risk of patient–ventilator asynchrony, which can be defined as a mismatch between the patient's neural output and the ventilator's inspiratory and expiratory times. A quarter of patients had high rates of asynchrony during assisted ventilation. Frequent asynchrony is associated with a longer duration of invasive ventilation. Compelling evidence accumulated over the past decade that also supports the use of V_T values that are lower than those traditionally used. Among the different forms of asynchrony, ineffective triggering (wasted effort) is the most common during invasive ventilation. Ineffective efforts are explained both by patient characteristics and by ventilator settings. PEEPi increases the patient effort required to trigger the ventilator and the likelihood that the patient's inspiratory effort eventually fails to trigger a ventilator breath. A weak inspiratory effort, which may occur during situations of low respiratory drive such as excessive ventilation, is also a risk factor and is common in patients receiving high assist levels or sedation. An excessive level of PSV is also associated with prolonged insufflation, thus promoting DPH and PEEPi. Reduction of ineffective efforts is often possible through a careful optimisation of the ventilator settings, at least in short-term studies. Reducing V_T during PSV can improve most factors contributing to ineffective efforts. Because high PSV is associated with prolonged insufflation beyond the end of the patient's neural inspiratory time, another useful way to decrease wasted efforts involves reducing inspiratory time by increasing the flow threshold of the cycling criterion.

Monitoring Monitoring should include expired V_T (in the 6–8 mL·kg^{-1} predicted body weight range), total respiratory rate (which is not provided by the ventilator) and patient effort. The latter is difficult to assess. Diaphragm contraction can be measured by using an electromyogram probe attached to a dedicated ICU respirator. However, accessory inspiratory muscles are also involved and are not measured with this probe. Oesophageal pressure reflects the overall contraction of the respiratory muscles. The measurement of the drop in airway pressure 100 ms after having occluded the airways ($P_{0.1}$) is useful, easy to perform and readily available on any ICU ventilator. It assesses intensity of respiratory drive and is a surrogate of the WOB. It can allow titrating pressure support level.

Further reading

- Davidson AC, *et al.* (2016). BTS/ICS guideline for the ventilatory management of acute hypercapnic respiratory failure in adults. *Thorax*; 71: Suppl. 2, ii1–ii35.

- Derenne JP, *et al.* (1996). Acute respiratory failure of COPD. *In*: Lenfant C, ed. Lung Biology in Health and Diseases Series. New York. Marcel Dekker.

- Guerin C, *et al.* (1997). Small airway closure and positive end-expiratory pressure in mechanically ventilated patients with chronic obstructive pulmonary disease. *Am J Respir Crit Care Med*; 155: 1949–1956.

Invasive ventilation in interstitial lung diseases

Sunil Patel, Ricardo Estêvão Gomes and Antonio M. Esquinas

The multiple subtypes and heterogeneity of interstitial lung diseases (ILDs) often means that recognition, diagnosis and treatment can be difficult. Interstitial abnormalities can be characterised as focal or widespread and predominantly inflammatory or fibrotic. All such changes cause architectural distortion and/or airspace infiltration leading to dyspnoea, cough and reduced exercise tolerance. Objectively, the presence of ILD is defined by radiological findings and abnormal pulmonary function tests, *i.e.* a restrictive pattern with a reduced total lung capacity or vital capacity, which correlates with poor pulmonary compliance if invasive ventilation is then required, and/or reduced gas transfer factor. Once there are established fibrotic changes, the parenchyma is permanently damaged and there is even greater focus on preventing progression. Predicting decline is difficult, as discussed further in box 1.

Acute presentations in patients with known ILDs are common. Once acute respiratory failure (ARF) or acute-on-chronic respiratory failure is apparent, prompt

Key points

- The mortality in mechanically ventilated patients with interstitial lung disease is extremely poor, particularly in those with idiopathic pulmonary fibrosis.

- Selection of patients for invasive ventilation is difficult and should be on a case-by-case basis and in a multidisciplinary setting. Treatment decisions should ideally be made in advance during stable phases of the patient's disease, with consideration of the patients' and/or caregivers' wishes regarding goals of current and future care.

- Invasive ventilation in interstitial lung disease patients may be indicated when potential lung transplantation is a possibility or when there is a clear reversible precipitant such as infection.

- Patients with established fibrotic lung disease have markedly increased elastance but a suggested protective strategy during invasive ventilation includes targeting a low V_T (6–7 mL·kg^{-1} ideal body weight) and a reduced PEEP (<10 cmH$_2$O).

> *Box 1. The "percolation" concept of functional decline*
>
> ILD patients require frequent follow-up, specialist input and prompt initiation of treatment, ideally before any significant decline characterised by either progressive symptoms, decline in lung function or aggravation of radiological features. However, prediction of decline is difficult. An interesting "percolation" concept has been proposed by Bates *et al.* (2007). It refers to a threshold at which lung function deterioration and symptoms become evident. Focal areas of fibrotic lung are subjected to serial stretching and/or repeated insults, leading to a "density threshold" being reached. The net effect is that an uninterrupted path of fibrosis occurs, in which the lung function will remain unchanged. It is only when the so-called "percolation threshold" is passed that the functional change becomes measurable.

discussion of management options should occur. If invasive ventilation is being considered as a therapeutic strategy then the aetiology, recent disease trajectory and potential for treatment and recovery should be carefully considered; the latter most likely holds the greatest importance. Therefore, identifying the correct patients for invasive ventilation is challenging. Fundamental to a management plan is whether intubation and ventilation are appropriate in the first instance or, in fact, may prove traumatic and futile. Due to the poor prognosis of ILD patients receiving invasive ventilation, the decision about whether they should receive this therapy should centre around the common medical ethical principles of beneficence, non-maleficence and justice.

Unfortunately, when invasive ventilation is initiated in patients with ILD, evidence-based ventilatory strategies are lacking. However, the application of lung-protective ventilation (see details later in this chapter) may be assumed to be the best strategy and this is well recognised and associated with better patient outcomes, albeit in an ARDS cohort. Furthermore, optimisation of the patient during invasive ventilation should be according to the usual practice for invasive ventilation patients, *i.e.* with careful monitoring of fluid balance, minimised sedation and prompt recognition and treatment of infection.

In patients with ILD and acute worsening of respiratory symptoms and lung function, three possible scenarios may be distinguished:

1) acute worsening in patients with known chronic ILD,
2) patients with an unknown ILD or suspected ILD but without a formal diagnosis, and
3) ILD developing *de novo* and presenting with acute respiratory symptoms.

With respect to the acute deterioration of a patient with an unknown ILD or without a formal diagnosis and concurrent severe ARF, intubation and invasive ventilation may be needed to allow for appropriate evaluation and to ensure no reversible causes of respiratory failure are present. The ILD diagnosis may then be confirmed during invasive ventilation. The same principle may be assumed for patients with *de novo* acute ILD presenting with acute respiratory symptoms and ARF.

In this chapter, we refer to an acute exacerbation of ILD (AE-ILD) as meaning an acute deterioration of <1 month in the context of a known, diagnosed, ILD. Furthermore, other radiological changes and other diagnoses that would give a similar presentation and radiological appearance should have been excluded (*i.e.* acute congestive heart failure, overt infection, drug-induced change). The discussion of diagnosis and specific treatment options in the individual ILDs is beyond the scope of this chapter.

Idiopathic pulmonary fibrosis *versus* other ILDs

Idiopathic pulmonary fibrosis (IPF) carries a significantly worse prognosis compared to other ILDs. The median survival of IPF patients is 2–3 years following diagnosis. Among ILDs, sarcoidosis is the one with the best prognosis. Similarly, during AE-ILD, there is a higher mortality in IPF patients (AE-IPF) when compared to other ILDs. This extends to patients with IPF and receiving invasive ventilation, where survival decreases to <10% following an acute exacerbation that requires ICU admission. Retrospective studies have shown that prognosis of AE-IPF is extremely poor, with an in-hospital mortality of 50% in less severe patients. Exacerbations typically occur in advanced stages of the disease and often a specific precipitant is not identified. However, infection is commonly assumed and should be empirically treated.

Management strategies before invasive ventilation

Noninvasive ventilation NIV represents a sensible strategy in the acute phase. The reduction in the work of breathing and re-balancing of respiratory muscle load can provide symptomatic relief in the immediate period. However, supportive evidence in a setting outside of COPD is lacking. If NIV is used, alternative strategies should be discussed concurrently. The general findings of studies looking at NIV use in ARF in AE-ILD have shown some evidence to support improved oxygenation, and some studies demonstrate a reduced 30-day mortality if NIV is applied early, an objective response is observed and intubation is avoided. Furthermore, NIV responsiveness is associated with less severe ARF and disease and is favourable in those who tolerate interruptions of NIV. Mortality at 1 year, however, remains high; thus, the application of NIV does not seem to alter the underlying disease or even benefit one particular ILD type.

High-flow nasal oxygen This technique allows delivery of humidified oxygen at flow rates >15 and up to 60 L·min⁻¹. Its exact mechanism of action is unclear, but it is thought to reduce dead space ventilation, improve oxygenation and provide a degree of PEEP (and hence offset auto-PEEP), and thus serves as a useful strategy to relieve the symptoms of dyspnoea. RCTs and meta-analyses comparing high-flow nasal cannula oxygen (HFNC) against other oxygenation techniques in non-ILD pre-intubation and post-extubation scenarios are well described. While the current literature suggests no significant difference in intubation rates when HFNC is used in ARF, there is a paucity of evidence of its use within AE-ILD. However, HFNC can be a particularly useful management strategy for AE-ILD patients with advanced decisions against intubation in the event of significant decline. In 2018, a study in Japan retrospectively analysed the use of HFNC and NIV in patients with AE-ILD and an advanced decision against intubation and invasive ventilation. While they found no difference in 30-day mortality (31% *versus* 30%) or in-hospital mortality (79% *versus* 83%), a particularly interesting finding was that those patients using HFNC had a lower incidence of treatment interruptions at the patient's request, as well as more frequent conversations and ability to have a meal (factors that are imperative in the palliative care of a patient with ILD not appropriate for invasive ventilation). HFNC is generally well tolerated and should be considered early in the management of ARF secondary to ILD, particularly in those who are deemed not suitable for invasive ventilation. Conversely, in those patients where HFNC has been applied but has not been successful, contingency plans should be made when HFNC is first applied. These should include a suitable place of monitoring (likely to be a higher-dependency unit or ICU), target values for $S_{p}O_2$, $P_{a}O_2$ and respiratory rate that would alert the clinician to treatment failure, and whether NIV should be trialled before intubation. Unfortunately, there are very few prospective RCTs investigating HFNC compared to other oxygenation methods (including NIV) in AE-ILD; thus, a pragmatic, patient-focused management plan should be applied.

Using invasive ventilation in ILD patients

Invasive ventilation may have a role in patients with fibrotic ILDs. While the majority of retrospective studies to date have shown a high mortality rate, there may be a role in those that are eligible for potential lung transplantation or it could allow for treatment of reversible causes of ARF (e.g. pneumonia). The high mortality (reported as high as 100% in some studies) seems to be independent of ILD aetiology. Retrospective analysis of ILD patients who died while receiving invasive ventilation showed that a significant proportion of deaths did not have a formal ILD diagnosis; thus, the disease behaviour while on invasive ventilation is poorly understood. A retrospective study in the USA found that in >70% of cases, the cause of respiratory failure was unknown and the in-hospital mortality was 53% with a 1-year survival of 43%. Higher mortality rates have been reported in other studies, which included a significantly higher number of patients with IPF.

The deleterious consequences of invasive ventilation, such as VILI, may be amplified in patients with ILDs. ILD with established fibrotic changes leads to increased elastance (the pressure change that is required to cause a unit change in volume). Fibrotic lung units are not recruitable and applied pressure or volume is merely directed towards normal lung units and increases the risk of VILI. Simply put, the lungs in ILD are stiff and resistant to applied pressures; thus, higher pressures are often required but do not necessarily result in improved ventilatory mechanics. VILI, partially caused by repeated stretching of alveolar units, is often accompanied by accumulation of intra-alveolar pro-inflammatory cytokines. Reactive oxygen species, cellular exudates and endothelial damage can cause subsequent systemic "leak" of these pro-inflammatory mediators, leading to multi-organ failure, which has an associated high mortality.

Unfortunately, the number of robust, prospective clinical trials in ILD patients receiving invasive ventilation is low, most likely due to the acuteness of deterioration among ILD patients. Therefore, no appropriate, evidence-based strategies for invasive ventilation in ILD patients have been established and optimal ventilation approach, mode and weaning are often generalised from other patient cohorts. However, one retrospective study found that high PEEP (>10 cmH$_2$O), APACHE III (Acute Physiology, Age, Chronic Health Evaluation)-associated mortality, age and a low $P_{a}O_2/F_{IO_2}$ ratio were independent determinants of poor patient survival. It therefore seems sensible to employ a ventilation strategy that reduces stretch and atelectotrauma. Lung-protective ventilation, using volume assist-controlled ventilation with low V_T (6–7 mL·kg^{-1} ideal body weight) and reduced PEEP (<10 cmH$_2$O), seems to be the most appropriate strategy. Moreover, due to the poor lung compliance, elevated P_{plat} (>30 cmH$_2$O) is often necessary to adequately ventilate patients with ILD requiring invasive ventilation, and higher respiratory rates can be used in order to achieve adequate minute volume ventilation. In terms of patient monitoring, minimisation of inhaled oxygen content, with goals of haemoglobin saturation >88%, and a restrictive fluid balance are advised in these patients, although this is not evidence based.

Extubation parameters for ILD patients are not defined. However, if the patient is comfortable, not hypercapnic and the appropriate F_{IO_2} can be supplied noninvasively, using HFNC for example, a trial of invasive ventilation liberation may be attempted after a spontaneous breathing trial. The role of tracheostomy in ILD patients has not been documented and no recommendations can be made on its use.

One clinical scenario that may support the need for invasive ventilation is for those patients that are candidates for lung transplantation. Rapid assessment and listing for transplant may occur; however, the principles of protective ventilation should continue. In this situation, ECMO is often considered very early on, in order to provide suitable "lung rest". However, the use of ECMO of course does not guarantee a good prognosis and carries significant risks specific to the support, *e.g.* bleeding risk. Patients who undergo cannulation for ECMO while awake, with a primary intention of avoiding intubation and ventilation, may avoid the deleterious effects of invasive ventilation altogether. However, a study that observed patients who received ECMO as a bridge to transplant found that a significant proportion of the patients died while waiting for a transplant and only 29% went on to transplant. Thus, ECMO alongside conventional measures does not result in an improved survival.

Summary

ILD patients receiving invasive ventilation have an extremely high risk of death (particularly those with established fibrotic disease). It is imperative to optimise conventional factors before and during invasive ventilation to prevent detrimental effects and prolonged invasive ventilation. In the context of AE-ILD, invasive ventilation should be considered if patients are potential candidates for lung transplantation or where a clear reversible cause is identified. The ventilator strategy is poorly defined. However, the use of lung-protective ventilation has shown better disease outcomes and should be applied. Finally, the initiation of invasive ventilation should be explored with experienced teams and involve the patient and their family, well in advance, to ascertain treatment wishes and avoid futile interventions.

Further reading

- Bates JH, *et al.* (2007). Linking parenchymal disease progression to changes in lung mechanical function by percolation. *Am J Respir Crit Care Med*; 176: 617–623.

- Raghu G, *et al.* (2015). An official ATS/ERS/JRS/ALAT clinical practice guideline: treatment of idiopathic pulmonary fibrosis. An update of the 2011 clinical practice guideline. *Am J Respir Crit Care Med*; 192: e3–e19.

- Tobin MJ, ed. (2013). Principles and Practice of Mechanical Ventilation. 3rd Edn. New York, McGraw-Hill Medical.

- Travis WD, *et al.* (2013). An official American Thoracic Society/European Respiratory Society statement: update of the international multidisciplinary classification of the idiopathic interstitial pneumonias. *Am J Respir Crit Care Med*; 188: 733–748.

Monitoring oxygenation

Marco Giani and Giacomo Bellani

Pulse oximetry constitutes one of the fundamental monitoring tools for critically ill patients, together with ECG and noninvasive blood pressure. It allows immediate detection of changes in haemoglobin oxygen saturation, thus leading to timely clinical interventions to avoid severe hypoxaemia. Outside the critical care setting, it improves patient surveillance monitoring, and it can reduce the need for rescues and ICU admission. The clinical benefits of this monitoring tool appear so obvious as to justify widespread use even in the absence of evidence supporting its positive impact on outcomes.

The birth of oximetry dates to the nineteenth century, when spectrometers were invented. In the 1930s, physiologists developed the first two-wavelength ear oxygen saturation meter. The main limitation was the need for calibration, as light absorbance depends on pathlength and tissue optical density. In 1972, Takuo Aoyagi, a Japanese electrical engineer, developed the first pulse oximeter that could be used as a clinical monitor by combining the pulsatile signal with spectroscopy. His intuition was to use the rhythmic arterial pulsatility to isolate the signal arising from arterial blood, excluding other artefacts, such as light absorbance due to venous blood or tissue optical density.

Pulse oximetry relies on the pulsatile variations in tissue absorbance, assessed as permeability to red and infrared light waves. Deoxygenated haemoglobin (DeoxyHb) preferentially absorbs red light (630–660 nm), whereas oxygenated haemoglobin (OxyHb) absorbs more infrared light (900–950 nm). When saturation is 100%,

---

Key points

- Pulse oximetry represents an essential monitoring tool for critically ill patients.

- S_{pO_2} might be used as a surrogate of arterial blood gas measurement to monitor oxygenation in patients with respiratory failure.

- The plethysmographic trace of the pulse oximeter, similar to the arterial pressure trace, may be used to assess respiratory rate, fluid responsiveness and the presence of pulsus paradoxus.

a)

b)

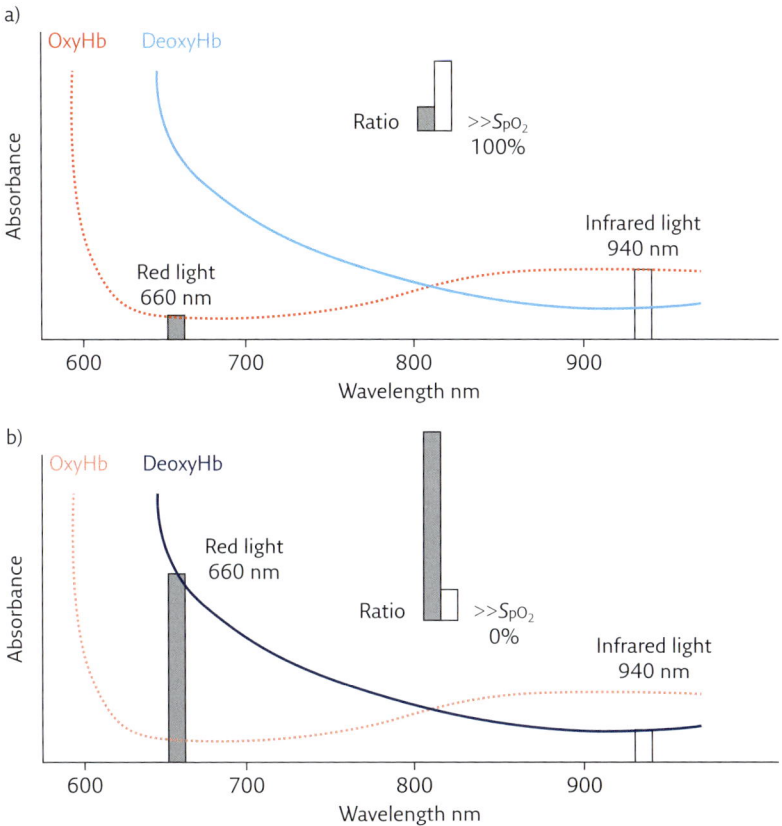

Figure 1. Pattern of light absorbance of a) oxygenated (OxyHb; red dashed line) and b) deoxygenated (DeoxyHb; blue line) haemoglobin.

the absorbance ratio (*i.e.* the ratio of red light to infrared light absorption) will reflect that of the OxyHb absorbance curve (figure 1a). By contrast, when saturation decreases towards 0%, the absorbance ratio will approach the DeoxyHb absorbance curve (figure 1b). Thus, oxygen saturation can be computed *in vivo* by analysing the rate of absorption of these two wavelengths.

Sensors and measurement sites

Pulse oximeters feature transmission or reflection sensors. In the transmission modality, the light goes through the measurement site (*e.g.* a finger) and reaches the photodiode. If peripheral perfusion is maintained, this method provides an accurate and stable measurement. Studies have compared different measurements sites in terms of precision and accuracy. Probes applied on fingers and toes were found to be more precise and accurate compared with the ear lobe, even if the error is usually not clinically significant (1–2%). In reflection-mode oximeters, which have been developed in the past few years, the light sources and the photodiode are on the same side, and the light is reflected by the measurement site. Despite some technical issues, recently overcome by developments in the technology, this modality is promising: sensors can be applied to central sites (*i.e.* the forehead), thus avoiding most of the problems connected with peripheral vasoconstriction. Forehead reflectance sensors proved to be more accurate to assess oxygen saturation in patients taking high dose vasopressors compared with peripheral transmission sensors. Moreover, this technique allowed a quicker detection of desaturation compared with transmission finger sensors.

Pitfalls

Low-quality signal Checking correspondence between the pulse oximeter signal and an invasive blood pressure measurement or ECG tracing is essential. A low-quality plethysmographic signal is often associated with incorrect calculation of arterial saturation.

Motion artefacts, hypothermia and hypoperfusion Under normal conditions, the pulsatile absorbance due to arterial blood only accounts for about 2% of the total absorbance. Therefore, the pulse oximeter is very susceptible to error if the probe is not placed correctly or in the case of motion. This percentage decreases further when peripheral arterial perfusion is reduced, as occurs during hypothermia or hypoperfusion. For this reason, during motion or reduced peripheral perfusion, many oximeters may not separate the arterial pulsation from moving venous blood. New pulse oximeters feature special signal processing algorithms, such as signal extraction technology (SET), that reduce misreading due to movements or other artefacts.

Interferences The following factors interfere with pulse oximetry measurement.

- Oxyhaemoglobin and carboxyhaemoglobin absorb equal amounts of light at 660 nm, thus conventional pulse oximeters cannot distinguish between these two haemoglobin species. Therefore, haemoglobin saturation may be overestimated in patients with carboxyhaemoglobinaemia. Methaemoglobin causes the pulse oximeter readout to trend towards 85%.
- Intravenous dyes (such as methylene blue and indocyanine green) interfere with pulse oximetry readings.
- Nail polish and artificial nails may interfere with pulse oximetry when finger sensors are used. Different colours affect the oxygen saturation reading to different extents. This effect is rarely clinically significant; however, routine removal of nail polish and artificial nails may be considered.
- Skin pigmentation influences the oximetry reading: a study showed that the risk of missing desaturation is increased in people with black skin.
- Fluorescent light may interfere with pulse oximetry. Opaque side shielding around the probe may be recommended to reduce the amount of ambient light reaching the light detector.

The following factors do not interfere with pulse oximetry measurement.

- Anaemia does not significantly affect pulse oximetry, with accurate results obtained even in patients with an extremely low haematocrit.
- Increased concentration of bilirubin does not interfere with measured oxygen saturation.

Multiwavelength pulse oximetry

The use of multiple light wavelengths allows measurement of more than two forms of haemoglobin, including carboxyhaemoglobin and methaemoglobin. Moreover, it may help in solving several problems that commonly affect pulse oximetry, such as accuracy, motion artefacts, low-pulse amplitude, response delay, and improve overall reflection oximetry.

Monitoring oxygenation through pulse oximetry

The relevance of S_pO_2 monitoring comes from the well-known relationship between P_aO_2 and haemoglobin saturation. Due to the nonlinear shape of the relationship; however, S_pO_2 measurement will be sensitive and meaningful only to P_aO_2 values below 70–80 mmHg (9.3–10.6 kPa), since above this value the haemoglobin will be fully saturated. The accuracy of pulse oximetry is known to be low below 80%, although it is difficult (also for ethical reasons) to calibrate pulse oximeters in patients or volunteers with oxygen saturation <80%. However, values of S_pO_2 <80% invariably indicate severe hypoxaemia, prompting immediate action.

Arterial blood gas sampling allows the collection of several pieces of clinical information in addition to the oxygenation status, such as P_aCO_2, acid–base status and electrolytes.

With regards to oxygenation alone, S_pO_2 might be used instead of arterial blood gas sampling to monitor oxygenation in ventilated patients. Maintaining a S_pO_2 between 92 and 95% was proposed as a target to provide a safe oxygenation (P_aO_2 >60 mmHg (8.0 kPa)) while minimising the risk of oxygen toxicity. Despite the well-known risks of hyperoxia, far greater attention is usually payed to low S_pO_2 compared with high S_pO_2. To minimise the exposure to hypoxia or hyperoxia automated closed-loop control systems have been developed: ventilators which feature these systems continuously adjust the F_IO_2 to maintain oxygen saturation within the "safe" range. The use of automated systems results in better control of a predefined oxygen target.

Pulse oximetry may prove helpful in clinical situations where continuous monitoring of oxygenation might be used as a proxy for lung recruitment.

S_pO_2/F_IO_2 ratio Several studies have shown that the S_pO_2/F_IO_2 ratio can be a valuable surrogate for the P_aO_2/F_IO_2 ratio in hypoxaemic patients, reducing or avoiding the need for an arterial blood gas sample. S_pO_2/F_IO_2 ratios of 235 and 315 correspond to P_aO_2/F_IO_2 ratios of 200 and 300 mmHg (26.6 and 39.9 kPa), respectively. To overcome the flattening of the oxygen saturation curve described above, low F_IO_2 should be used and values obtained at S_pO_2 >97% should be discarded. A modified definition of ARDS, specifically devised for low-resource settings, based on lung ultrasound and S_pO_2/F_IO_2 ratio has been developed and validated.

Beyond oxygen saturation

- The plethysmographic trace of the pulse oximeter, similar to the invasive arterial pressure trace, can be used to assess the haemodynamic response to intrathoracic pressure variations during breathing. Therefore, respiratory rate, pulse pressure variation and the presence of pulsus paradoxus may be assessed by analysing this trace. A good agreement between respiratory rate determined by this algorithm and capnography has been recorded. Respiratory variations in pulse oximetry plethysmographic waveforms allow prediction of fluid responsiveness, with similar cut-offs to invasive blood pressure tracing (13–15% of pulse amplitude variation).

- Newer pulse oximeters with multiple light wavelengths can measure haemoglobin levels. Despite good accuracy, these devices still lack precision: the wide limits of agreement might not allow definitive decisions on transfusions.

Further reading

- Bilan N, *et al.* (2015). Comparison of the S_pO_2/F_IO_2 ratio and the P_aO_2/F_IO_2 ratio in patients with acute lung injury or acute respiratory distress syndrome. *J Cardiovasc Thorac Res*; 7: 28–31.

- Ebmeier SJ, *et al.* (2018). A two centre observational study of simultaneous pulse oximetry and arterial oxygen saturation recordings in intensive care unit patients. *Anaesth Intensive Care*; 46: 297–303.

- Funcke S, *et al.* (2016). Practice of hemodynamic monitoring and management in German, Austrian, and Swiss intensive care units: the multicenter cross-sectional ICU-CardioMan Study. *Ann Intensive Care*; 6: 49.

- Hess DR (2016). Pulse oximetry: beyond S_pO_2. *Respir Care*; 61: 1671–1680.

- Jubran A, *et al.* (1990). Reliability of pulse oximetry in titrating supplemental oxygen therapy in ventilator-dependent patients. *Chest*; 97: 1420–1425.

- Lee H, *et al.* (2016). Reflectance pulse oximetry: Practical issues and limitations. *ICT Express*; 2: 195–198.

- Pedersen T, *et al.* (2014). Pulse oximetry for perioperative monitoring. *Cochrane Database Syst Rev*; 3: CD002013.

- Pretto JJ, *et al.* (2014). Clinical use of pulse oximetry: official guidelines from the Thoracic Society of Australia and New Zealand. *Respirology*; 19: 38–46.

- Rice TW, *et al.* (2007). Comparison of the S_pO_2/F_IO_2 ratio and the P_aO_2/F_IO_2 ratio in patients with acute lung injury or ARDS. *Chest*; 132: 410–417.

- Taenzer AH, *et al.* (2010). Impact of pulse oximetry surveillance on rescue events and intensive care unit transfers: a before-and-after concurrence study. *Anesthesiology*; 112: 282–287.

Monitoring ventilation

Luis Morales-Quinteros, Lluís Blanch and Antonio Artigas

Noninvasive monitoring of respiratory function is common for mechanically ventilated patients. Monitoring expired carbon dioxide can easily be performed in this population by capnography. Nowadays, new devices can measure carbon dioxide kinetics in real time. These are useful tools to assess how carbon dioxide behaves on its passage from the bloodstream through the alveoli to the ambient air. By knowing how this works, physicians can obtain meaningful information about ventilation and perfusion. Transcutaneous carbon dioxide monitoring provides an alternative to capnographic carbon dioxide monitoring.

This chapter will describe the basics of capnography and transcutaneous carbon dioxide monitoring, and their potential clinical applications in the critically ill. We will not discuss the physiology of hypercarbia, as this will be discussed elsewhere in this book.

Capnography

Capnography is the measurement and graphical display of fractional carbon dioxide concentration in the respired gases. There are two types of capnography:

- Conventional capnography, which focuses on exhaled carbon dioxide plotted over time (TCap) and is the most frequently used modality
- Volumetric capnography (VCap), where exhaled carbon dioxide is plotted against exhaled volume

Key points

- Capnography provides substantial information about respiratory and cardiovascular function, and has many potential applications in the critically ill.

- Its applications include assessment of the effectiveness of ventilation, exclusion of pulmonary embolism, prognostication of ARDS, optimisation of alveolar recruitment and noninvasive measurement of cardiac output.

- Transcutaneous monitoring of carbon dioxide may offer an alternative method for assessing tissue perfusion. However, more studies in critical adult patients need to be performed to make more robust recommendations for its use.

Although both techniques can be used to measure end-tidal carbon dioxide, there are significant differences. During TCap, dead space and carbon dioxide output cannot be calculated. TCap cannot differentiate between the end of inspiration and the beginning of expiration, making the analysis of time capnograms during inspiration difficult and resulting in an inaccurate assessment of rebreathing, which is grossly underestimated.

VCap focuses on exhaled carbon dioxide plotted relative to exhaled volume. VCap provides more precise carbon dioxide elimination kinetics allowing volume-based variables, such as the volumes of the physiological, airway and alveolar dead space, and several dead space-to-volume ratios.

Single-breath carbon dioxide curve The volumetric capnogram, also called the single-breath test of carbon dioxide, is the dynamic representation of the kinetics of carbon dioxide elimination measured by VCap. The single-breath carbon dioxide ($SBCO_2$) curve is produced by the integration of airway flow and carbon dioxide concentration, and is presented as a breath-to-breath analysis. The graph provides information on anatomical dead space ($V_{D_{aw}}$), alveolar dead space (V_{D_A}) and carbon dioxide elimination ($V'CO_2$) for each breath. With invasive ventilation, the added volume between the Y-piece and the patient airway is considered the instrumental dead space (*e.g.* that of the endotracheal tube, filters, capnograph and nebuliser). VCap provides continuous monitoring of $V'CO_2$, ventilation (V')/perfusion (Q') status, and airway patency.

The volumetric capnogram is divided into three phases (figure 1).

- Phase I: anatomical dead space. $V_{D_{aw}}$ results from the exhaled V_T and the conducting airways emptying. Since this gas did not reach the alveoli during inspiration and did not participate in gas exchange, exhaled carbon dioxide amounts are near to zero. A prolonged phase I indicates an increase in $V_{D_{aw}}$. The presence of carbon dioxide during this phase indicates rebreathing or that the sensor needs to be recalibrated (table 1).
- Phase II: transition phase. Carbon dioxide increases almost linearly, reflecting the mixing of the remaining gas content between the anatomic and the alveolar gas from fast-emptying alveoli. It provides information about Q' changes and airway resistance.
- Phase III: plateau phase. The carbon dioxide curve has a positive rising slope. It reflects the carbon dioxide tension (PCO_2) of pure alveolar gas during expiration. The final carbon dioxide value of this phase is called the end-tidal carbon dioxide tension ($PETCO_2$). This slope reflects V'/Q' mismatch.

The volumetric capnogram is also divided into three areas.

- Area X: carbon dioxide elimination. This represents the amount of carbon dioxide exhaled in the breath, assuming that no exhaled air is rebreathed. The area under the $SBCO_2$ curve is the volume of carbon dioxide in a single breath, namely the alveolar gas volume, and this area represents the volume that participates in gas exchange. Adding all the single breaths in a minute gives $V'CO_2$. Thus, VCap can describe not only the volume of carbon dioxide in one breath (VCO_2) but also the $V'CO_2$ in one minute. Area q area would be included in area X if area p is excluded.
- Area Y: V_{D_A}.
- Area Z: $V_{D_{aw}}$.

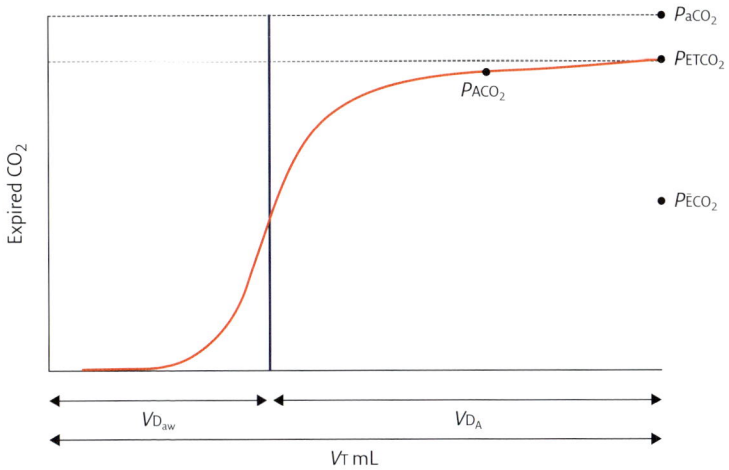

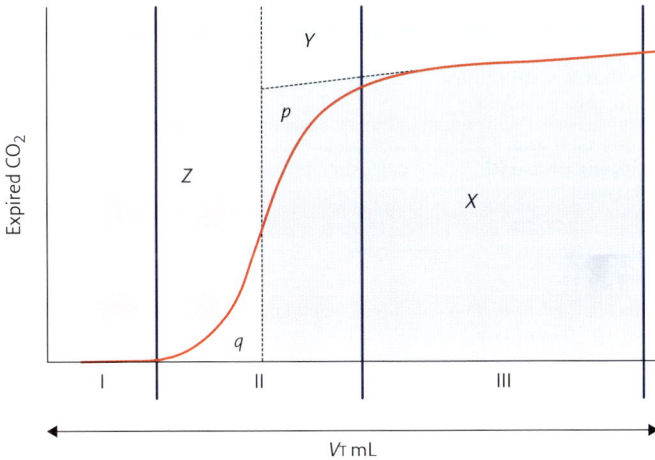

Figure 1. *Typical capnography curve. Phase I: emptying of the conducting airways. Phase II: emptying of distal airways and alveoli close to the airways. Phase III: emptying of the alveolar gas compartment. Phase II is bisected by a dotted line where area q is equal to area p. Area X (blue) is the alveolar gas volume. Area Z is $V_{D_{aw}}$ (purple). Area Y is the V_{D_A} (green). P_{ACO_2}: alveolar carbon dioxide tension.*

Table 1. Capnography trace characteristics

Waveform characteristic	Interpretation
Sudden drop in P_{ETCO_2} to near zero or zero	Circuit disconnection Dislodged, occluded or kinked endotracheal tube Oesophageal intubation Massive CO_2 embolism during laparoscopy Cardiac arrest
Sudden decrease in P_{ETCO_2}	Reduced pulmonary blood flow: pulmonary embolism, hypotension, sudden cardiac arrest with active CPR
Persistently low P_{ETCO_2} with normal plateaus	Hypothermia Hyperventilation Deep anaesthesia/sedation Increased dead-space ventilation
Increase in P_{ETCO_2} with normal plateaus	Hypoventilation Increased CO_2 production (hyperthermia, malignant hyperpyrexia) Absorption of CO_2 from peritoneal insufflation
Increase in P_{ETCO_2} with failure to return to zero baseline	CO_2 rebreathing
Prolonged phase II and upward sloping phase III (loss of plateau)	Incomplete expiration related to partial airway occlusion, bronchospasm or mucus plugging

CPR: cardiopulmonary resuscitation. Modified from Foot *et al.* (2012), Examination Intensive Care Medicine, 2nd Edn, Elsevier, with permission.

Measurements derived from the volumetric capnogram Mean alveolar P_{CO_2} is the averaged P_{CO_2} of all ventilated alveoli. Graphically, it is the mid-point of phase III of the capnogram.

P_{ETCO_2} is the highest final value at the end of phase III. It represents the emptying of alveoli with the longest expiratory time. It can be obtained from both time- and volume-based capnograms. In healthy subjects or in patients with mild lung disease, P_{ETCO_2} is, on average, 2–5 mmHg (0.3–0.7 kPa) less than P_{aCO_2}, making TCap a useful tool in this population. However, the difference between P_{aCO_2} and P_{ETCO_2} in the mechanically ill-ventilated patient is often large and has poor correlation, moving in the opposite direction; therefore, P_{ETCO_2} should be used with caution to assess ventilation.

Mixed-expired carbon dioxide tension ($P_{\bar{E}CO_2}$) is the P_{CO_2} in the expired gas during a tidal breath. This value is essential for calculating physiological dead space after having introduced all the parameters for its computation.

Clinical applications of capnography in intensive care Capnography is a reliable tool to confirm correct placement of endotracheal tubes or supraglottic devices and to allow immediate recognition of inadvertent extubation during transport. False negatives are found, such as in a cardiac arrest or due to technical issues (leaks, kinking or ventilator failure). False positives are encountered if the stomach contains carbon dioxide (*e.g.* in NIV). Despite recommendations for its systematic use, it is still underused in the ICU.

Physiological dead-space volume ($V_{D_{phys}}$) can be calculated using the Bohr–Enghoff equation:

$$\frac{V_{D_{phys}}}{V_T} = \frac{P_{a}CO_2 - P_{\bar{E}}CO_2}{P_{a}CO_2}$$

However, $V_{D_{phys}}$ assessed by this approach overestimates the true $V_{D_{phys}}$, since venous admixture and low V'/Q' areas increase the difference between $P_{a}CO_2$ and $P_{A}CO_2$.

Measurements of dead space have been studied in the following clinical settings in ICU patients.

- To assess prognosis in ARDS patients: an elevated $V_{D_{phys}}$ computed by the Bohr–Enghoff equation is a strong independent predictor of mortality in the early and intermediate phases of ARDS.
- Alveolar recruitment optimisation in ARDS: it has been shown that the best PEEP (*i.e.* that associated with the highest oxygen delivery and respiratory system compliance) is associated with the lowest $V_{D_{phys}}/V_T$; however, there are limited data in humans to suggest that the lowest levels of $V_{D_{phys}}/V_T$ during PEEP titration correspond with peak compliance of the respiratory system.
- Pulmonary embolism (PE) exclusion: PE interrupts blood flow to ventilated alveoli, increasing $V_{D_{phys}}$ and V_{D_A}; however, no studies have evaluated the use of VCap to exclude PE in mechanically ventilated patients.

Recently, methods for estimating $V_{D_{phys}}$ not requiring VCap have been evaluated. The ventilatory ratio is a bedside index of ventilatory efficiency computed by using routinely measured respiratory variables that correlates well with $V_{D_{phys}}$ in ARDS and could function as a surrogate for it.

VCap can provide quantitative measurements of cardiac output using a technique called partial carbon dioxide rebreathing based on a Fick principle modification using measurements of V_{CO_2} and $P_{ET}CO_2$ on a breath-by-breath basis before and during a carbon dioxide rebreathing manoeuvre. This technique has been tested with good reliability in cardiac surgery patients. However, it has several limitations:

- Lack of reliability in conditions of high intrapulmonary shunt
- Carbon dioxide is not continuous (one measurement every 3 min)
- Contraindicated in patients requiring strict $P_{a}CO_2$ control (brain-injured patients)
- Haemodynamic and respiratory instability may decrease its reliability

Transcutaneous carbon dioxide monitoring

$P_{tc}CO_2$ measurement is another noninvasive method for carbon dioxide monitoring. It uses a calibrated probe placed on the trunk, thigh, abdomen or earlobe (figure 2). Calibration is performed by exposing the probe to a known concentration of carbon dioxide (5%, 10% or room air). The probe is continuously heated to a temperature between 42ºC and 44ºC, allowing the skin's blood vessels to dilate and serve as passive conduits for blood flow.

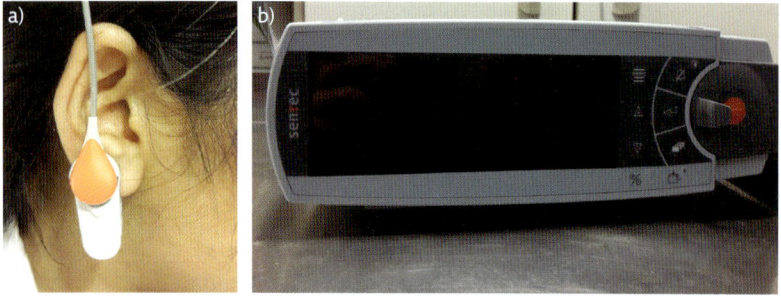

Figure 2. a) Earlobe sensor for P_{tcCO_2} and b) noninvasive device for monitoring through a single sensor. Images courtesy of M. Galdeano (Sagrat Cor University Hospital, Dept of Respirology, Barcelona, Spain).

Box 1. Limitations of P_{tcCO_2} monitoring

- Frequent calibration required every 4–6 h; accuracy directly linked to skin perfusion
- Skin site change every 4 h to avoid burning at the sensor site
- P_{tcCO_2} at one skin segment may not be reflective of all tissues
- Relatively long equilibration time following electrode placement
- Performance may be suboptimal over poorly perfused areas
- P_{tcCO_2} tends to overestimate P_{aCO_2}
- Haemodynamic instability overestimates P_{aCO_2}
- Frequent membrane/electrolyte changes and electrode maintenance required
- Performance more reliable in neonates than adults

P_{tcCO_2} measurement detects the carbon dioxide that escapes through the skin surface coming from capillary blood in the dermis and epidermis. P_{tcCO_2} has good correlation with P_{aCO_2} in healthy subjects and in patients with stable haemodynamics; however, P_{tcCO_2} may not be a good reflection of P_{aCO_2} in the critically ill. P_{tcCO_2} has also been tested in the assessment of tissue perfusion in ICU. It is seldom used in adult ICU patients (box 1).

Further reading

- Ferluga M, *et al*. (2018). Dead space in acute respiratory distress syndrome. *Ann Transl Med*; 6: 388.

- Kreit JW (2019). Volume capnography in the intensive care unit: physiological principles, measurements, and calculations. *Ann Am Thorac Soc*; 16: 291–300.

- Kreit JW (2019). Volume capnography in the intensive care unit: potential clinical applications. *Ann Am Thorac Soc*; 16: 409–420.

- Restrepo RD, *et al*. (2012). AARC clinical practice guideline: transcutaneous monitoring of carbon dioxide and oxygen: 2012. *Respir Care*; 57: 195–62.

- Sinha P, *et al*. (2019). Physiologic analysis and clinical performance of the ventilatory ratio in acute respiratory distress syndrome. *Am J Respir Crit Care Med*; 199: 333–341.

Monitoring respiratory mechanics

Cong Lu, Nicole Philips and Lu Chen

Invasive ventilation is an essential, life-saving treatment for patients with respiratory failure. However, inappropriate management with invasive ventilation can result in secondary lung injury and inflammation (VILI). The principle behind invasive ventilation is the application of external forces on the respiratory system while achieving optimal safety and efficiency. However, it appears that there is no single solution that works for all patients since the mechanical properties of an individuals' respiratory system may differ substantially. These differences can be significant even among patients with a similar respiratory pathology, such as ARDS. Therefore, monitoring individual respiratory mechanics can aid in the identification of a patients' pathophysiological changes and allows the application of personalised ventilator settings. In this chapter we will discuss how to assess the fundamental parameters of respiratory mechanics at the bedside, with or without spontaneous breathing effort. We also give some empirical suggestions for interpreting those parameters. Of note, the assessment of respiratory effort will be covered elsewhere in this book (see the chapter entitled "Monitoring breathing effort").

Monitoring mechanics during passive ventilation

Classical mechanics studies the motion of macroscopic objects, characterised by force, displacement and its derivatives. In respiratory mechanics, this translates to the study of motion of the respiratory system, characterised by pressure, volume and flow. During invasive ventilation, breath can be driven by two pressures applied on the respiratory system:

1) pressure applied by the ventilator, known as airway pressure (P_{aw}); and
2) pressure generated by the respiratory muscles (P_{mus}).

Key points

- Intrinsic PEEP and P_{plat} should be routinely monitored, allowing simple calculation of compliance and resistance of the total respiratory system.

- Monitoring oesophageal pressure can differentiate lung from chest wall mechanics.

- It is difficult, but not impossible, to monitor mechanics in patients with spontaneous breathing.

Pmus can be challenging to measure, particularly if the patient is actively expiring. It is therefore much easier to monitor respiratory mechanics when the respiratory muscles are inactive (during deep sedation or paralysis), this is called passive ventilation. In this case, the only external force is provided by the ventilator (Paw); allowing us to investigate the relationship between force, volume and flow. To better understand this relationship, imagine an object lying on the floor, attached to the wall by a spring. The force we need to push the object is equal to the sum of the recoil force of the spring and the friction force between the object and the floor. The magnitude of this pushing force depends on the displacement of the spring and the speed of the object. Similarly, Paw is the sum of the elastic recoil pressure of the respiratory system (spring) and the resistive pressure of gas flow (friction). The elastic recoil pressure (Pel) depends on the change in volume (ΔV); therefore, this relationship can be quantified as elastance (Pel$/\Delta V$) or compliance ($\Delta V/\Delta P$el). By contrast, the resistive pressure depends on flow. This relationship is quantified as resistance (resistive pressure/flow). We can then use the elimination method described below, and illustrated in figure 1, to measure the magnitude of elastic and resistive pressures using their sum, Paw. For quick reference, the common calculations during passive ventilation are summarised in table 1.

Total PEEP When performing an end-expiratory hold on the ventilator, flow is zero and the resistive pressure is eliminated. Assuming the airways remain open, Paw measured in the absence of flow is equivalent to Pel at end-expiration (*i.e.* alveolar pressure). This elastic pressure is also known as PEEPtot, which is the sum of the external PEEP (applied by the ventilator) and PEEPi. During resting breathing in healthy subjects, end-expiratory lung volume (EELV) reaches functional residual capacity (FRC), where the inward recoil pressure of the lung is counterbalanced with the outward recoil pressure of the chest wall. In ventilated patients, EELV can be greater than FRC, where the inward recoil pressure of the lung is greater than the outward recoil pressure of the chest wall. This increase in lung volume can result from the application of external PEEP or from the interaction between ventilator settings and intrinsic properties of the patient. For example, insufficient

Table 1. Common calculations in respiratory mechanics

Parameters	Calculations	Unit
PEEPi	PEEPtot−PEEP	cmH_2O
Ers[#]	(Pplat−PEEPtot)/VT	$cmH_2O·L^{-1}$
Crs	VT/(Pplat−PEEP$_{tot}$)	$mL·cmH_2O^{-1}$
Rrs	(Ppeak−Pplat)/flow	$cmH_2O·s·L^{-1}$
Ecw[#]	(Poes,end-insp−Poes,end-exp)/VT	$cmH_2O·L^{-1}$
EL[#]	(PL,end-insp−PL,end-exp)/VT	$cmH_2O·L^{-1}$
Ccw	VT/(Poes,end-insp−Poes,end-exp)	$mL·cmH_2O^{-1}$
CL	VT/(PL,end-insp−PL,end-exp)	$mL·cmH_2O^{-1}$

PEEPi: intrinsic PEEP; Ers: elastance of the respiratory system; Crs: compliance of the respiratory system; Rrs: resistance of the respiratory system; Ecw: elastance of the chest wall; EL: lung elastance; Ccw: chest wall compliance; CL: lung compliance. [#]: note that elastances are merely the reciprocal of compliances, we often scale the units of volume during calculations to avoid too many decimals.

expiratory time and expiratory flow limitation are common reasons that a patient generates PEEPi. Insufficient expiratory time is relative, as any patient can generate PEEPi if the respiratory rate is set too high. A patient with COPD may require more time for expiration compared with a patient with ARDS, due to differences in compliance and resistance. By assessing PEEPtot, we now have an estimate of elastic or alveolar pressure at end-expiration. This estimate may be biased, however, since we assume open airways, which may not always be the case (see the paragraph on "Airway closure").

Plateau pressure The elastic pressure at end-inspiration can be measured by performing an end-inspiratory hold. This is known as P_{plat} and represents the alveolar pressure at end-inspiration. We can measure P_{plat} by performing a manual hold of 1–2 s or set an inspiratory pause of 0.3 s. A set, short inspiratory pause can provide continuous monitoring of P_{plat} and may facilitate carbon dioxide elimination. We do not recommend performing a long hold (>2 s) since the measured pressure can be confounded by potential microleakage (*i.e.* through the cuff of the endotracheal tube). Furthermore, we often limit P_{plat} to <28–30 cmH_2O to avoid overdistension, unless we measure P_L (see the paragraph on "Transpulmonary pressure").

Respiratory system compliance We can use the two simple manoeuvres described above to derive the change in elastic pressure:

$$\Delta P_{el}=P_{plat}-PEEP_{tot}$$

This can then be used to calculate C_{rs}, provided V_T is known:

$$C_{rs}=V_T/\Delta P_{el}$$

C_{rs} is not always linear, although it can provide an estimate of the relationship between change in volume and the change in elastic pressure in clinical practice. A reference range of C_{rs} for ventilated patients is provided in table 2, derived from a small sample-size of anaesthetised, paralysed patients for minor surgery in the supine position (not healthy awake subjects). In addition, C_{rs} measures total respiratory system compliance and can be modified by both lung and chest wall. The chest wall represents all of the parts in the wall surrounding the lungs, including the intrathoracic extrapulmonary structures such as the heart and mediastinum, as well as the rib cage, diaphragm, abdominal contents and abdominal wall. To assess lung and chest wall compliance, respectively, we need to measure P_{oes}, a surrogate of local pleural pressure (discussed later in this chapter). Furthermore, it is important to note that we commonly assess C_{rs} during tidal breathing. Other methods exist for calculating C_{rs} (ΔEELV/ΔPEEP) and may have a different physiological meaning, providing more insight into respiratory mechanics of the individual.

Respiratory system resistance R_{rs} is the ratio of resistive pressure to flow. Resistive pressure during inspiration can be calculated by subtracting P_{el} from P_{aw}, and inspiratory flow can be fixed using volume-controlled ventilation (figure 1). For example, peak airway pressure (P_{peak}) is the sum of P_{el} and resistive pressure when V_T is reached, whereas P_{plat} is equal to P_{el} at V_T. Therefore, the difference between P_{peak} and P_{plat} is the resistive pressure. Because the resistive pressure is flow-dependent, resistance can then be obtained by dividing resistive pressure

Table 2. Clinical reference ranges for the fundamental parameters of respiratory mechanics

	Reference range[#]	Frequent causes for reduction	Frequent causes for elevation
Crs	60–80 mL·cmH$_2$O^{-1}	Lung volume loss such as ARDS High intra-abdominal pressure Pneumothorax Massive pleural infusion Pulmonary fibrosis	Pulmonary emphysema Post open-thorax surgery
CL	90–120 mL·cmH$_2$O^{-1}	Lung volume loss such as ARDS Pulmonary fibrosis	Pulmonary emphysema
Ccw	100–200 mL·cmH$_2$O^{-1}	High intra-abdominal pressure Pneumothorax Massive pleural infusion	Post open-thorax surgery
Rrs	<10 cmH$_2$O·s·L^{-1} at 60 L·min^{-1} of flow[¶]		Small endotracheal tube size Airway obstruction (at endotracheal tube, primary or distal airways) Bronchospasm

[#]: reference range represents mechanically ventilated patients. Data were derived from anaesthetised patients undergoing minor surgery in the supine position. All compliance reference values may depend on height. [¶]: Rrs is flow-dependent. Higher flow can generate greater resistive pressure, which is not linear.

by the preset flow. The unit of flow on the ventilator is "L·min^{-1}" and should be converted into "L·s^{-1}" for calculations. For example, we can set 60 L·min^{-1} of constant flow, which is exactly 1 L·s^{-1} of flow. By monitoring P_{peak} and P_{plat} we immediately know the magnitude of R_{rs}. A lower flow, such as 30 L·min^{-1}, can easily lead to an inversed inspiratory–expiratory ratio and can increase the risk of flow starvation and pendelluft once the patient resumes their spontaneous effort. However, we do not recommend setting a flow >60 L·min^{-1}, as this may lead to insufficient humidification. Moreover, we simplified the relationship between flow and resistive pressure by a linear coefficient, R_{rs}; however under turbulent conditions this is no longer linear. In other words, R_{rs} varies depending on the preset flow.

Airway closure We often assume the airways remain open when we eliminate flow with an end-expiratory or end-inspiratory hold. Under this assumption, P_{aw} is equivalent to alveolar pressure, because there is no pressure difference at zero flow. This assumption may be true at end-inspiration but should be verified at end-expiration. In the presence of airway closure, communication between the proximal airways and alveoli are interrupted. Airway closure has been previously reported in asthma or COPD, or restrictive disease, such as ARDS, where lung

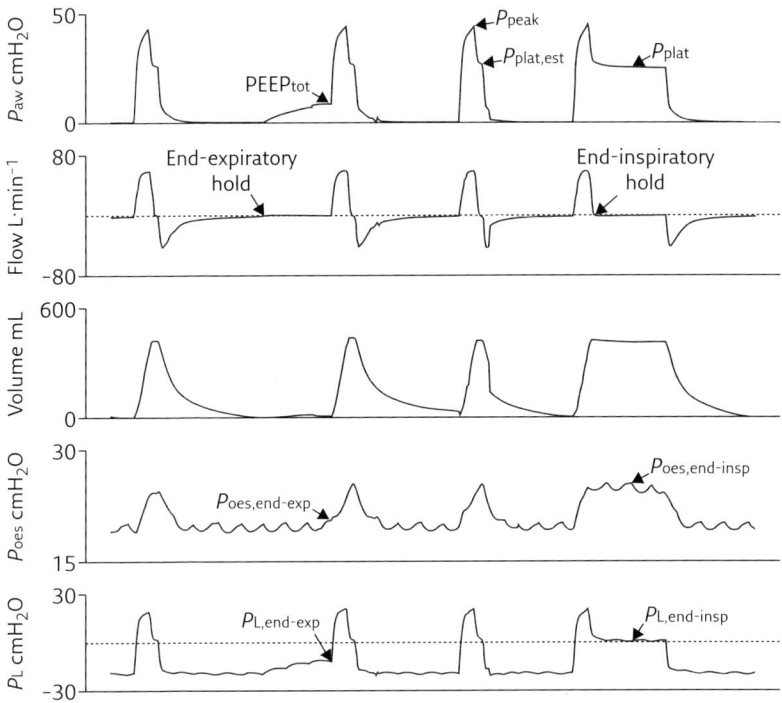

Figure 1. Measurement of respiratory mechanics during passive ventilation using volume-controlled mode with constant flow. Measurements can also be made in pressure-targeted mode, but may be less feasible. PEEPtot: total PEEP; Pplat,est: estimated Pplat; Poes: oesophageal pressure; Poes,end-exp: oesophageal pressure measured at end-expiration; Poes,end-insp: oesophageal pressure measured at end-inspiration; PL: transpulmonary pressure; PL,end-exp: transpulmonary pressure at end-expiration; PL,end-insp: transpulmonary pressure at end-expiration.

volume is significantly reduced. We recently showed that about one-third of patients with ARDS have complete occlusion of the airways with an airway opening pressure (P_{AO}) >5 cmH$_2$O. This means that any pressure delivered below P_{AO} is insufficient to open the closed airways. We demonstrated this phenomenon by comparing the pressure–volume curve of a patients' respiratory system with a blocked ventilator circuit. Airway closure can also be detected at the bedside using pressure–time curves (figure 2). Ignoring the phenomenon of airway closure can lead to misinterpretation of a patients' respiratory mechanics. Detecting airway closure is also potentially important for minimising the risk of cyclic airway closure and reopening, which may cause bronchial trauma.

Oesophageal pressure and transpulmonary pressure The measurements described above require only P_{aw} and flow to calculate, and provide information on global respiratory mechanics. Separating mechanics of the chest wall from the lung

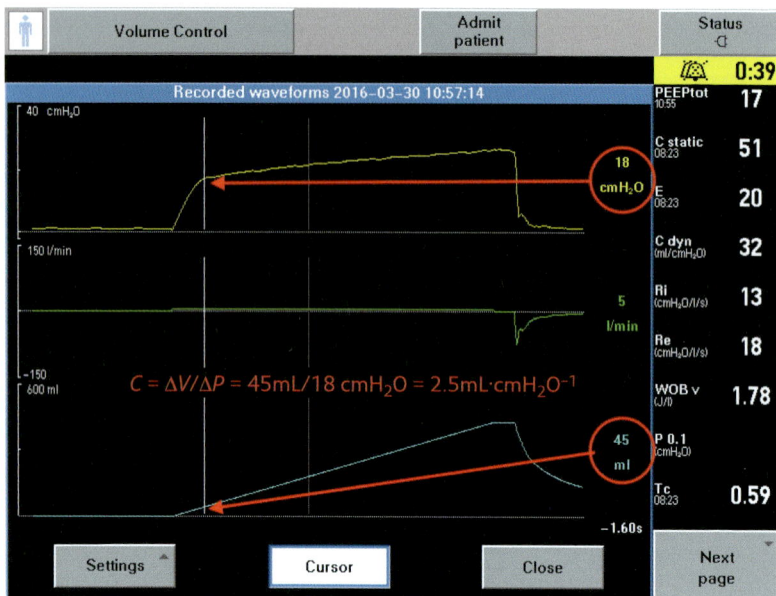

Figure 2. Detection of complete airway closure using the pressure–time curve during low-flow (5 L·min⁻¹) inflation. A low-flow (green line) inflation was conducted using volume-controlled mode. Airway pressure (yellow line) increased rapidly from 0 to 18 cmH₂O at the beginning of inflation when only 45 mL of volume (blue line) was delivered. The compliance of this initial period of inflation was only 45 mL/18 cmH₂O=2.5 mL·cmH₂O⁻¹. This extremely low compliance denotes the exact circuit compliance (which can be measured during pre-test of the ventilator). In other words, there is no actual lung inflation until the airway pressure exceeded 18 cmH₂O (PAO). Note that there is no fluctuation of Paw during this initial period.

requires monitoring pleural pressure, which can be estimated by monitoring P_{oes}. Generally speaking, P_{oes} during passive ventilation reflects chest wall mechanics, whereas P_L (the difference between P_{aw} and P_{oes}) reflects lung mechanics (figure 1). For example, the change in P_{oes} during tidal breathing ($\Delta P_{oes} = P_{oes,end-insp} - P_{oes,end-exp}$) represents the pressure of the chest wall, whereas the change in P_L ($\Delta P_L = P_{L,end-insp} - P_{L,end-exp}$) represents the pressure of the lungs. This general concept is helpful for understanding the physiology of P_{oes} and P_L. However, we should keep in mind that P_{oes} only reflects local pleural pressure close to the oesophagus (mid-lung or dorsal-lung level) as there is no global pleural pressure due to the pleural pressure gradient. The directly measured P_L ($P_L = P_{aw} - P_{oes}$), therefore, represents local transpulmonary pressure of the lung. A negative directly measured P_L is usually considered an indicator of lung collapse, although not all lung regions may be collapsed. What we might conclude is that the dorsal lung (close to the oesophagus) is probably collapsed. In this case, the P_L of the non-dependent lung (or the portion of aerated lung, termed "baby lung") remains unknown. Fortunately, we can use the ratio of

Table 3. Directly measured and elastance-derived PL

	Directly measured P_L at end-expiration	Elastance-derived plateau P_L
Definition	$P_{L,end-exp}=PEEP_{tot}-P_{oes,end-exp}$	$P_{L,plat}=P_{plat}\times$ $(E_L/E_{RS})=P_{plat}\times(\Delta P_L/\Delta P_{aw})$
Assumption	At the end of expiration, local pleural pressure is equivalent to intra-oesophageal pressure	At the end of expiration, local P_L in the absence of PEEP is zero
Physiological meaning	Reflects P_L at the dorsal lung (close to the oesophagus)	Reflects P_L at the ventilated lung (or "baby lung")
Application	Set PEEP to recruit dorsal lung	Prevent overdistension of the "baby lung"
Intervention target	>0 cmH$_2$O	<22–25 cmH$_2$O

$P_{L,plat}$: elastance-derived transpulmonary plateau pressure; ΔP_L: directly measured transpulmonary pressure at end-inspiration minus pressure at end-expiration; ΔP_{aw}: airway P_{plat} minus total PEEP.

ΔP_L to ΔP_{aw} (the same as $\Delta E_L/\Delta E_{rs}$) to estimate the P_L of the ventilated "baby lung", also known as elastance-derived P_L. Table 3 summarises the definitions, physiological meanings, and potential clinical applications of the directly measured P_L and elastance-derived P_L.

Chest wall compliance and lung compliance Once ΔP_{oes} and ΔP_L have been measured by end-expiratory and end-inspiratory holds (figure 1), we can calculate the C_{CW} and C_L by dividing each by V_T. C_{CW} can be treated as the elastic characteristics of a single compartment system; the C_L, however, is more complex. C_L is predominately determined by the amount of functional lung units rather than the intrinsic elastic characteristic of the lung. If we block ventilation to one lung, we halve lung compliance. Therefore, C_L is often proportional to FRC. This phenomenon can be seen in ARDS patients who have a remarkable reduction in C_L due to lung volume loss (alveolar collapse, flooding and consolidation). Frequent causes of alteration in C_{CW} and C_L are summarised in table 2.

Monitoring mechanics during spontaneous breathing

Monitoring respiratory mechanics during spontaneous breathing is more challenging due to the generation of pressure from respiratory muscles (P_{mus}). However, the approach to the measurements is similar to those used in passive breathing. For example, we can measure P_{plat} by doing an end-inspiratory hold (this manoeuvre is allowed in pressure support ventilation in some brands of ventilators). When P_{aw} or P_{oes} is stabilised, as demonstrated in figure 3, the P_{plat} as well as P_{oes} at end-inspiration and P_L at end-expiration can be measured. Notice that we visually inspect if P_{aw} and P_{oes} have reached a plateau stage. A dramatic drop in P_{aw} during the end-inspiratory hold suggests inspiratory effort. A significant elevation in P_{aw} is also possible, and suggests active expiratory effort. Although it remains unclear which parameter can better indicate the risk of VILI during spontaneous

117

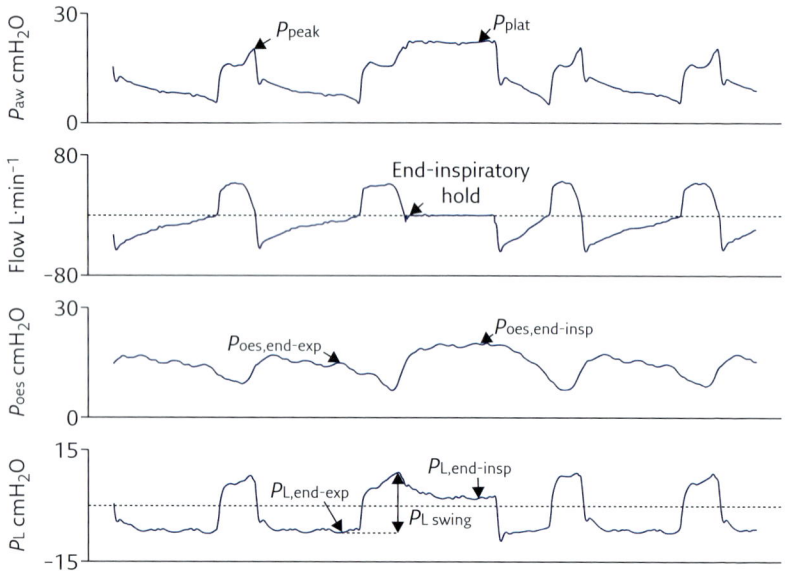

Figure 3. Measurement of respiratory mechanics during spontaneous breathing. Airway Pplat is obtained by performing an end-inspiratory hold.

breathing, data from physiological studies suggest that airway driving pressure (P_{plat}–PEEP) or P_L swing (maximal tidal change in P_L) can be useful to limit the risk of VILI during spontaneous breathing.

Further reading

- Calverley PMA, *et al.* (2005). Flow limitation and dynamic hyperinflation: key concepts in modern respiratory physiology. *Eur Respir J*; 25: 186–199.

- Chen L, *et al.* (2018). Airway closure in acute respiratory distress syndrome: an underestimated and misinterpreted phenomenon. *Am J Respir Crit Care Med*; 197: 132–136.

- Henderson WR, *et al.* (2017). Fifty years of research in ARDS. Respiratory mechanics in acute respiratory distress syndrome. *Am J Respir Crit Care Med*; 196: 822–833.

- Mauri T, *et al.* (2016). Esophageal and transpulmonary pressure in the clinical setting: meaning, usefulness and perspectives. *Intensive Care Med*; 42: 1360–1373.

- Yoshida T, *et al.* (2018). Esophageal manometry and regional transpulmonary pressure in lung injury. *Am J Respir Crit Care Med*; 197: 1018–1026.

Monitoring breathing effort

Heder J. de Vries and Leo Heunks

Monitoring breathing effort might improve outcomes for mechanically ventilated patients. This chapter describes techniques to monitor breathing effort in mechanically ventilated patients, provides recommendations to conduct and interpret the measurements, and discusses how monitoring can affect ventilator management.

Physiology of breathing effort

Breathing effort is the combined work (or energy expenditure) of the respiratory muscles to drive alveolar ventilation. The magnitude of breathing effort is tightly matched to the metabolic demand, *i.e.* pH and P_{aCO_2} (and to a lesser extent, to P_{aO_2}).

The diaphragm is the main muscle of inspiration. Contraction of the diaphragm increases the size of the thorax. This lowers pleural pressure and leads to lung inflation. The accessory inspiratory muscles (mostly intercostal muscles and neck muscles) can be recruited to increase inspiratory capacity. Expiration is generally

Key points

- Inappropriate breathing effort during invasive ventilation has several downsides.

- Prolonged low breathing effort can lead to respiratory muscle atrophy and weakness, while prolonged excessive breathing effort can cause injury to the respiratory muscles and lungs.

- Monitoring breathing effort can be used to guide ventilator management and may limit the detrimental effects of inappropriate breathing effort.

- Several techniques are available to monitor breathing effort: some are readily available on the ventilator, but more accurate parameters may require additional instrumentation.

- We recommend using airway occlusion pressure at 100 ms ($P_{0.1}$) to screen for inappropriate breathing effort, and to consider more sophisticated monitoring tools when $P_{0.1}$ is outside the reference range.

a passive process. The abdominal wall muscles can be recruited to increase expiratory capacity.

Respiratory failure develops when the respiratory muscles are unable to meet the metabolic demands of the body. Unloading an unendurable work of breathing to restore adequate ventilation is one the principle reasons to initiate invasive ventilation.

Breathing effort during invasive ventilation

In controlled ventilator modes (*e.g.* volume-controlled ventilation), the total work of breathing is performed by the ventilator; while in partially supported modes (*e.g.* pressure support ventilation, assist-control ventilation), the work of breathing is shared between the patient and the ventilator.

It is difficult to quantify the magnitude of patient breathing effort without using dedicated monitoring techniques. While clinical examination may reveal that the patient triggers the ventilator in a partially supported mode, their breathing effort may be close to zero. This can occur at higher support levels (overassist), higher arterial pH and/or higher levels of sedation. By contrast, a patient might appear to breathe comfortably on a partially assisted ventilator mode while their breathing effort is close to unendurable. This occurs most often at lower support levels (underassist), lower arterial pH and/or low levels of sedation.

Rationale for monitoring breathing effort

Maintaining adequate patient breathing effort during invasive ventilation improves recruitment of basal lung fields, which facilitates oxygenation and reduces global lung stress.

In addition, monitoring might limit the detrimental effects of inappropriate breathing effort. Like all skeletal muscles, the respiratory muscles are prone to atrophy and contractile dysfunction upon disuse (see also the chapter "Effects of invasive ventilation on the respiratory muscles"). Weakness of the respiratory muscles can contribute to ventilator weaning failure and can increase the duration of invasive ventilation. However, excessive breathing effort can injure the respiratory muscles and lungs. Vigorous patient breathing effort increases lung stress and can lead to patient self-inflicted lung injury (P-SILI). Furthermore, the negative intrathoracic pressure can compromise cardiac function and result in pulmonary oedema.

Monitoring techniques

Monitoring can be defined as the near-continuous measurement of physiological parameters in a patient to guide clinical management. Although clinical examination and ultrasound do not meet this definition, we will briefly discuss these entities, given their clinical importance. Several parameters of breathing effort are readily available on the ventilator monitor, others require dedicated equipment (table 1).

Visual inspection Visual inspection of the ventilated patient can provide a quick, noninvasive assessment of breathing effort.

Multiple signs can point towards elevated breathing effort:
- facial expression of distress
- diaphoresis
- visible recruitment of the accessory inspiratory muscles or expiratory muscles
- intercostal and supraclavicular retractions

Table 1. *Techniques for monitoring breathing effort*

Parameter	Benefits	Downsides	Physiological range
Visual inspection	Can alert clinicians to consider high breathing effort	Cannot reliably detect low breathing effort	No accessory muscle recruitment, no expiratory muscle recruitment
Ventilator variables (flow, airway pressure, breathing frequency)	Readily available on all ventilators	Depend greatly on ventilator settings, poor correlations to breathing effort	Not available
$P_{0.1}$	Continuously available on most ventilators Fair correlation to breathing effort Suitable screening tool	Calculation depends on ventilator type	$P_{0.1}$ is 0.5–1.5 cmH_2O in healthy subjects at rest $P_{0.1}$ between 1.5 cmH_2O and 3.5 cmH_2O is a reasonable target in ICU patients
Oesophageal pressure	Strong correlation to patient effort Breath-by-breath monitoring Allows for more advanced analysis	Invasive: requires placement of a dedicated catheter Requires training before measurements are reliable	Drop of ±5–10 cmH_2O during inspiration is reasonable in partially supported ventilation No rise during expiration
Advanced oesophageal pressure monitoring	Very strong correlation to energy consumption of the respiratory muscles Can quantify how much energy is spent on PEEPi, resistance, and compliance	Invasive: requires placement of a dedicated catheter Requires extensive understanding of respiratory physiology and dedicated software	See reading list
Diaphragm electromyography	Breath-by-breath monitoring of respiratory drive	Not equal to force generation Not sensitive to accessory muscles	At least 3 µV per breath Upper boundary currently unknown
Ultrasound	Steep learning curve, available in most ICUs Moderate to fair correlation to breathing effort Quick screening of breathing effort	Sensitive to measurement errors Displacement is not valid during ventilator support	In healthy subjects at rest, thickening fraction is 15–30% and caudal displacement is 10–15 mm per breath Thickening fraction of 20–40% is reasonable during partially supported ventilation

PEEPi: intrinsic PEEP.

Detecting low or absent patient breathing effort by visual inspection of the ventilated patient is unreliable. Triggering the ventilator requires almost no effort (depending on the settings), and movement of the chest wall cannot distinguish between work performed by the patient or the ventilator.

Ventilator variables Volume, breathing frequency, airway pressure and flow depend greatly on the settings of the ventilator. This hampers their usefulness to monitor breathing effort.

- If the observed breathing frequency is higher than the set frequency (assist-control ventilation) there is evidence of patient effort, although auto-triggering (for example by cardiac activity) must be excluded. The amount of effort cannot be quantified reliably based on ventilator pressure/flow waveforms.
- If patient breathing effort is low (or absent), the flow and pressure curves might become very "smooth" and uniform, similar to the patterns observed during controlled ventilation (figure 1a).
- If effort is vigorous, the ventilator might be unable to deliver preset inspiratory pressures. This is called "flow starvation" or "outsucking the machine". It is a sign of a high respiratory drive combined with low inspiratory support (underassist) (figure 1c).

Airway occlusion pressure at 100 ms ($P_{0.1}$) The $P_{0.1}$ is an important parameter for monitoring patient breathing effort, because it requires no additional equipment, is easy to interpret and reacts quickly to changes in a patient's breathing effort.

The initial drop in airway pressure prior to a ventilator-supported breath is caused by the patient's own breathing effort. This drop occurs in semi-static conditions, and is therefore relatively insensitive to the ventilator settings, to the resistance of the airways and to the compliance of the respiratory system. This initial drop can be measured or estimated by the ventilator (figure 2). Most modern ventilators will display the $P_{0.1}$ continuously on a breath-by-breath basis during partially supported invasive ventilation.

- $P_{0.1}$ has a strong linear correlation with the work-of-breathing (r=0.75–0.87) of the respiratory muscles (see below) during invasive ventilation.
- $P_{0.1}$ reacts quickly to changes in patient breathing effort, which makes the $P_{0.1}$ a useful parameter to evaluate the effect of ventilator adjustments.
- $P_{0.1}$ has been shown to remain an adequate reflection of patient breathing effort during expiratory flow limitation and high PEEPi.
- In ventilated patients, a $P_{0.1}$ between 1.5 and 3.5 cmH$_2$O generally indicates that breathing effort is within the physiological limit (as observed in healthy subjects).
- A $P_{0.1}$ below 1.5 cmH$_2$O can indicate low patient breathing effort, while a $P_{0.1}$ above 3.5 cmH$_2$O can indicate elevated patient breathing effort.

Ultrasound Ultrasound is a noninvasive diagnostic tool that is available in most ICUs. As ultrasound is not a monitoring technique, but rather a diagnostic tool, it will only be briefly discussed in this chapter. For more extensive discussion see the chapter "Monitoring respiratory muscles: respiratory muscle ultrasound".

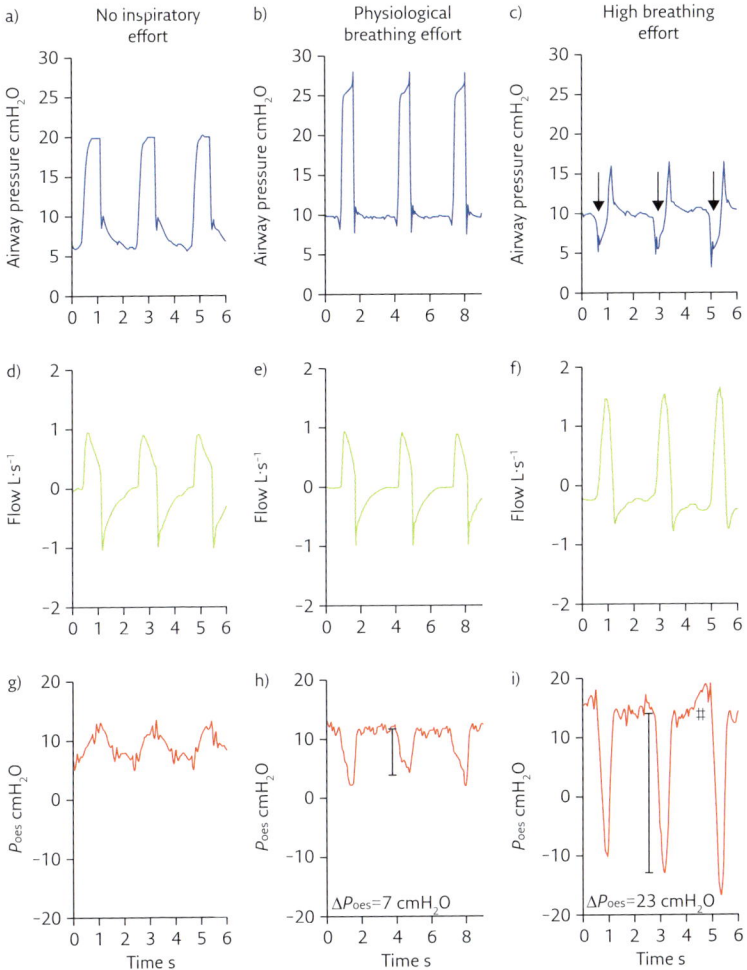

Figure 1. Airway pressure, flow and oesophageal pressure (Poes) traces in patients on partially supported ventilation during no inspiratory effort (a, d, g), physiological effort (b, e, h) and excessive effort (c, f, i). a, d, g) Patient on pressure support ventilation with 14 cmH₂O inspiratory support at 6 cmH₂O of PEEP. The Poes (g) rises during most of the inspiration, which indicates that patient breathing effort is close to zero. b, e, h) A different patient on pressure support ventilation with 15 cmH₂O inspiratory pressure support at 10 cmH₂O of PEEP. Poes (h) decreases by ~5–10 cmH₂O with each inspiration, consistent with physiological breathing effort. c, f, i) The same patient as in the middle column, but inspiratory pressure support has been reduced to 5 cmH₂O. This leads to elevated patient breathing effort: Poes (i) now falls by >20 cmH₂O per breath. Furthermore, Poes rises at the end of expiration, suggestive of expiratory muscle recruitment (⌗). The breathing effort is so vigorous that the patient lowers the pressure in the airway circuitry (c) below the set PEEP level during most of the inspiration ("outsucking the machine", arrows).

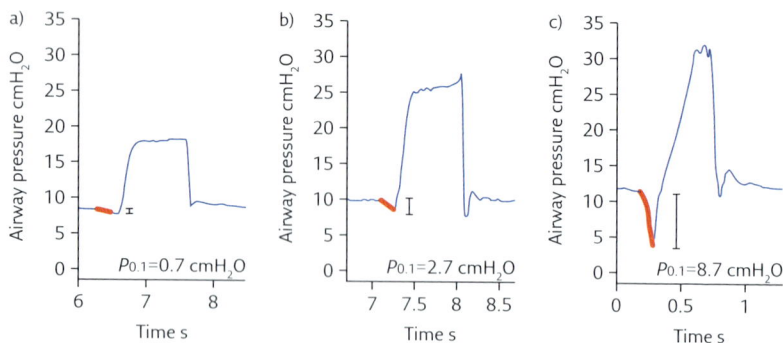

Figure 2. P0.1 *during a) low, b) adequate and c) high patient breathing effort. Airway pressure tracings during a single breath in three different patients are shown. The initial drop in airway pressure is caused by the patient's respiratory muscles (red area). The ventilator quantifies (or estimates) this drop in the first 100 ms of the inspiration (bars next to the red area). a) Low breathing effort, the airway pressure barely deviates from baseline. b) Adequate effort, airway pressure drops between 1.5 and 3.5 cmH$_2$O prior to ventilator insufflation. c) High patient effort, the airway pressure drops more than 8 cmH$_2$O per breath in the first 100 ms.*

Diaphragm excursion during tidal breathing can be quantified by subcostal positioning of the probe and visualising the diaphragm dome (figure 3).

- Diaphragm excursion during tidal breathing is poorly correlated with more advanced parameters of breathing effort, such as the pressure–time product of the diaphragm (r=0.5).
- Diaphragm excursion ranges from 10 to 15 mm per breath in healthy subjects at rest and can increase up to 75 mm during vigorous breathing.
- Using diaphragm excursion to detect patient effort is only reliable in the absence of ventilator support, as ventilator insufflation will also cause caudal movement of the diaphragm irrespective of patient effort.

A cross-section of the diaphragm can be visualised by placing a high-frequency probe in the in the mid-axillary line. The diaphragm appears as a thin (2 mm) two-layered structure, bound by the thoracic and abdominal pleura and a fibrous plate. The thickness of the diaphragm can be measured during inspiration and expiration, and used to calculate the thickening fraction (figure 3). Usually, obtaining adequate visualisation of the diaphragm on the left side is more difficult compared to the right side.

- The thickening fraction shows a fair correlation with more advanced parameters of patient breathing effort such as the pressure–time product (r=0.7-0.8).
- The thickening fraction can reliably detect breathing effort during ventilator support.
- Thickening fraction is 15–30% during tidal breathing in healthy subjects.
- In ventilated patients, a thickening fraction of 20–40% was correlated with preserved muscle thickness in ICU patients.
- Because the diaphragm is very thin, small measurement errors (0.1 mm) can result in large differences in estimated breathing effort when using ultrasound.

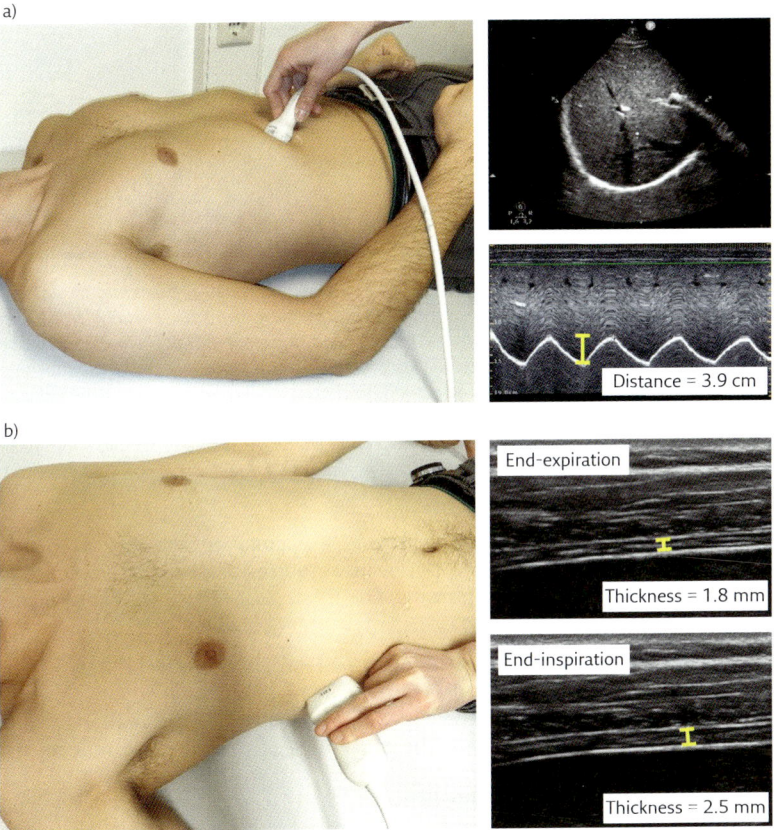

Figure 3. Ultrasound assessment of the diaphragm. a) Assessment of diaphragm displacement during inspiration. The diaphragm is visualised as a white echo-dense structure on top of the liver. It moves downward during inspiration ("towards the probe"). The displacement can be quantified in M-mode. Displacement = position on inspiration − position on expiration. b) Assessment of diaphragm thickening fraction during tidal breathing. The diaphragm thickens during contraction (inspiration). The increase in thickness is quantified with the thickening fraction. Thickening fraction = (thickness at end-inspiration − thickness at end-expiration)/thickness at end-expiration)×100% = (2.5−1.8)/1.8×100% = 38%.

Oesophageal pressure measurement Oesophageal pressure measurement is the state-of-the-art technique to monitor breathing effort in clinical practice. Because the respiratory muscles act by changing intrathoracic pressure, the changes in the oesophagus (a compliant structure within the thorax) reflect patient breathing effort (figure 1).

Measurement requires placement of a small balloon-tipped catheter or a feeding tube equipped with a balloon. Some ventilators are equipped with pressure transducers and can display oesophageal pressure on the monitor. If not available, a disposable

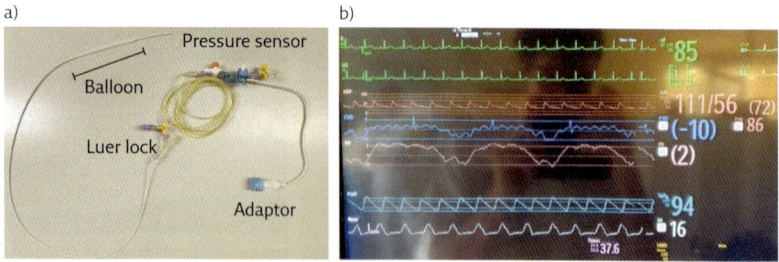

Figure 4. Connecting an oesophageal balloon to a monitor. a) An oesophageal balloon catheter has been connected to a standard blood pressure transducer using Luer locks. The tubing connecting the balloon to the pressure sensor are air-filled. The adaptor can be connected to a standard ICU monitor. b) Oesophageal pressure is visible on the monitor as a pink curve (fifth tracing from top). The oesophageal pressure has an end-expiratory value of about 7 cmH$_2$O and drops to –7 cmH$_2$O during inspiration, meaning that the total drop in oesophageal pressure is 14 cmH$_2$O per breath, consistent with elevated breathing effort. Note that values on the monitor are in mmHg; a conversion factor of 1.36 is required to obtain values in cmH$_2$O (5 mmHg×1.36=6.8 cmH$_2$O).

pressure transducer can be used as well (figure 4). Appropriate calibration is required before measurements are reliable, but online resources describing the practice of oesophageal pressure monitoring are available (Mauri *et al.* (2016) and Akoumianaki *et al.* (2014)).

- If oesophageal pressure rises during inspiration, patient effort is very low or absent (figure 1g).
- Oesophageal pressure will decrease during inspiration if breathing effort is physiological (or excessive). The magnitude of this decrease reflects the magnitude of breathing effort.
- A drop in oesophageal pressure between 5 and 10 cmH$_2$O per breath is within the physiological level of effort in healthy subjects. It seems reasonable to aim for a similar pressure in most ventilated patients. This should protect against disuse atrophy while preventing load-induced muscle injury.
- A drop in oesophageal pressure over 15 cmH$_2$O per breath indicates elevated patient breathing effort.
- A rise in oesophageal pressure during expiration can point to recruitment of the expiratory muscles, and is a sign of elevated breathing effort or pulmonary hyperinflation (figure 1i).

Advanced oesophageal pressure analysis Advanced monitoring of breathing effort is possible by combining the oesophageal pressure with time and volume dimensions to calculate the pressure–time product, the work-of-breathing and the mechanical power. These parameters relate strongly to energy consumption of the respiratory muscles, and to the development of respiratory muscle fatigue and lung injury. In addition, these parameters can distinguish between work used to overcome PEEPi, resistance or elastance.

However, acquiring and interpreting these parameters requires extensive physiological knowledge, specialised equipment and dedicated software (de Vries *et al.*, 2018). Please see the list of further reading for more information.

Diaphragm electromyography Electromyography of the diaphragm reflects diaphragm recruitment and is closely related to neural respiratory drive. It can be displayed continuously, and is especially useful to screen for ventilator overassist and patient–ventilator asynchrony. It is also used to control the ventilator in the neurally adjusted ventilator assist (NAVA) mode (see the chapter entitled "Proportional modes"). The electrical activity of the diaphragm (EAdi) can be obtained with oesophageal electrodes (by using a dedicated catheter) or with surface electrodes.

- The EAdi signal is not synonymous with pressure generation. This is comparable to an ECG, which does not reflect cardiac contractions.
- The efficiency of the diaphragm (*i.e.* the amount of pressure generated per microvolt electrical activity) varies greatly between subjects. Therefore, an EAdi peak of 10 µV may be consistent with a diaphragmatic muscle pressure of 5 cmH_2O in one patient and 25 cmH_2O in another patient. This makes it difficult to provide an optimal range.
- However, an increase in EAdi within a patient reflects increased respiratory drive, and probably increased breathing effort.
- If there is no EAdi during inspiration, the diaphragm is inactive. This can point to low patient effort and ventilator overassistance.

Target population Today, it is not known which patient categories potentially benefit from monitoring breathing effort. The $P_{0.1}$ is a suitable screening technique for inappropriate breathing effort because it is available on all modern ventilators.

We suggest monitoring the $P_{0.1}$ in all patients on partially supported ventilator modes. In patients with a $P_{0.1}$ outside of the reference range, more sophisticated tools to monitor breathing effort should be considered. Depending on local experience and availability this could be either an oesophageal balloon (preferred), diaphragm ultrasound or EAdi.

Clinical management

Clinical management recommendations in case of inappropriate breathing effort are listed below. Currently, no clinical trials have evaluated the impact of adapting ventilator inspiratory support or sedation level based on patient breathing effort. However, animal studies and physiological reasoning provide a strong rationale to try and optimise breathing effort until clinical trials are available.

Low breathing effort and ventilator overassist

1) Reduce level of sedation, unless this leads to more agitation and discomfort. This might take several minutes to hours before it has an effect.
2) Reduce inspiratory pressure support in steps of 2–4 cmH_2O. Carefully monitor the minute volume to ensure ventilation remains adequate. Reassess breathing effort after ~5 min.
3) Obtain an arterial blood gas sample when target effort has been reached to ensure adequate oxygenation and P_{aCO_2} clearance.

High breathing effort and ventilator underassist

1) Consider (and treat) pain, delirium, and agitation.

2) Increase inspiratory pressure support with 2–4 cmH$_2$O. Reassess breathing effort after 5 min. If this causes prolonged high V_T or high P_{plat}, reduce support.
3) Consider increasing the level of sedation. Titrate carefully until effort is acceptable.
4) If effort remains injuriously high, and the patient has severe lung injury (P_{aO_2}/F_{IO_2} <150 mmHg (<20.0 kPa)), consider administering a neuromuscular blocking agent to abolish patient effort. Reassess after 24 h.

Further reading

- Akoumianaki E, *et al.* (2014). The application of esophageal pressure measurement in patients with respiratory failure. *Am J Respir Crit Care Med*; 189: 520–531.

- American Thoracic Society/European Respiratory Society (2002). ATS/ERS Statement on respiratory muscle testing. *Am J Respir Crit Care Med*; 166: 518–624.

- de Vries H, *et al.* (2018). Assessing breathing effort in mechanical ventilation: physiology and clinical implications. *Ann Transl Med*; 6: 387.

- Heunks LMA, *et al.* (2015). Monitoring and preventing diaphragm injury. *Curr Opin Crit Care*; 21: 34–41.

- Jonkman AH, *et al.* (2017). Novel insights in ICU-acquired respiratory muscle dysfunction: implications for clinical care. *Crit Care*; 21: 64.

- Mauri T, *et al.* (2016). Esophageal and transpulmonary pressure in the clinical setting: meaning, usefulness and perspectives. *Intensive Care Med*; 42: 1360-1373.

- Schepens T, *et al.* (2019). Diaphragm-protective mechanical ventilation. *Curr Opin Crit Care*; 25: 77–85.

- Telias I, *et al.* (2018). The airway occlusion pressure ($P_{0.1}$) to monitor respiratory drive during mechanical ventilation: increasing awareness of a not-so-new problem. *Intensive Care Med*; 44: 1532-1535.

- Yoshida T, *et al.* (2016). Spontaneous effort during mechanical ventilation. *Crit Care Med*; 44: e678-e688.

Electrical impedance tomography

Inéz Frerichs, Tobias Becher and Norbert Weiler

Invasive ventilation is an established and often a life-saving therapy in patients with respiratory failure. Nonetheless, it is not a physiological form of ventilation and may cause VILI. The occurrence and severity of this injury depends on how well the ventilator settings match with the individual mechanical properties of the patient's respiratory system and the underlying lung disease. Different patients need different ventilator modes and settings, which ideally should be personalised to each patient's needs.

Inadequate ventilator settings may increase the risk of deleterious regional alveolar overdistension, tidal recruitment and/or collapse, which promote the development of biotrauma. Therefore, the monitoring of ventilator therapy should preferably not only assess the pulmonary gas exchange efficiency but also detect the presence of the aforementioned injurious events. EIT is a method capable of providing this clinically relevant information. In combination with the results of other established methods, described in this section on Monitoring the ventilated patient, EIT findings can be applied to optimise invasive ventilation.

This chapter briefly describes the basics of EIT and how EIT examinations are carried out in mechanically ventilated patients with some practical hints. Further,

Key points

- Electrical impedance tomography (EIT) is a bedside, radiation-free imaging method for continuous assessment of regional lung function.

- EIT measures the distribution of regional V_T and changes in regional end-expiratory lung volumes in mechanically ventilated patients.

- EIT detects asymmetric ventilation distributions caused by pneumothorax or tube malposition, and identifies deleterious phenomena like regional overdistension, tidal recruitment and atelectasis.

- EIT provides guidance for personalised selection of ventilator settings.

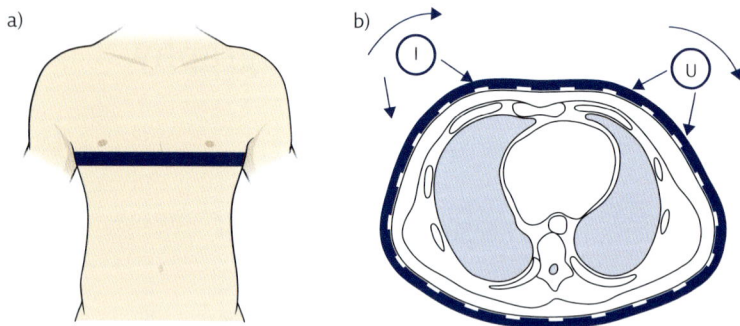

Figure 1. Schematic drawings showing a) the placement of the EIT electrode interface around the chest and b) the measurement principle, with rotating electrical current (I) application and voltage (U) measurement. Figure partially created using BioRender.

the analysis of EIT data is explained and EIT findings relevant for monitoring and guidance of invasive ventilation are provided. This chapter focuses mainly on the measurement of regional lung ventilation and changes in aeration.

Basics

EIT determines the electrical properties of thoracic tissues, including the lung tissue, by applying very small unperceivable alternating currents through an array of electrodes placed around the chest (figure 1). The current applications rotate around the body at a very high speed. Electrical bioimpedance is the measure of the opposition of tissues to the current flow. Regional values of electrical bioimpedance within the chest can be calculated by EIT from voltage values measured through the same array of electrodes during each current application. Modern EIT devices determine changes in electrical bioimpedance in comparison to reference data (baseline) and not absolute impedance values.

The set of voltage values acquired during one complete circular cycle of current applications renders one primary EIT image. Such primary images are sampled at a scan rate of up to about 50 images per second. EIT images have the conventional radiological tomographic orientation with right chest side on the left side of the image and with ventral at the top. Electrical bioimpedance of lung tissue rises with increasing air volume, for instance periodically during each inspiration, and it falls when regional air volume falls, for instance during expiration or alveolar collapse. These changes in regional pulmonary electrical bioimpedance can be continuously measured by EIT.

EIT examination

Patient examinations with EIT can be performed directly at the bedside because EIT devices are small and can be placed on trolleys (figure 2). EIT can be used as a stand-alone medical technology or integrated into ventilators or monitors. It is usually combined with simultaneous recording of other biological signals and/or ventilator-related parameters and settings. EIT can be applied during controlled and assisted invasive ventilation, and also during NIV and spontaneous breathing.

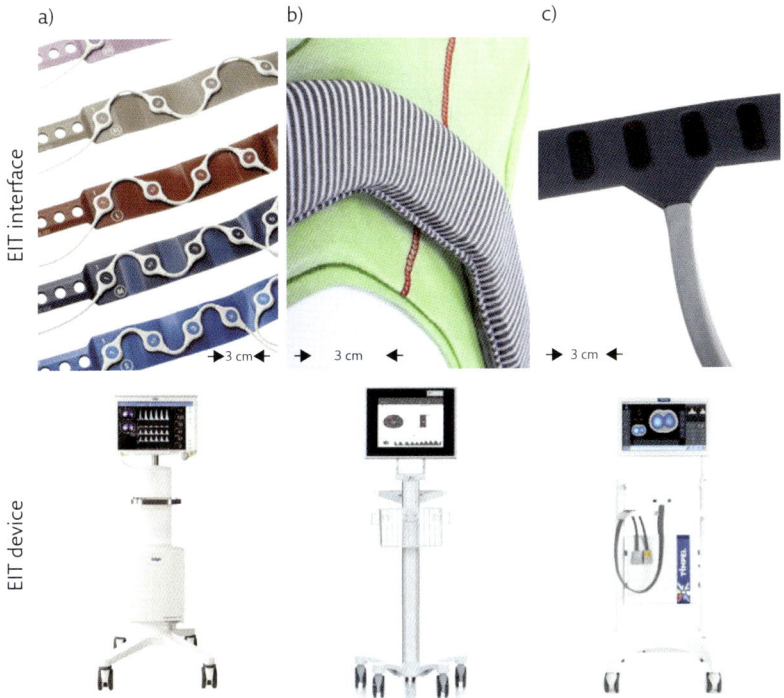

Figure 2. Commercially available EIT devices: a) PulmoVista 500 (Drägerwerk AG & Co. KGaA, Lübeck, Germany, image © Drägerwerk AG & Co. KGaA, all rights reserved), b) BB² Monitor (SenTec AG (formerly Swisstom AG), Landquart, Switzerland) and c) Enlight 1800 (Timpel, São Paulo, Brazil). The corresponding vendor-specific EIT electrode interfaces are shown in the upper panels. The photos were kindly provided and are reproduced with permission from Drägerwerk AG & Co. KGaA, SenTec AG and Timpel.

Because the method has no known risks there are hardly any exclusion criteria for EIT use. It is only recommended not to apply EIT:

- in patients with electrically active implants, or
- in patients with large chest wounds or multiple chest drainage tubes that preclude the placement of an electrode interface around the chest.

The EIT electrode interfaces are designed as belts, vest-like garments or strips (figure 2, upper panels) and are available in different sizes. They are placed around the chest in a transverse or slightly oblique plane. Good skin contact is essential. When the chosen size of the interface matches the patient's chest dimension then skin–electrode contact is generally not a critical issue. Visual feedback on the contact quality is provided. Some vendors recommend the use of specific contact agents to further improve the contact. The users are advised to wait for a few minutes before EIT data acquisition is started.

The interface should not be located caudally to approximately the sixth intercostal space (in the parasternal line). Otherwise the diaphragm may periodically enter the electrode plane and affect the measurement, especially in patients that are lying down. If the users need to reattach the EIT electrode interface after its removal, anatomical landmarks on the chest should be used to place it in the same location to guarantee measurement reproducibility and allow comparison between separate measurements.

The duration of patient examination using EIT is variable. It depends on the decision of the user and is guided by the clinical question. EIT data may be acquired for just a few minutes or for up to several hours or days. The maximum duration depends on the device specifications. EIT may offer immediate feedback on the short-term effect of an intervention or it can follow the long-term effects and provide monitoring.

It is recommended that the EIT electrode interface should not be touched or moved during a running examination as this may induce disturbances and affect the results. Because EIT data are sampled continuously, temporary disturbances are not critical as the disturbed phases may be discarded and still leave enough data for reliable analysis. The use of event markers is recommended, especially when EIT data analysis is planned at a later date, in addition to online monitoring. Users are advised not to change the body position of the patient during the examination, unless the posture change is the intervention whose effect is to be examined by EIT.

EIT findings

EIT generates a time series of primary EIT images during the examination. These consecutive images can be presented online on the screen of the EIT device. They show the instantaneous changes in regional electrical bioimpedance in the chest cross-section. In addition, the image values are instantaneously summed up in the whole image or in predefined arbitrary, anatomical or functional regions of interest (ROI), and plotted as global (whole image) and regional (ROI) waveforms. During ongoing ventilation, these waveforms show the ventilation-related variation in electrical bioimpedance. The tidal variation, *i.e.* the difference between the end-expiratory trough and end-inspiratory peak values, is proportional to V_T. The end-expiratory values represent the end-expiratory pulmonary air filling, *i.e.* the end-expiratory lung volume (EELV).

The distribution of regional tidal EIT signal variation and regional changes in end-expiratory lung impedance are highly relevant for monitoring the adequacy of ventilator settings. They enable the assessment of regional V_T and regional changes in EELV that depend on the set V_T, PEEP and other ventilator parameters.

The breath-by-breath measurement of regional V_T using EIT is robust and reliable. However, under certain circumstances, the measurement of EELV may reflect other effects in addition to true changes in regional air content. For example, if an EIT examination is carried out during rapid administration of a large volume of electrically conductive electrolyte solution then end-expiratory values in the EIT signal will fall by a mechanism not related to local pulmonary air content. Massive blood loss will have the opposite effect and result in rising end-expiratory values. If the contact between the patient's skin and some of the electrodes fluctuates when the patient is lying on an inflating mattress this will induce slow quasi-periodic waves in the acquired EIT signal. Under all such circumstances the assessment of EELV based on end-expiratory lung impedance is not reliable.

The calculation of tidal impedance variation in all image pixels allows the characterisation of ventilation distribution within the chest cross-section, which can be described using functional EIT images or numerical values. Examples of functional EIT images are shown in figure 3. The top row of images in figure 3b show the spatial distribution of V_T. Ventilation was detected only in the left lung region in this patient due to massive one-sided chest trauma. Such high ventilation asymmetry may also be caused by one-sided pneumothorax or tube malposition with one-sided lung ventilation. Continuous monitoring of ventilation distribution showing the development of such ventilation asymmetry may facilitate the early diagnosis of such adverse events and speed up the initiation of therapeutic measures.

The bottom row EIT images in figure 3b show another type of functional image. Such images can be generated from EIT data acquired during a decremental PEEP trial conducted during pressure-controlled ventilation and under the condition that end-inspiratory and end-expiratory flows reach a value of zero. The images highlight areas exhibiting regional overinflation and collapse, with separate colour-coding of each, based on the calculation of regional respiratory system compliance. Simultaneous recording of airway pressure with EIT data acquisition is recommended for correct measurement of regional respiratory system compliance. The resulting information can be applied to identify the PEEP level at which the degree of overinflation and atelectasis is best balanced (see the "cross-over point" in figure 3d). Some users set the PEEP value exactly at the cross-over point, while others prefer to set the nearest PEEP step value to the left of the cross-over point or they add the value of the PEEP step to the PEEP value at the cross-over point. The latter two approaches aim to prevent atelectasis development. In the example patient in figure 3, the cross-over point occurred at a PEEP of about 14 mbar and PEEP was set at 16 mbar (*i.e.* the PEEP value at the cross-over point plus the 2 mbar PEEP step size used).

Several other types of functional EIT images exist. Two examples of these images are generated by:

- Categorisation of regional tidal impedance variation that can then be applied to show regions with very low variation in colour-coded silent ventilation spaces.
- Analysis of regional nonlinearity of electrical bioimpedance increase between end-expiration and end-inspiration that allows generation of functional EIT images visualising the heterogeneity of intra-tidal dynamics of air filling.

In addition to functional images, various numerical measures can be calculated from EIT data. Some of these EIT measures, like the global inhomogeneity index and the coefficient of variation, characterise the overall degree of ventilation heterogeneity. Other measures, like the centre of ventilation or the fractions of ventilation in the right, left, ventral and dorsal image halves, provide some positional information on the distribution of ventilation between the right and left and/or ventral and dorsal lung regions.

Functional EIT images and numerical measures are complementary. They are all derived from the same time series of primary EIT images. They describe different aspects of regional lung function traceable in the EIT data.

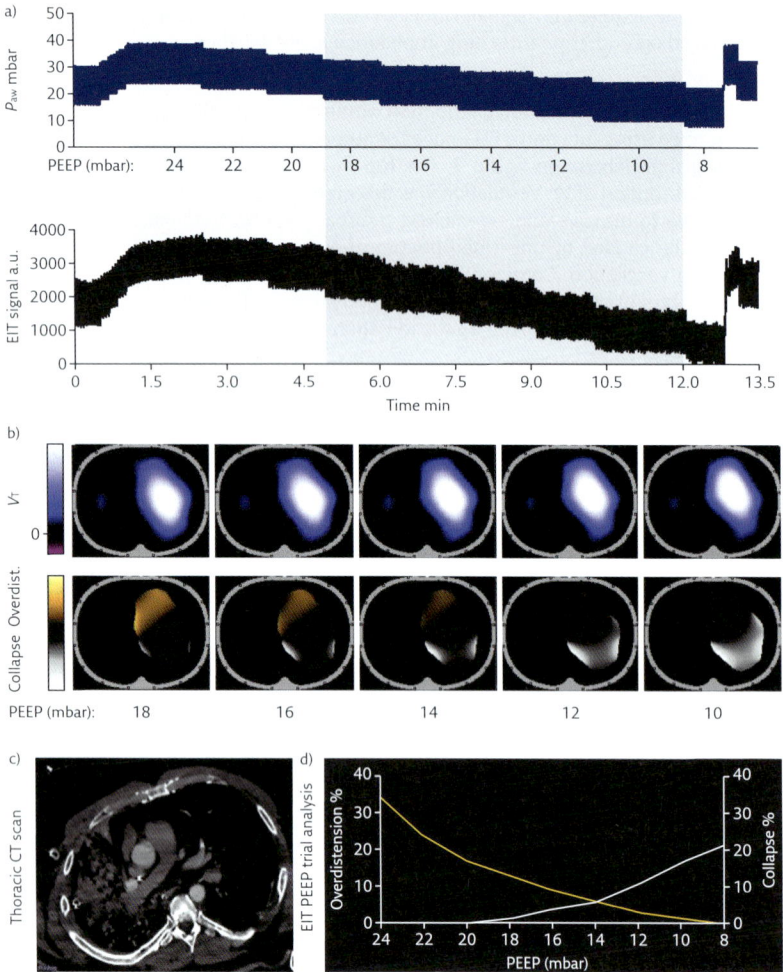

Figure 3. EIT examination of a 49-year-old patient with moderate-to-severe ARDS during a decremental PEEP trial. The patient suffered from right-sided lung contusion and left-sided pneumonia after polytrauma (see the CT scan in panel c). a) The waveforms of airway pressure (Paw) and global EIT signal in arbitrary units (a.u.). b) Functional EIT images obtained at five out of nine decremental PEEP steps, they show the distribution of VT in the chest cross-section as white–blue areas (top row of images) and regional overdistension (overdist.) as brown–orange areas in the nondependent lung regions and collapse as white–light grey areas in the dependent regions (bottom row of images). d) The progressive fall in regional overdistension and rise in regional collapse with decreasing PEEP led to a cross-over of the respective lines. Based on these EIT data, PEEP was increased from 10 mbar before the trial to 16 mbar. The corresponding Pplat were 22 mbar and 29 mbar, ΔP 12 mbar and 13 mbar, and VT 426 mL and 453 mL, respectively. The ratio of P_{aO_2}/F_{IO_2} rose from 105 to 163 mmHg (14.0 to 21.7 kPa).

The built-in tools for online and offline analysis of EIT data are device specific. However, most of the functional images and measures described in this chapter can easily be obtained. Other less frequent or experimental EIT parameters can be analysed using dedicated research tools.

Summary

EIT is an approved medical technology mainly used for monitoring of regional lung function during invasive ventilation in ICUs and operating theatres. EIT examinations are carried out during ongoing ventilation and also during specific ventilation manoeuvres, like decremental PEEP trials or quasi-static low-flow inflation. EIT continuously measures the distribution of inspired air in the lungs. It determines changes in regional EELV and regional parameters of respiratory system mechanics. EIT also identifies regional overinflation, tidal recruitment or alveolar collapse and other adverse events, like pneumothorax. EIT findings during specific ventilation manoeuvres or other interventions increase the information content of EIT results and facilitate the optimisation of ventilator settings to the individual patient. In the future, the clinical decision-making based on EIT may be further improved by standardised examination and data analysis procedures and unified interpretation schemes including findings from other diagnostic and monitoring methods.

Further reading

- Adler A, *et al.* (2012). Whither lung EIT: where are we, where do we want to go and what do we need to get there? *Physiol Meas*; 33: 679–694.

- Bachmann MC, *et al.* (2018). Electrical impedance tomography in acute respiratory distress syndrome. *Crit Care*; 22: 263.

- Frerichs I (2015). Bedside lung imaging methods (Electrical impedance tomography). *In*: Rimensberger PC, ed. Pediatric And Neonatal Mechanical Ventilation. Berlin Heidelberg, Springer-Verlag, pp. 457–471.

- Frerichs I, *et al.* (2014). Electrical impedance tomography imaging of the cardiopulmonary system. *Curr Opin Crit Care*; 20: 323–332.

- Frerichs I, *et al.* (2017). Chest electrical impedance tomography examination, data analysis, terminology, clinical use and recommendations: consensus statement of the TRanslational EIT developmeNt stuDy group. *Thorax*; 72: 83–93.

- Kobylianskii J, *et al.* (2016). Electrical impedance tomography in adult patients undergoing mechanical ventilation: a systematic review. *J Crit Care*; 35: 33–50.

- Shono A, *et al.* (2019). Clinical implication of monitoring regional ventilation using electrical impedance tomography. *J Intensive Care*; 7: 4.

Monitoring lung aeration: lung ultrasound

Ezgi Ozyilmaz and Annia Schreiber

Critically ill patients need rapid access to accurate and reproducible imaging methods for diagnosis and monitoring. Lung ultrasound has numerous advantages in the critically ill, since it is a safe, easy-to-learn, fast, accurate, repeatable, real-time method that avoids exposure to ionising radiation and transfer-related risks. This chapter provides an outline of the technique and interpretation of lung ultrasound in critically ill patients.

Although ultrasonography has been used to evaluate solid organs for almost half a century, until 30 years ago, lung ultrasound was traditionally considered off limits due to the poor penetration of ultrasound beams through air and the impossibility of passing through bones. Eventually, it became clear that, although normal lungs cannot be directly assessed by ultrasound, the artefacts resulting from the sound beams interacting with the air-filled alveoli still contain valuable information and >70% of the pleural surface is still visible between the ribs.

Key points

- Lung ultrasound is an excellent bedside diagnostic tool in critically ill patients, as it is safe, easy to learn, fast, accurate and repeatable, and gives real-time data.

- There is evidence in the literature of the usefulness and accuracy of lung ultrasound in diagnosing interstitial syndrome, consolidation, pneumothorax, pleural effusion and acute respiratory failure.

- Lung ultrasound is also appropriate for monitoring aeration changes deriving from any treatment or procedure. It is possible to use a standardised and comparable method to monitor alveolar recruitment/derecruitment in the critically ill patient.

- Lung ultrasound is of limited usefulness in cases of deep lesions not reaching the pleural surface, hyperinflation, and subcutaneous emphysema.

How to perform lung ultrasound

The machine, the probe and where to scan A simple machine is suitable for lung ultrasound, since using filters may erase artefacts. There is no evidence of the superiority of one probe over another. A combination of a linear high-frequency probe with a convex low-frequency probe, or a single high-resolution micro-convex probe with a wide frequency range, may be used. The linear probe will better assess the pleural surface, while the convex probe will show deeper structures.

Lung ultrasound can be performed on the whole chest by positioning the probe along the intercostal spaces. There are several scanning methods. The Bedside Lung Ultrasound in Emergency (BLUE) protocol defines two BLUE points and one posterolateral alveolar and/or pleural syndrome (PLAPS) point per lung. The International Consensus Conference on Lung Ultrasound (Volpicelli *et al.*, 2012) recommends an approach using four chest areas per side (eight zones), while in the ICU a more exhaustive 12-region examination is frequently used (figure 1).

The basics of interpretation In a normally aerated lung, the only detectable structure is the pleura, which is visualised as a hyperechoic horizontal line located 0.5 cm below the ribs at each side (figure 2a). The pleura and the two rib shadows together indicate the bat sign. If the lung is also normally ventilated, the pleural line moves horizontally, rhythmically and synchronously with respiration, generating the so-called lung sliding. In normal conditions, the pleura acts as a mirror of the lung, reflecting the chest wall below, generating multiple, horizontal, equally spaced, hyperechoic artefacts called A-lines. When the air content of the lung decreases, the pleura no longer acts as a mirror and some reverberation vertical artefacts appear, called B-lines (figure 2b). The number and coalescence of B-lines is proportional to the amount of aeration loss. When the air content further decreases, sound can easily propagate and for the first time a real image of the lung can be seen, which is called lung consolidation.

Although chest radiography is considered the first-line diagnostic imaging modality in the critically ill, its diagnostic accuracy is relatively low. Chest CT has been considered the gold standard method but has limitations, such as the transportation of critically ill patients, contrast fluid and radiation exposure and high cost, which result in low repeatability. In the ICU, lung ultrasound has proven to be useful in the evaluation of many different acute and chronic conditions, including pneumothorax, pleural effusion, pneumonia and atelectasis, and differentiating interstitial lung disease from cardiogenic pulmonary oedema and acute lung injury. The diagnostic accuracy is over 80%, higher than for chest radiography and CT scans.

A bedside diagnostic tool for the critically ill patient

Lung ultrasound is an excellent bedside diagnostic tool in critically ill patients. This section will discuss how it can be used to diagnose interstitial syndrome, consolidation, pneumothorax, pleural effusion and acute respiratory failure.

Interstitial syndrome The B-lines are generated by the juxtaposition of alveolar air and septal thickening due to any cause. The ultrasound feature of interstitial syndrome is having three or more B-lines in a longitudinal scan (or three or more

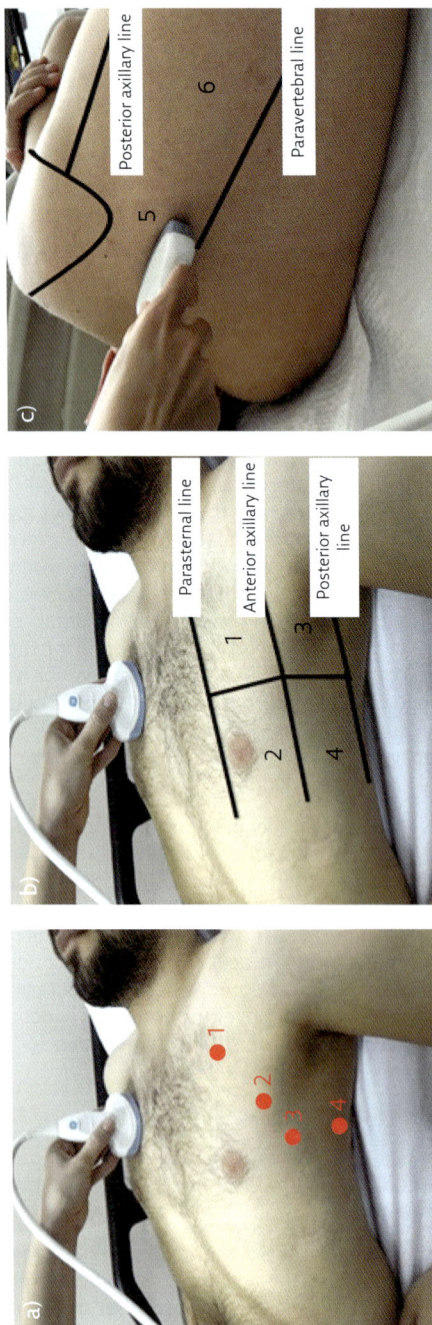

Figure 1. Lung ultrasound scanning methods. a) Points 1 and 2 correspond to the anterior BLUE points: the upper BLUE point (1) is located 2 cm below the clavicle on the midclavicular line; the lower BLUE point (2) is lateral to the nipple. The third point (3) corresponds to the phrenic point and is located at the intersection between the mid-axillary line and the phrenic line. The fourth point (4) is called the PLAPS point and is located at the intersection between the posterior axillary line and the transverse line continuing posteriorly from the lower BLUE point. A simple approach is to start with the anterior region (upper and lower BLUE points): this is named stage 1, which is the most informative on respiratory life-threatening conditions such as pneumothorax and interstitial syndrome secondary to pulmonary oedema. The investigation is then extended to the lateral and posterior region of the chest (stages 2 and 3, phrenic and PLAPS points, respectively). Stages 2 and 3 give information on either effusion or consolidations. b) Lung ultrasound score assessment using four zones for each lung, with upper and lower regions delineated by parasternal, anterior axillary and posterior axillary lines. c) Posterior view, showing the 12-region approach.

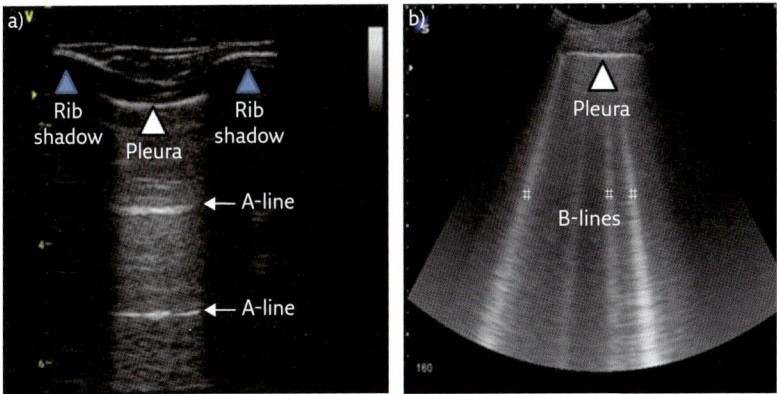

Figure 2. The basics of lung ultrasound. a) The pleura, the bat sign (pleura plus two rib shadows) and A-lines. b) The pleura and B-lines ([#]).

close B-lines in an oblique scan). The B-lines are often characterised by the following seven features:

- Comet tail
- Vertical well-defined bright lines (laser like)
- Hyperechoic
- Arising from the pleural line
- Extending to the bottom of the screen without fading
- Erasing A-lines
- Moving in concert with lung sliding

Occasional B-lines can be seen in normal lungs, especially at the bases; however, having three or more B-lines between two adjacent ribs is considered pathological. Localised and unilateral B-lines (focal interstitial syndrome) can be observed in pneumonia, pneumonitis or neoplasms in the peri-lesional area. Multiple bilateral B-lines (diffuse interstitial syndrome) can be an expression of the following lung diseases that affect the lung interstitium: pulmonary oedema, either haemodynamic or permeability induced (ARDS); interstitial pneumonia or pneumonitis; or lung fibrosis. Ultrasound may guide the differential diagnosis of B-lines by considering their distribution, gradient of concentration, treatment response and possible associated irregularity of the pleural line (table 1).

Consolidation The characteristic sonographic signs of a consolidation are hypoechoic tissue or liver-like areas beneath the pleura and air bronchograms (figure 3). A dynamic air bronchogram, which moves centrifugally with inspiration, excludes bronchial obstruction and is helpful to distinguish between pneumonia and atelectasis since a static air bronchogram is a feature of atelectasis. The margins of the consolidation, presence of comet tail artefacts, vascular pattern and the presence of associated effusion/abscess are also helpful to determine the cause of the consolidation, which can include infection, pulmonary embolism, atelectasis, cancer/metastasis and contusion.

Table 1. *Differential diagnosis of B-lines in interstitial syndrome*

	Acute cardiogenic pulmonary oedema	ARDS	Pulmonary fibrosis
Clinical scene	Acute	Acute	Chronic
B-lines	Multiple, diffuse, bilateral, symmetric	Multiple, diffuse, bilateral, more likely to be asymmetric	Varies according to the extent of the disease
Distribution	Homogeneous	Nonhomogeneous, with the presence of spared areas close to highly damaged areas	Nonhomogeneous
Predominant localisation	Lateral in the early phase, then progress anteriorly	Posterior dependent	Varies according to the localisation of collagen tissue accumulation
Lung sliding	Normal	Varies	Varies
Pleural line	Normal	Irregular, thickened, coarse	Varies
Pleural effusion	Common	Less common	Rare
Correlation of ultrasound findings with clinical symptoms	Not correlated	Highly correlated	Not correlated

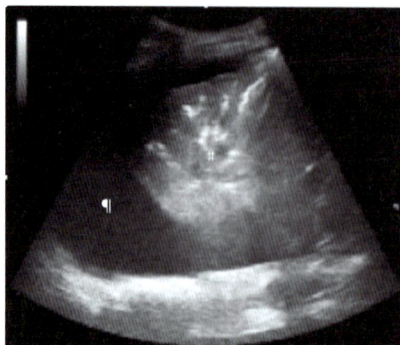

Figure 3. *Lung ultrasound showing consolidation with air bronchogram (‡) and pleural effusion (¶).*

Pneumothorax Lung ultrasound is an excellent method for the diagnosis of pneumothorax, with approximately 100% sensitivity (comparable to CT). In a supine patient, the air will collect at the anterior chest wall. Thus, placing the probe on the upper anterior point will reveal the following sonographic signs of pneumothorax:

- Absence of lung sliding (not specific to pneumothorax), also seen in M-mode as a replacement of the normal seashore sign with the stratosphere sign.
- Predominant A-lines (not specific to pneumothorax).
- Absence of B-lines.
- The lung point: the point at which the two pleural layers rejoin one another. This will be more lateral with increasing pneumothorax size so the probe should be moved laterally until the lung point is observed. Specificity on the diagnosis of pneumothorax is 100%; however, sensitivity is lower since it is not always found.
- No lung pulse: abolished pleural movement with the cardiac oscillations.

The pneumothorax decision tree is presented in figure 4.

Lung ultrasound in the critically ill can also predict the size of the pneumothorax. Even if the exact volume cannot be measured, a lung point anterior to the mid-axillary line predicts a lung collapse volume of <15%, while a lung point posterior to that line predicts >15% lung collapse with high sensitivity and specificity (83.3% and 82.4%, respectively).

Pleural effusion Up to 500 mL of fluids can be missed with chest radiography. Pleural effusion is observed as anechoic or hypoechoic with lung ultrasound

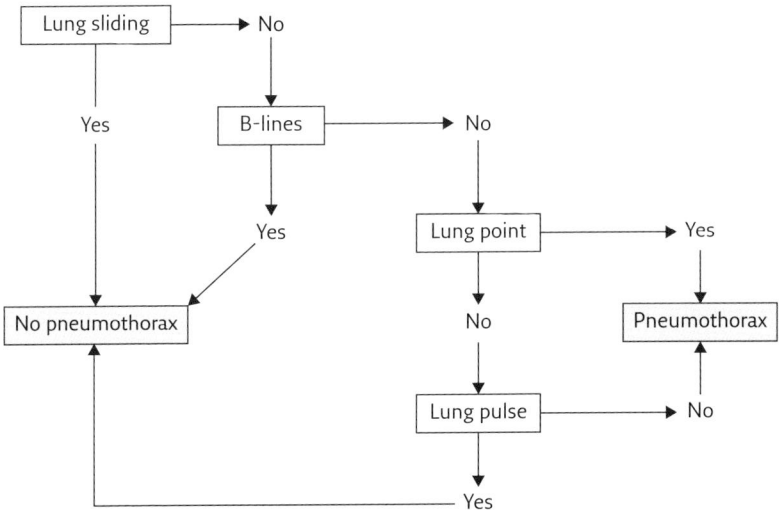

Figure 4. The pneumothorax decision tree, a flow chart for diagnosing pneumothorax. This suggests the correct sequence and combination of the four sonographic signs useful to rule out or rule in pneumothorax. Reproduced and modified from Volpicelli et al. *(2012) with permission.*

(figure 3). Lung ultrasound may reliably identify even 20 mL of fluid with almost 100% accuracy, as well as its size and nature, and may guide thoracentesis. After starting at the level of the diaphragm, the transducer should be placed in a longitudinal plane on the posterior axillary line with the transducer orientation marker pointed cephalad. Five structures must be identified to diagnose a pleural effusion: liver/spleen, diaphragm, pleural fluid, lung and ribs. The quad sign is an anechoic pocket of fluid contained between these borders. The sinusoid sign is a dynamic clue on M-mode when respiratory variation decreases the difference between parietal and visceral pleura in the presence of a pleural effusion.

Based on its sonographic appearance, the nature of the pleural effusion can be predicted and categorised. Simple pleural effusions (*i.e.* transudates) are anechoic, whereas exudates (such as complex pleural effusions and subacute haemothoraces) are subcategorised as homogeneously or heterogeneously echogenic, with/ without septations.

The size of a pleural effusion can also be determined. Although it is difficult to predict the precise volume, an effusion depth of >4–5 cm at the widest point will mean an effusion of at least 1000 mL. Another method is to multiply the maximal depth of fluid by a factor of 20.

Acute respiratory failure: the BLUE and FALLS protocols The BLUE protocol is an approach using lung and venous ultrasound to diagnose the main causes of acute respiratory failure. It uses a micro-convex probe at the standardised BLUE points and seven different profiles have been defined. The limitations of the protocol include its inability to exclude rarer diagnoses and that it has not been validated in the ICU. Lung ultrasound is also used in the assessment of patients with shock and as a guide for fluid management, as defined in the Fluid Administration Limited by Lung Sonography (FALLS) protocol. Further information, including the details of these protocols, is provided in the recommended reading list.

The differential diagnosis of acute respiratory failure is often challenging in the ICU. Lung ultrasound is a fast, accurate and valuable diagnostic tool in the critically ill with acute respiratory failure. A systematic diagnostic approach for evaluating acute respiratory failure with lung ultrasound is presented in figure 5.

A monitoring tool for the critically ill

The utility of lung ultrasound for monitoring the critically ill derives from the observation that repeated ultrasound evaluations can provide quantifiable measures of progressive aeration changes. Lung ultrasound is able to monitor aeration changes and the effect of therapy in the critically ill.

Monitoring pulmonary congestion Since a tight relationship has been detected between the number of B-lines and pulmonary congestion, lung ultrasound is a promising tool for monitoring pulmonary congestion. Quantification of pulmonary congestion may be obtained by dividing the anterolateral chest wall into eight or 11 regions, assigning a score of 1 to each region if multiple B-lines (at least three) are detected, and then comparing the observed changes over time. Another technique based on the assessment of 28 intercostal spaces can be used in the setting of outpatients with chronic cardiac diseases. A score of 0, 5 or 10 is

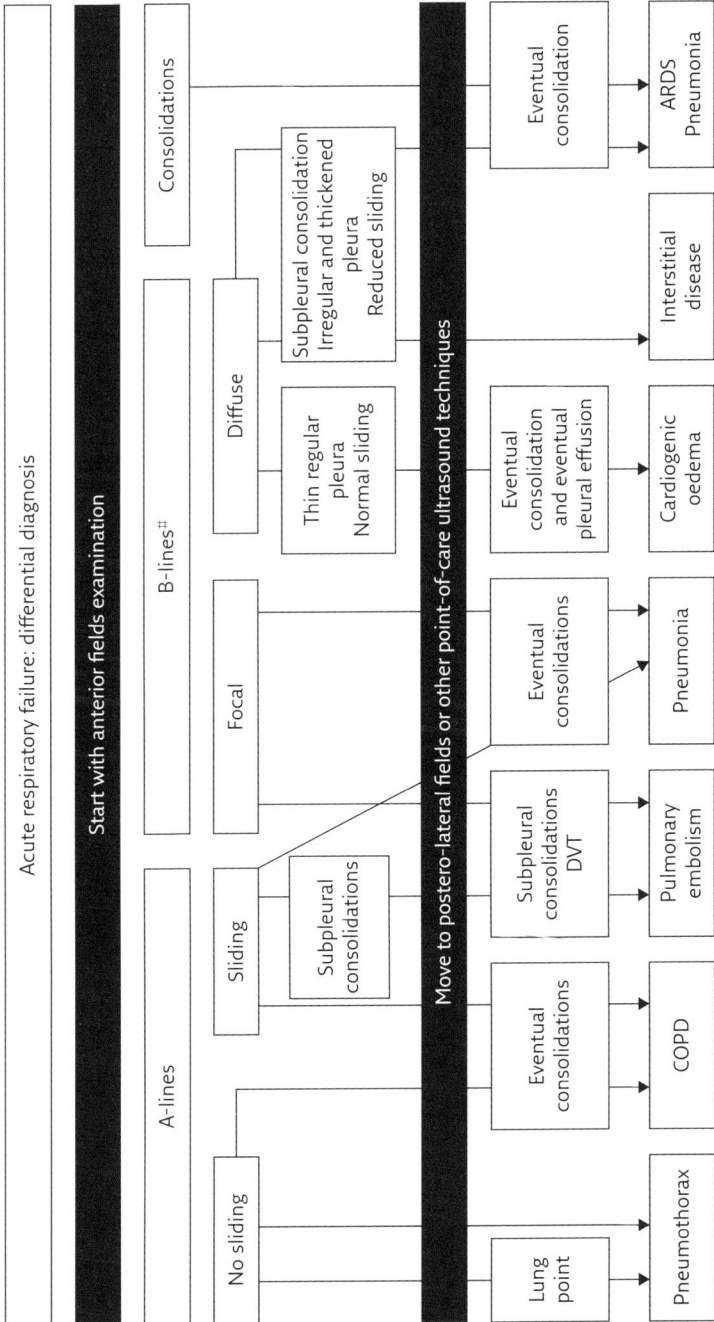

Figure 5. A systematic diagnostic approach for evaluating acute respiratory failure with lung ultrasound. DVT: deep venous thrombosis. #: at least three B-lines per scan. Reproduced and modified from Mojoli et al. (2019) with permission.

assigned to each scan, based on the absence of significant B-lines, the presence of multiple B-lines only visible in a part of the screen image, or multiple B-lines visible in most of or the whole image, respectively. This technique correlates well with radiological signs of extravascular lung water, lung density measured by means of CT scanning, transpulmonary thermodilution and gravimetric studies.

Monitoring pulmonary aeration A decrease in pulmonary aeration can be related to other conditions in the critically ill, so monitoring pulmonary aeration should also include the analysis of consolidations and the exploration of posterior regions. With this aim, two different lung ultrasound scores have been proposed and validated: the aeration score and the re-aeration/de-aeration score.

The aeration score measures the degree of lung aeration at a precise moment. It results from the conversion of lung aeration patterns into numeric values in each of the 12 regions defined at the International Consensus Conference on Lung Ultrasound. The score is allocated according to the worst ultrasound pattern observed in each region and can range from 0 to 3 (the higher the numeric value, the worse the aeration pattern), giving a final score from 0 to 36. For each region, a score of 0 corresponds to normal aeration (lung sliding and A-lines), 1 point to moderate loss of lung aeration related to interstitial syndrome (multiple spaced B-lines only visible in a limited area of the intercostal space), 2 points to severe loss of lung aeration related to alveolar-interstitial syndrome (multiple coalescent B-lines observed in the entire intercostal space) and 3 points to complete loss of lung aeration caused by alveolar consolidation.

The re-aeration/de-aeration score can be calculated by adding or subtracting changes in ultrasound pattern detected in each region of interest. This dynamic score allows us to compare changes in aeration between two different situations over time. The score is obtained for each region by adding a score of 1, 3 or 5 in case of a slight, moderate or substantial increase in lung aeration, respectively, or subtracting the same values in case of a decrease in aeration.

Both scores provide quantifiable and comparable measures of aeration and have been applied and validated in critically ill ventilated patients in different clinical conditions and at different times during their stay in the ICU. For example:

- When monitoring the evolution and assessing the effects of treatments in ventilator-acquired pneumonia, the re-aeration/de-aeration score was accurate in detecting significant variations following antimicrobial therapy and was thus able to differentiate a successful response from failure and appeared to be as accurate as CT scanning.
- When guiding PEEP titration and recruitment manoeuvres, the re-aeration score accurately assessed PEEP-induced alveolar recruitment in ARDS, and was equivalent to the pressure–volume curve method. The score also provided regional assessment of lung recruitment.
- In the setting of weaning, the aeration score was able to predict post-extubation failure/success. A score >17 was associated with failure in 85% of the cases, while <13 was associated with success. When lung ultrasound is combined with diaphragm and heart ultrasound during the weaning process, it gives even more valuable information.

- In patients monitored after cardiothoracic surgery, lung ultrasound can detect more post-operative pulmonary complications (seen as aeration changes) than chest radiography, particularly the clinically relevant complications and at an earlier time-point. Recent reports suggest that lung ultrasound may be used as the primary imaging technique to search for post-operative pulmonary complications after cardiothoracic surgery.
- When monitoring patients supported by ECMO, lung aeration scores can be used to predict mortality in ARDS patients requiring veno-venous ECMO, since a significant improvement in lung aeration was evident in survivors.

Limitations of lung ultrasound in the critically ill patient

Lung ultrasound evaluation in the critically ill patient has several limitations. Since ultrasound is a surface imaging technique, every alteration of the lung surrounded by normally aerated lung will not be visible with lung ultrasound. This is only partially relevant in critically ill patients as the diseases they are affected by are generally severe enough to extend to the visceral pleura. Lung ultrasound is extremely sensitive in assessing any worsening of lung aeration, regardless of whether this is related to an increase in fluids or to a pure deflation. However, it cannot be used to assess an increase in the amount of air starting from a condition of normal aeration, such as overdistension related to invasive ventilation or COPD. In addition, the technique may be problematic, especially in obese patients, since ICU patients are commonly in the supine position, under sedation and unable to follow commands for the posterior regions. The presence of subcutaneous emphysema, subcutaneous oedema, large dressings, bandages and drains may limit access to the chest wall and result in a suboptimal view. Lastly, despite its excellent sensitivity, it is unclear how to manage small lesions detected by lung ultrasound. Bearing these limitations in mind, lung ultrasound remains a fundamental tool to assess, diagnose and monitor the critically ill.

Further reading

- Doerschug KC, *et al.* (2013). Intensive care ultrasound: III. Lung and pleural ultrasound for the intensivist. *Ann Am Thorac Soc*; 10: 708–712.

- Gargani L (2011). Lung ultrasound: a new tool for the cardiologist. *Cardiovasc Ultrasound*; 9: 6.

- Jankowich M, *et al.*, eds. (2015). Ultrasound in the Intensive Care Unit. New York, Humana Press.

- Laursen CB, *et al.*, eds. (2018). Thoracic Ultrasound (ERS Monograph). Sheffield, European Respiratory Society.

- Lichtenstein DA (2015). BLUE-protocol and FALLS-protocol: two applications of lung ultrasound in the critically ill. *Chest*; 147: 1659–1670.

- Lichtenstein DA, ed. (2016). Lung Ultrasound in the Critically Ill: The BLUE Protocol. Cham, Springer.

- Mayo P, *et al.* (2016). Ultrasonography evaluation during the weaning process: the heart, the diaphragm, the pleura and the lung. *Intensive Care Med*; 42: 1107–1117.

- Mojoli F, *et al.* (2019). Lung ultrasound for critically ill patients. *Am J Respir Crit Care Med*; 199: 701–714.

- Volpicelli G (2013). Lung sonography. *J Ultrasound Med*; 32: 165–171.

- Volpicelli G, *et al.* (2012). International evidence-based recommendations for point-of-care lung ultrasound. *Intensive Care Med*; 38: 577–591.

- Volpicelli G, *et al.* (2014). Semi-quantification of pneumothorax volume by lung ultrasound. *Intensive Care Med*; 40: 1460–1467.

Monitoring respiratory muscles: respiratory muscle ultrasound

Pieter R. Tuinman and Nic Tjahjadi

Dysfunction of the main respiratory muscle, the diaphragm, is a frequently seen complication in critically ill patients. In patients receiving invasive ventilation, diaphragm dysfunction is associated with increased mortality and difficult weaning from invasive ventilation. A range of factors may cause diaphragm dysfunction in these patients, including disuse of muscles leading to atrophy. Also, patients with unexplained shortness of breath might have diaphragm dysfunction, which can be unilateral or bilateral. In these patients, the underlying causes of diaphragm dysfunction can be traumatic, neurological, inflammatory, due to myopathy, or idiopathic.

Current available diagnostic modalities to detect diaphragm dysfunction, such as chest radiography, diaphragm electromyography or pressure–flow recordings, have several limitations in terms of practicality, invasiveness and cost-effectiveness.

Key points

- Ultrasound is emerging as a diagnostic tool for the assessment of the respiratory muscles. It is radiation-free, noninvasive and easily available, and allows repeated measurements.

- The major indications of diaphragm ultrasound are assessment of dyspnoea of unknown origin, evaluation of diaphragm functionality and assessment of weaning outcome.

- Measurements of diaphragm thickness, thickening fraction and diaphragm excursion are used to quantify diaphragm atrophy, function and respiratory effort.

- Diaphragm ultrasound should be used in concert with clinical findings and other ultrasound findings, *e.g.* from lungs and heart.

- Pitfalls/limitations are that its use is restricted to specific clinical settings and there is potential for measurement error.

- Ultrasound of the expiratory muscles needs further validation before it can be used in clinical practice.

Over the past decade, diaphragm ultrasound has become a well-established tool to assess diaphragm function. Diaphragm ultrasound allows real-time visualisation of the diaphragm. Measurements of diaphragm thickness, thickening fraction (TF$_{di}$) and diaphragm excursion are used to quantify diaphragm function, atrophy and respiratory effort. The advantages of diaphragm ultrasound lie in the ability for it to be performed at the bedside, its cost-effectiveness and its noninvasiveness.

This chapter provides the bedside clinician with a succinct and pragmatic guide for the applications of diaphragm ultrasound. In addition, we give a short introduction on expiratory respiratory muscle ultrasound, along with its limitations and evidence gaps.

What is diaphragm ultrasound used for?

To diagnose diaphragm dysfunction Diaphragm ultrasound can be used to diagnose diaphragm function, and measurements are best obtained during assisted or spontaneous ventilation. Diaphragm thickening reflects the activity of this muscle during breathing and provides an estimate of its strength. The current gold standard method to detect diaphragm dysfunction is the phrenic stimulation technique, which quantifies the function of the diaphragm by measuring the negative pressure generated by the diaphragm (change in twitch pressure generated at the outside tip of the endotracheal tube ($P_{et,tw}$)). Diaphragm dysfunction is defined as $P_{et,tw}$ <11 cmH$_2$O. In patients under pressure support ventilation, TF$_{di}$ was strongly correlated to diaphragm function when compared to $P_{et,tw}$. For TF$_{di}$, a cut-off value of <30–36% is defined as the threshold for diaphragm dysfunction. More importantly, TF$_{di}$ has been shown to be a predictor of duration of invasive ventilation and adverse outcome.

M-mode ultrasound is used to quantify diaphragm excursion. Excursion can only be measured during spontaneous breathing (see the section on image acquisition for explanation). During quiet breathing, diaphragm dysfunction is defined as an excursion of <10–14 mm. At maximal inspiratory effort, an excursion of <25 mm corresponds with severe diaphragm dysfunction.

Diaphragm ultrasound is also of value in diagnosing diaphragmatic paralysis. When visualising the diaphragm in M-mode in healthy subjects, the diaphragm moves caudally and shows a steep lift during the sniffing test. In patients with diaphragmatic paralysis, the M-mode trace shows less or completely absent caudal movement during inspiration and paradoxical or cranial movement when performing the sniffing test.

Regardless of the ultrasound technique, diaphragm ultrasound has been shown to outperform traditional techniques such as fluoroscopy and chest radiography in diagnosing diaphragm dysfunction.

To assess weaning outcome Diaphragm ultrasound can be used to predict weaning outcome in mechanically ventilated patients. This is relevant, since failure of extubation is associated with longer time on invasive ventilation, clinical deterioration and a higher mortality rate. Cut-off values to predict weaning failure using TF$_{di}$ range from <30% to <36% and for excursion range from <10 to 14 mm for quiet breathing and <25 mm for deep breathing. TF$_{di}$ as an index for discontinuation from ventilation is superior to clinical parameters. Diaphragm ultrasound is especially useful to identify the mechanism explaining spontaneous breathing trial (SBT) outcome. Therefore, TFdi is best performed before the SBT, with the lowest level of assistance. Once an SBT is successful, the diaphragm may no longer be the major determinant of extubation outcome. In line with this, we advise not to use diaphragm ultrasound as a single parameter to assess weaning outcome, but to use a structured and integrated approach, combining clinical parameters, laboratory parameters and ultrasound parameters of diaphragm, heart and lungs.

To assess work of breathing Another potential application of diaphragm ultrasound is to measure work of breathing or the pressure–time product (PTPdi) during invasive ventilation (PTPdi per breath = average inspiratory pressure × time/number of breaths). Currently, measurement of both indices requires invasive pressure recordings. Work of breathing and PTPdi provide information about loading of the diaphragm and therefore allow the clinician to accurately control the ventilator support and to prevent over- and underassist of the diaphragm and potentially limit muscle injury or disuse atrophy. Several studies have been conducted demonstrating the relationship between ultrasound-measured TFdi and PTPdi or work of breathing. However, these studies have substantial limitations and show that ultrasound is not yet validated to quantify breathing effort and further research is needed.

Assessment of expiratory muscles: the abdominal muscle wall

The abdominal muscle wall is part of the expiratory respiratory muscle system. During quiet breathing, expiration is the result of relaxation of the diaphragm, which causes a positive intrathoracic pressure, and this causes the lungs to expel the air. There is little or no muscle contraction involved. During forceful expiration, the abdominal muscle wall and other accessory respiratory muscles cause an increase in intra-abdominal and intrathoracic pressure, which forces expiration. One could surmise that these muscles might play a more important role during respiratory dysfunction or respiratory disease that requires a higher work of breathing. Several studies have accurately described the sonographic measurement technique for the different muscles of the abdominal muscle wall, including the Musculus transversus abdominis (TA), Musculus obliquus internus (OI) and Musculus obliquus externus (OE). Measurement of abdominal muscle thickness is highly repeatable. The TA plays a major role during a progressive increase of expiratory effort and thus intra-abdominal pressure generation. There are no studies of sonographic measurement of abdominal wall muscles in critically ill patients and no studies on abdominal muscle wall ultrasound and outcome. Despite the increase of studies on the relationship between diaphragm thickness, excursion and outcome, research focused on the abdominal muscles is scarce. However, there is a possible value in studying the relationship between sonographic measurement of abdominal muscle and respiratory disease.

Image acquisition

Intercostal approach: diaphragm thickness and thickening fraction Thickness and TFdi can be measured in both B- and M-mode by using a high-frequency linear array probe (≥10 MHz). The probe is positioned in the so-called "zone of apposition", which is located between the 8th and 11th rib at the mid-axillary line or antero-axillary line (figure 1a). The zone of apposition is the area where the diaphragm and abdominal contents can be visualised in the same window. It is important to remember that this approach allows visualisation of one hemidiaphragm and not

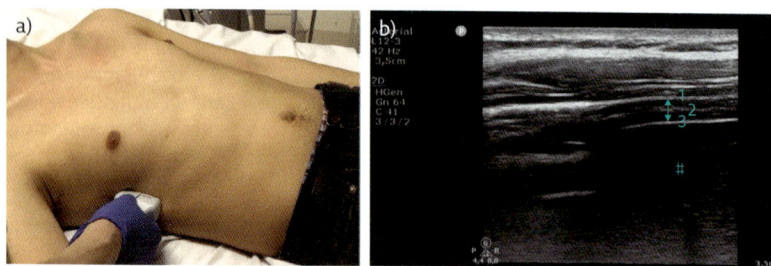

Figure 1. a) Measurement of diaphragm thickness in the zone of apposition using a linear transducer. b) B-mode ultrasound of the diaphragm. 1) Pleura; 2) fibrous layer in the centre of the diaphragm; 3) peritoneum. #: liver.

the whole diaphragm itself. Images obtained from the right hemidiaphragm offer better quality, since the liver provides an excellent ultrasound window. In the mid-axillary line, the diaphragm is visualised as a structure composed of three separate echogenic layers: the pleural membrane, a central tendinous layer and the peritoneal membrane (figure 1b). The diaphragm is the least echogenic structure in between the three layers. Reported mean diaphragm thickness in healthy volunteers is 1.6 mm (95% CI 1.5–1.7 mm). TF$_{di}$ can be calculated when diaphragm thickness is measured in M-mode at maximal inspiration and expiration (TF$_{di}$ = (end-inspiratory thickness – end-expiratory thickness)/end-expiratory thickness). There is a wide range of TF$_{di}$ values: it is 0–5% in patients under neuromuscular blockade, whereas it ranges between 20% and 50% in spontaneously breathing patients.

Subcostal approach: diaphragm excursion Diaphragm excursion is measured by using a low-frequency cardiac or abdominal probe (1–5 MHz). The low frequency of the probe provides measurement at a greater depth, at the expense of less spatial resolution. The probe should be positioned below the left or right costal arch on the midclavicular line, with the probe directed cranially and slightly tilted dorsally, aiming the ultrasound beam at the highest point of the diaphragmatic dome (figure 2a). At first, the two-dimensional mode is used to obtain the best view and to select an exploration line. Then the machine is switched to M-mode to display the motion of anatomical structures alongside the selected line (figure 2b). The sweep speed has to be carefully set (10 mm·s^{-1}) and it is important to keep the cursor as perpendicular as possible. The liver provides an acoustic window when imaging the right hemidiaphragm, whereas the spleen offers one for the left hemidiaphragm. The operator should identify a bright line right below the liver (or spleen) that moves caudally. Inspiration is displayed as caudal movement as the diaphragm moves towards the ultrasound probe (so the bright line moves up on the screen). Expiration is displayed as cranial movement as the diaphragm moves away from the probe. Diaphragm excursion can only be measured in individuals during spontaneous breathing, since active or passive displacement of the diaphragm cannot be distinguished during assisted ventilation. Therefore, when measuring diaphragm excursion in mechanically ventilated patients, all the assistance needs to be removed in order to obtain measurements. In cases where the patient is able to cooperate, ask the patient to provide maximal breathing effort. In healthy volunteers, diaphragm excursion is known to vary with sex, body

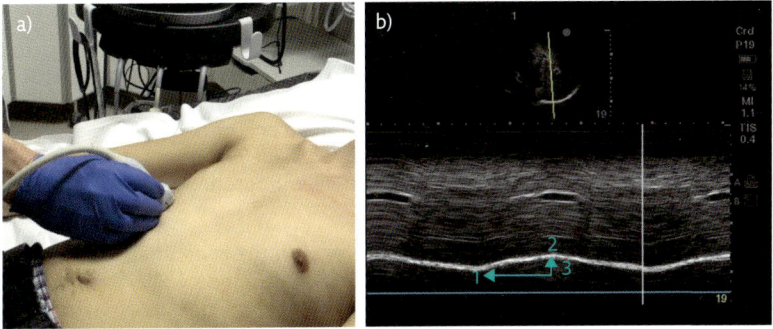

Figure 2. a) Measurement of diaphragm excursion using a cardiac transducer. b) M-mode ultrasound of the diaphragm. 1) Diaphragm at end expiration; 2) diaphragm at end inspiration; 3) diaphragm excursion.

height and weight, breathing state, intra-abdominal pressure and in the presence of respiratory illness.

For detailed descriptions of diaphragm ultrasound measurement techniques, we refer the reader to the further reading list at the end of this chapter.

Ultrasound of (abdominal) expiration muscles Abdominal wall muscle thickness is measured by using a linear array probe. Probe frequencies that have been used in several studies range from 5 to 10 MHz. The machine has to be put in B-mode. The patient is placed in a supine position and pillows are placed under the patient's knees for support. For measurement of antero-lateral muscles of the abdominal wall (TA, OI and OE), the probe is placed transversally and either on the right or left side of the abdominal wall, on the antero-axillary line, midway between the 12th rib and the anterior superior iliac spine (figure 3a and b). For measurement of the anterior abdominal wall muscle (Musculus rectus abdominis), the probe is placed 2–3 cm above the umbilicus and moved laterally from the midline until the muscle cross-section is visualised.

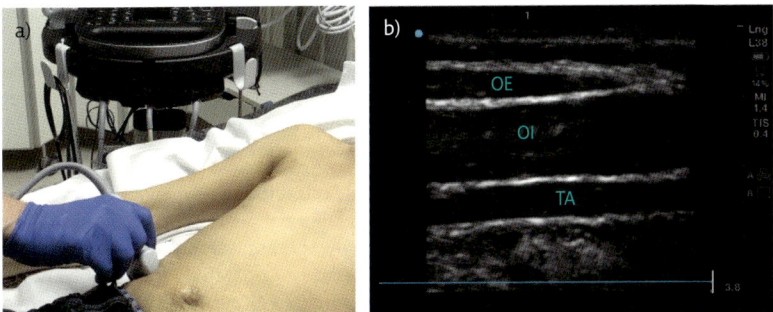

Figure 3. a) Measurement of antero-lateral abdominal muscle wall. The probe is placed on the antero-axillary line. b) Ultrasound of the abdominal wall muscles.

Pearls and pitfalls

During deep breathing and when visualising the right hemidiaphragm, the descending lung could mask the sonographic images and impede the measurement of total diaphragm excursion. In these circumstances, the probe could be tilted slightly caudally to maintain a perpendicular approach of the (right) diaphragm motion. Adjustment of the probe has no added value when measuring the left hemidiaphragm, since the spleen offers a smaller ultrasound window compared to the right hemidiaphragm.

When visualising and measuring the diaphragm in the zone of apposition, the diaphragm appears as a thin muscle with a mean thickness of 1.9 mm for men and 1.4 mm for women. When measuring diaphragm thickness in order to calculate the TF$_{di}$, changes <0.5 mm have to be accurately measured while the majority of ultrasound probes have a smallest measurable distance of <0.1 mm. This equals 5–7% of total diaphragm thickness. As previously mentioned, there is a wide range in cut-off values of TF$_{di}$ to predict the success rate of extubation; this means that small differences in measurement of thickness could influence the assessment of this parameter and ultimately influence clinical decision-making. Therefore, we advise that measurements have to be carefully performed. Possible pitfalls in measurement technique are the placement of the probe, probe position and angulation. Marking of the skin can improve reproducibility and repeatability.

Several factors influence diaphragmatic excursion measured by ultrasound, *e.g.* sex, age, patient position and both intrathoracic and intra-abdominal pressures. The transdiaphragmatic pressure is the result of the difference between the intrathoracic and intra-abdominal pressure. The diaphragm forces against the intra-abdominal pressure. The amount of transdiaphragmatic pressure is higher while in a supine position compared to while seated or semi-recumbent. This effect is stronger in patients with obesity, large pleural effusions or suffering from high intra-abdominal pressure, for instance as a result of COPD. Therefore, measurements have to be repeated in the same position to prevent measurement errors and variation in the evaluation of the diaphragm function. The timing of measurements during the SBT also influences results. Lastly, drainage of large pleural effusions can improve diaphragm excursions.

During invasive ventilation, diaphragm excursion cannot be used to assess diaphragm function and breathing effort. The caudal movement of the diaphragm may not only result from a negative intrathoracic pressure, but also from positive pressure enforced by the mechanical ventilator during inspiration. Hence, under these conditions, diaphragm excursion cannot be used to assess diaphragm function. Likewise, during controlled invasive ventilation, TF$_{di}$ cannot be assessed.

Most importantly, respiratory failure is a complex condition and its underlying cause is often multifactorial. It is generally a result of failure of heart, lungs and respiratory muscles or a combination of these. Accordingly, the assessment or follow-up of a patient with respiratory failure, diaphragm weakness or paralysis must not be done by ultrasound examination of the respiratory muscles alone. A holistic approach is of critical importance; hence, ultrasound of the diaphragm needs to be combined with ultrasound of the lungs and heart. In addition, ultrasound findings need to be assessed in concert with clinical examination, vital parameters and results from other diagnostic modalities such as laboratory tests or chest CT.

Summary

Diaphragm ultrasound is a noninvasive bedside test that allows real-time visualisation of diaphragm anatomy and function. Diaphragm dysfunction is diagnosed using diaphragm excursion with a cut-off of <10–14 mm and TF$_{di}$ with a cut-off of <30–36%. The literature suggests the use of diaphragm ultrasound in patients with dyspnoea of unknown origin and critically ill patients to diagnose diaphragm dysfunction or paralysis, to assess weaning outcome and to assess work of breathing. Although diaphragm ultrasound is promising, careful practice is essential, since there is a substantial risk of measurement error. In addition, diaphragm ultrasound should be used in concert with clinical findings and ultrasound findings from the lungs and heart. Ultrasound of the expiratory respiratory muscles needs further study before it can be used in clinical practice.

Further reading

- Dres M, *et al.* (2018). Diaphragm dysfunction during weaning from mechanical ventilation: an underestimated phenomenon with clinical implications. *Crit Care*; 22: 73.

- Dres M, *et al.* (2018). Diaphragm function and weaning from mechanical ventilation: an ultrasound and phrenic nerve stimulation clinical study. *Ann Intensive Care*; 8: 53.

- Goligher EC, *et al.* (2015). Measuring diaphragm thickness with ultrasound in mechanically ventilated patients: feasibility, reproducibility and validity. *Intensive Care Med*; 41: 642–649.

- Haaksma M, *et al.* (2017). Ultrasound to assess diaphragmatic function in the critically ill – a critical perspective. *Ann Transl Med*; 5: 114.

- Ishida H, *et al.* (2015). Correlation between abdominal muscle thickness and maximal expiratory pressure. *J Ultrasound Med*; 34: 2001–2005.

- Llamas-Alvarez AM, *et al.* (2017). Diaphragm and lung ultrasound to predict weaning outcome: systematic review and meta-analysis. *Chest*; 152: 1140–1150.

- Matamis D, *et al.* (2013). Sonographic evaluation of the diaphragm in critically ill patients. Technique and clinical applications. *Intensive Care Med*; 39: 801–810.

- Mayo P, *et al.* (2016). Ultrasonography evaluation during the weaning process: the heart, the diaphragm, the pleura and the lung. *Intensive Care Med*; 42: 1107–1117.

- Vivier E, *et al.* (2012). Diaphragm ultrasonography to estimate the work of breathing during non-invasive ventilation. *Intensive Care Med*; 38: 796–803.

- Zambon M, *et al.* (2017). Assessment of diaphragmatic dysfunction in the critically ill patient with ultrasound: a systematic review. *Intensive Care Med*; 43: 29–38.

Monitoring lung pathology: chest radiography and computed tomography

Lara Pisani, Giuseppe Francesco Sferrazza Papa and Davide Chiumello

Chest imaging in the ICU setting provides useful information for diagnosis, treatment and even, in some cases, prognosis. There are multiple imaging modalities available to the clinician caring for mechanically ventilated critically ill patients, including chest radiography, lung ultrasound, CT and less practical diagnostic studies, such as electrical impedance tomography and positron emission tomography or ventilation/perfusion scans. This chapter will discuss how chest radiography and CT may facilitate a patient's management during invasive ventilation. We will not discuss the role of bedside lung ultrasound, which is covered in the chapters "Monitoring lung aeration: lung ultrasound" and "Monitoring respiratory muscles: respiratory muscle ultrasound".

Key points

- Chest radiography plays a crucial role in monitoring ventilated critically ill patients, for whom the correct diagnosis, appropriate treatment and identification of complications are very important.

- Chest radiography is a readily available bedside diagnostic tool; however, supine position and other technical aspects can make its interpretation difficult.

- Chest radiography is often used to identify and quantify the presence of several conditions that may not be detected clinically, or contributes to the diagnostic approach by excluding alternative diagnoses.

- CT is the diagnostic gold standard of chest imaging and is an essential test for defining causes of acute respiratory failure in complicated or severe patients.

- Cost effectiveness of each CT request should be carefully balanced for invasively ventilated patients.

- CT should not be used as a routine monitoring tool; ultrasound and/or chest radiography may be more appropriate for this aim.

Chest radiography

Chest radiography is a readily available bedside diagnostic tool, making it more appealing than other imaging tests. For this reason, the conventional supine anteroposterior chest radiography plays a crucial role for monitoring ventilated critically ill patients, for whom the correct diagnosis, appropriate treatment and identification of complications are of considerable importance.

Role, principal aspects and limitations of chest radiography Although daily, routine chest radiography is no longer indicated in the ICU patient, it is often used for identifying and quantifying the presence of several conditions, and providing images of abnormalities in the heart, lung parenchyma, pleura, chest wall, diaphragm, mediastinum and hilum. It is also useful for detecting malposition and associated complications after insertion of an endotracheal tube, central venous catheters, pulmonary artery catheters, chest and nasogastric tubes (figure 1). In addition, chest radiography may also be used to follow the course of the abnormality, even in cases in which the initial diagnosis has been made using a CT scan.

In this regard, chest radiography is the preferred imaging modality in critical care settings both for the detection of new pulmonary infiltrates and for monitoring the response of pneumonia to therapy, with the possibility of identifying early complications including cavitations, abscesses, pneumothoraces and pleural effusions (figure 2).

However, it is also important to recognise that chest radiography cannot be used to confirm the diagnosis of all conditions. For example, in medical situations like pulmonary embolism (PE) or during an acute exacerbation in patients with COPD chest radiography is quite often completely normal. Therefore, chest radiography should only be used to contribute to the diagnostic approach by excluding

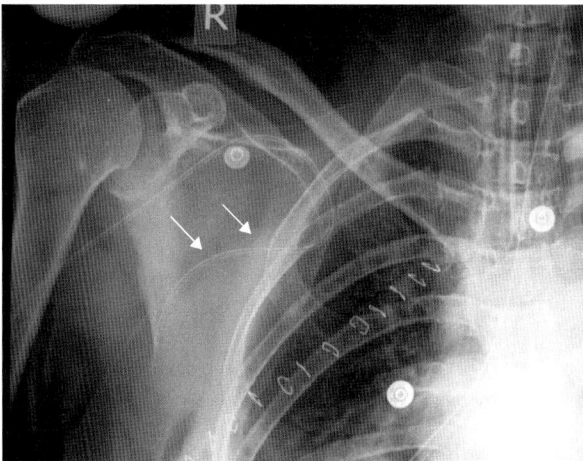

Figure 1. Chest radiograph showing malposition of the central venous catheter (path highlighted by white arrows) from right subclavian vein into axillary vein.

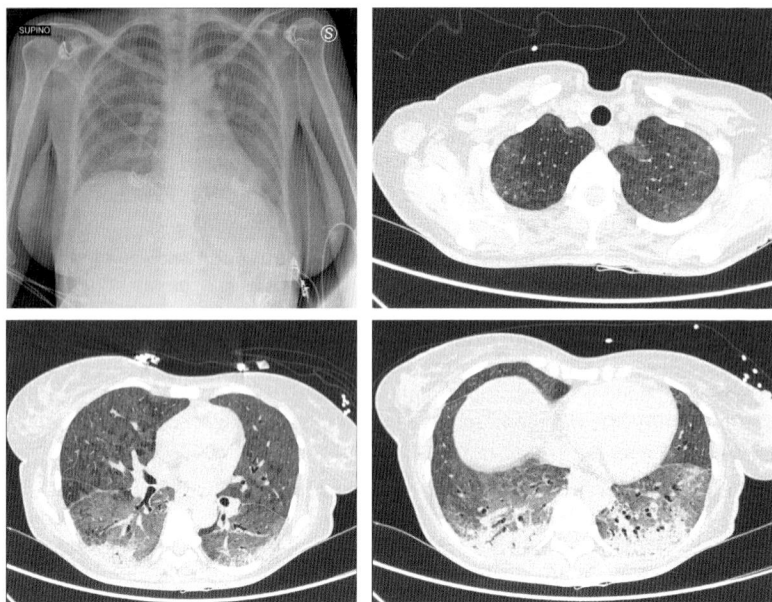

Figure 2. ARDS in a patient with a newly diagnosed HIV infection presenting with pneumocystis pneumonia. The CT scan shows bilateral, patchy consolidations with areas of ground-glass attenuation. An unremarkable chest radiography does not exclude parenchymal disease.

alternative diagnoses or ruling out conditions that mimic PE or such as atelectasis, pulmonary oedema, pleural effusions, pneumonia and pneumothorax.

Although many efforts have been made to improve the technical aspects, numerous limitations persist regarding the use of bedside chest radiography. These are related to:

- poor film quality,
- bedside attenuation factor,
- distance to the thorax, and
- synchronisation with invasive ventilation.

In addition, patients in the ICU are often not cooperative and this makes it difficult to position them correctly during the examination.

Even in optimal conditions, chest radiography is considered a moderately specific but not very sensitive examination in many conditions. This feature may explain the interobserver variability observed in many studies.

There are technical limitations in detecting pleural effusions on chest radiography, particularly when the pleural effusions are small and/or the patient is in the supine position. A previous report on the detection of pleural effusions on supine chest radiography showed an overall accuracy of 82%, with better results for larger pleural effusions (>300 mL). In this setting the role of imaging needs to be re-evaluated considering the increasing availability and safety of modalities such as ultrasound.

Finally, some underlying pathologies can mask concomitant problems. For example, although chest radiography is one of the criteria that defines ARDS (bilateral infiltrate on chest radiography that cannot be explained by effusion, a collapsed lung or lung nodule), the presence of a lung nodule can mask a concurrent new pulmonary infiltrate in ventilated critically ill patients.

Computed tomography

A CT scan is currently the gold standard for chest imaging. CT permits an anatomical study of the thorax including the lungs, mediastinum and hilum, and artificial airways. Notably, according to the clinical question, the airways maybe assessed by endoscopy. The diaphragm and other respiratory muscles are anatomically well defined with CT. However, the evaluation of respiratory muscle function requires tests that can easily capture movement, such as pulmonary function tests or ultrasound. In selected cases, magnetic resonance imaging (MRI) is also useful to study the chest wall and soft tissues; however, technical challenges mean MRI is currently impractical for routine study of ventilated patients.

Role, principal aspects and limitations of CT A key strength of CT is the great anatomical definition of virtually every region in the chest. Given the high amount of information, a detailed clinical question and the essential patient history is mandatory before referring a patient for a CT scan. Special consideration should be given to the challenge and risks of moving a mechanically ventilated patient to the radiology department for performing the examination.

In addition to the chest, CT of the neck should be requested to study artificial airways with granuloma, malacia or tube malpositioning.

To image the vascular system of the lung the injection of intravenous contrast media, mainly iodinated, is required. If PE is suspected, contrast CT angiography is a key test. Adequate renal function and the possibility of an adverse reaction to *i.v.* contrast media should be carefully checked before requesting a CT scan with contrast injection.

Practical limitations of CT CT requires a radiology room and the transportation of critically ill patients out of the ICU. Other costs of CT include exposure to ionising radiation and the risk of tube removal during transport. CT essentially provides an accurate picture of the chest. Therefore, to capture respiratory mechanics other dynamic tests are required.

Given the large amount of clinical information that a CT scan provides, an issue of modern medicine is the overuse of the technique. Notably, some clinical questions can be answered more easily with other, more cost-effective, imaging techniques.

Summary

In summary, chest radiography is an indispensable tool for critically ill ventilated patients in the ICU, while CT remains the reference diagnostic test to assess and monitor complicated, or severe, cases of acute respiratory failure. However, given its costs, CT should not routinely be used as first-line test if other imaging tests may be adequate to answer the clinical question. As logistical considerations are still a challenge, bedside-imaging techniques such as chest radiography and lung ultrasound should be considered.

Further reading

- Cardinale L, *et al.* (2012). Revisiting signs, strengths and weaknesses of standard chest radiography in patients of acute dyspnea in the emergency department. *J Thorac Dis*; 4: 398–407.

- Chiumello D, *et al.* (2019). ERS statement on chest imaging in acute respiratory failure. *Eur Respir J*; 54: 1900435.

- Eisenhuber E, *et al.* (2012). Bedside chest radiography. *Respir Care*; 57: 427–443.

- Gross BH, *et al.* (1994). Computed tomography of the chest in the intensive care unit. *Critical Care Clinics*; 10: 267–275.

- Raoof S, *et al.* (2012). Interpretation of plain chest roentgenogram. *Chest*; 141: 545-558.

Monitoring patient–ventilator interaction

Candelaria de Haro, Leonardo Sarlabous, José Aquino Esperanza,
Rudys Magrans and Lluís Blanch

Patient–ventilator asynchrony occurs when the phases of the breath delivered by the ventilator do not match the patient's respiratory centre output phases or when there is a mismatch between the patient's demand and the assistance offered by the ventilator. Poor patient–ventilator interaction could be associated with prolonged invasive ventilation, ICU and hospital stay, increased mortality, and could also be associated with higher rates of tracheostomy, discomfort, anxiety, dyspnoea and adverse events like self-extubation.

Poor patient–ventilator interaction is frequent in patients under controlled invasive ventilation, even during assisted ventilation, but is often underdiagnosed. Asynchronies are present during all periods of invasive ventilation (with minimal differences between day and night), in all modes and can occur in isolation or in clusters. Recognition requires clinical observation of the patient and ventilator waveforms at the bedside, but is not always possible throughout all periods of invasive ventilation. Treatment of patient–ventilator asynchrony requires comprehension of the physiological principles of respiratory mechanics and critical care practice to recognise the cause, in order to apply the optimal strategy to correct them.

Asynchronies can be classified depending on the phase of the respiratory cycle in which they appear. Thus, identification and treatment of patient–ventilator asynchrony is a complex process which involves the interaction of the ventilator with the lungs, respiratory muscles and respiratory centre output.

Key points

- Poor patient–ventilator interaction is associated with adverse outcomes.

- Asynchronies are frequent but underrecognised, and tend to occur in clusters over time rather than permanently.

- Asynchronies can be detected by analysis of waveforms from the ventilator, oesophageal pressure traces using an oesophageal balloon-tipped catheter, diaphragm electromyography or using automated algorithms.

Ineffective efforts

Ineffective inspiratory efforts (figure 1) are the most frequent asynchrony, and can be recognised during mechanical inspiration or expiration. Usually the causes are:

- inadequate trigger sensitivity,
- excessive assistance,
- pulmonary hyperinflation,
- low respiratory drive, or
- hypocapnia.

Depending on the cause, the treatment will involve an adjustment of the level of assistance and the cycling from inspiration to expiration, a decrease in sedation and/or an adjustment to adequate trigger sensitivity. Interestingly, clusters of ineffective

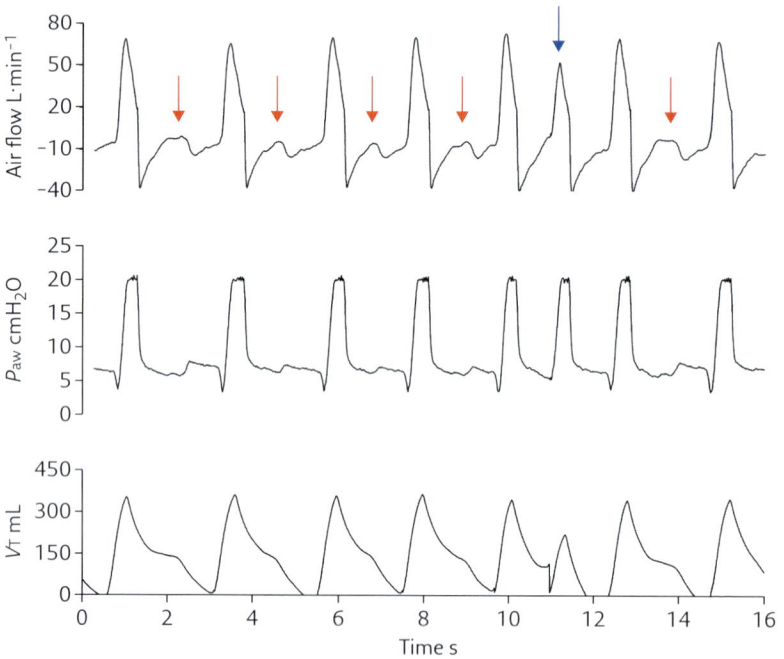

Figure 1. Traces of air flow, airway pressure (Paw) and VT in a mechanically ventilated patient on pressure support ventilation. Ineffective inspiratory efforts are present during expiratory periods. A decrease in Paw together with an increase in air flow not followed by a ventilator breath during expiration is suggestive of an ineffective inspiratory effort (red arrows). This asynchrony occurs when the patient's attempt to initiate a breath does not reach the ventilator's trigger threshold. In this example, the respiratory rate of the patient is almost double the mechanical breaths delivered by the ventilator. Autotriggering, defined as a cycle delivered by the ventilator and not triggered by the patient (no deflection in Paw trace), can also be observed (blue arrow). During pressure support ventilation, where all breaths are patient triggered, autotriggering occurs due to cardiogenic oscillations, condensed water inside the tubing circuit or leaks in the ventilator circuit.

inspiratory efforts are often present in mechanically ventilated critically ill patients and are associated with prolonged invasive ventilation and increased mortality.

Flow dyssynchrony

Inspiratory flow mismatching occurs when the ventilator fails to meet the patient's flow demand. This is usually because:

- ventilator flow delivery is set inappropriately low, or
- the combination of V_T and inspiratory time does not result in adequate air flow to fulfil the patient's demands (figure 2).

Inspiratory flow mismatching is more frequent in ventilation modes where it is impossible to modify the flow, such as volume assist-controlled mode with square flow. Inspiratory flow mismatching could be improved by increasing

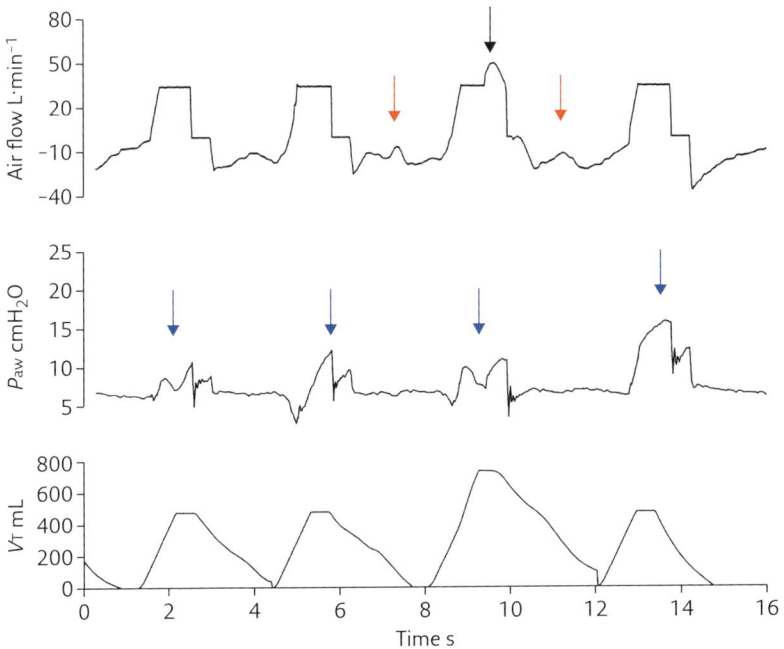

Figure 2. Example of inspiratory flow mismatching (also named flow starvation), which occurs when the ventilator fails to meet the patient's flow demand. In this case, ventilator air flow is set inappropriately low (34 L·min⁻¹) to fulfil the patient's high inspiratory flow demands which are different from breath to breath. The ventilator setting corresponds to volume assist-controlled mode with square flow. Different intensities of inspiratory efforts coexist during inspiration. P_{aw} appears pulled down (compared with an almost theoretical passive breath) because inspiratory effort persists during the inspiration period (blue arrows). Interestingly, when the inspiratory effort is strong enough, the patient can get some extra air flow at the end of inspiratory period in this particular ventilator (black arrow). Moreover, the patient's respiratory rate is greater than the set respiratory rate in the ventilator and some inspiratory ineffective efforts during expiration can be observed (red arrows).

ventilator flow delivery or by using the variable flow pressure-limited breath. Inspiratory flow mismatching could be particularly deleterious during lung-protective ventilation because vigorous inspiratory efforts could promote elevated transpulmonary pressures, overdistention and pulmonary oedema by increasing the transvascular pressure gradient. Moreover, inadequate pressurisation of the system could induce a respiratory sensation of flow starvation.

Double cycling

Double cycling occurs when the patient's neural time is longer than the ventilator inspiratory time. When the patient's effort is strong enough, a second breath can be triggered with no or minimal expiration (known as double cycling or breath stacking) (figure 3) resulting in a potentially dangerous higher V_T. Double cycling might be infrequent, but it occurs in all patients and its distribution and clustering

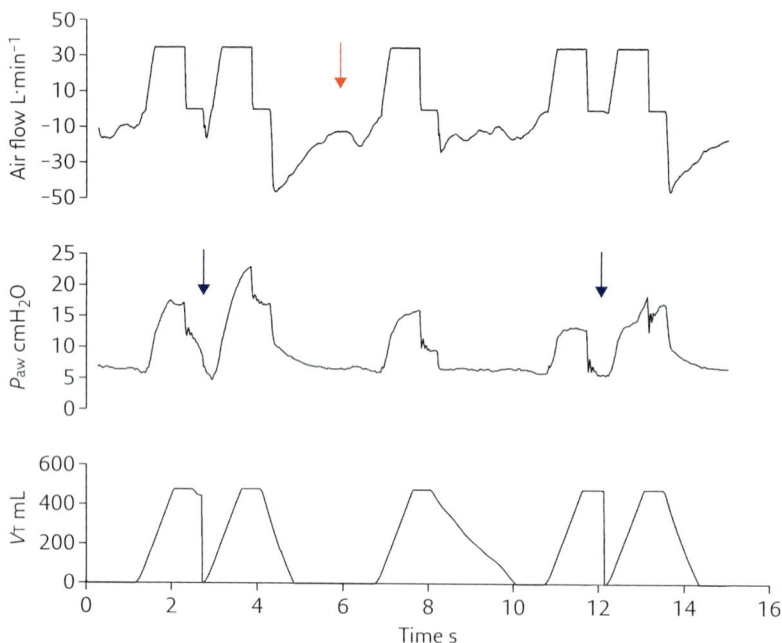

Figure 3. Traces obtained in the same patient shown in figure 2. In this clinical situation, the sustained inspiratory effort persists beyond the ventilator inspiratory time, cessation of inspiratory flow or the beginning of mechanical expiration, and thus triggers a second ventilator breath (blue arrows), which may or may not be followed by a short expiration. Breath stacking occurs when all or a portion of the volume from the previous breath is not entirely exhaled and is therefore added to the second breath. In the figure, a set inspiratory V_T of 476 mL is shown. The delivered volume accumulated during double triggering could be very high, possibly even doubling the set V_T in double-triggered breaths without expiration between them. This might result in overinflation, which can lead to VILI. This situation, which usually occurs in patients with poor patient–ventilator interaction, may coexist with other asynchronies such as ineffective expiratory efforts during expiration (red arrow).

over time varies widely among patients. The delivered volume accumulated during double cycling and breath stacking is very high, sometimes even doubling the V_T of normal breaths in volume-targeted modes resulting in overinflation and potential VILI. Moreover, clusters of double cycling could increase the mechanical power transferred from the ventilator to lungs.

Identification of double cycling requires optimisation of inspiratory flow to the patient's demand to correct it. An increase in mechanical inspiratory time or switching from assist volume- or pressure-controlled modes to pressure support or proportional modes might correct double cycling.

Reverse trigger (entrainment phenomenon)

Reverse triggering (figures 4 and 5) is a form of asynchrony reflecting an abnormal relationship between the ventilator and the patient, where mechanical insufflations generated by the ventilator elicit a reflexive neural response from the patient and triggers a muscular effort. Causes of this type of asynchrony include:

- oversedation,
- pulmonary hyperinflation, and
- entrainment phenomenon, which seems to be a reflex to external stimuli imposed by the ventilator respiratory rate that appears to match the patient respiratory centre.

Treatment will involve in a decrease in sedation and/or reducing overdistention. However, in some patients with reverse trigger reducing sedation may be inappropriate, in such cases, neuromuscular blocking agents may be necessary to abolish the reverse trigger. When the patient's effort is sufficiently deep and long, the decrease in P_{aw} can trigger a second ventilator breath with a nil or very short expiratory time. The consequences of the resultant double cycling with breath stacking can induce lengthening contractions and periodic lung overdistention with the of potential for VILI.

Phase dyssynchrony

Phase asynchronies occur when there is a mismatch between the start or the end of the patient's inspiratory time and the ventilator's inspiratory time. Short or premature cycling occurs when patient's inspiratory time is longer than ventilator's inspiratory time (figure 6). The patient's inspiratory muscles are still active when the ventilator starts expiration, impeding elastic recoil and peak expiratory flow is aborted. If the patient's inspiratory effort is strong enough a second breath can be triggered with no or minimal expiration (double cycling and breath stacking). Prolonged or delayed cycling occurs when patient's inspiratory time is shorter than ventilator's inspiratory time (figure 7). In this situation, the patient starts to exhale when the airway is still pressurised from ventilator inflow and tries to exhale activating the expiratory muscles.

Unplanned extubations

Poor patient–ventilator interaction is also seen as a prior event to an unplanned extubation, which has been recently recognised as a quality of care indicator, with very variable incidence worldwide. Different types of asynchronies, such as flow dyssynchrony, double cycling and phase asynchronies could be observed in the hours prior to an unplanned extubation (figure 8). The clinical value of these

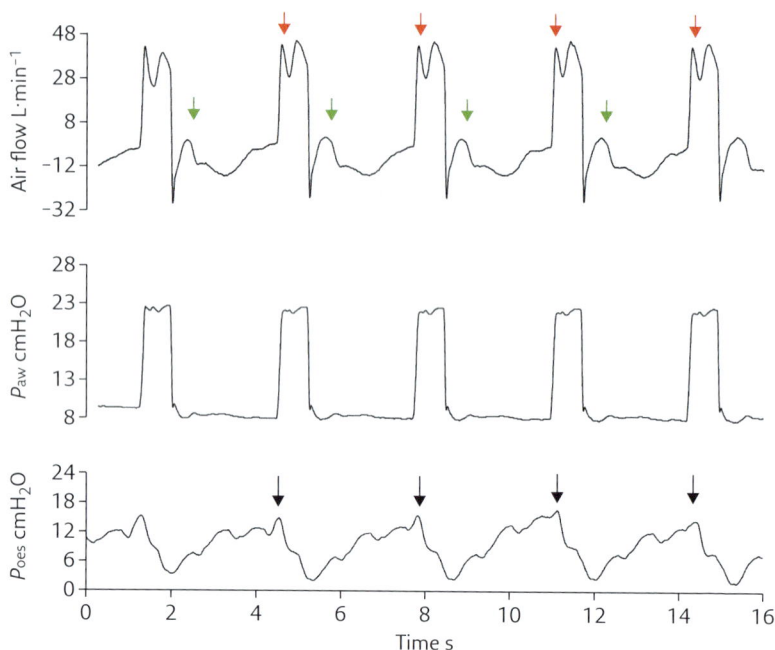

Figure 4.   Example of reverse triggering resulting in an ineffective effort in a patient ventilated with pressure assist-controlled mode. Ventilator insufflations trigger diaphragmatic muscle contractions in response to passive insufflations of the lungs. The oesophageal pressure (P_{oes}) trace shows a decrease in pressure indicating muscular contraction after the time-cycled ventilation insufflations (black arrows). In the absence of monitoring P_{oes} or electrical activity of the diaphragm, an increase in expiratory flow or decrease in inspiratory P_{aw} later in the respiratory cycle can indicate the event (red arrows). In this particular case, reverse triggering occurs at 190 ms after the beginning of mechanical insufflation. If patient's inspiratory effort persists beyond the machine breath, the patient's inspiratory muscles are still active at the beginning of expiration, impeding the elastic recoil of the respiratory system from increasing alveolar pressure, and peak expiratory flow is markedly reduced (green arrows). In this example, reverse triggering occurs as a fixed, repetitive and temporal relationship between mechanical insufflations and patient's neural inspiration (entrainment phenomenon). Image courtesy of L. Brochard (Interdepartmental Division of Critical Care Medicine, University of Toronto, Toronto, ON, Canada) and T. Pham (Keenan Research Centre and Li Ka Shing Knowledge Institute, St. Michael's Hospital, Toronto, ON, Canada).

types of patient–ventilator interactions during this critical moment have yet to be described.

Assessment of asynchronies

Detection of asynchronies can be made using several different techniques:

- analysis of waveforms provided from the ventilator of flow–time, pressure–time and integrated volume,
- the addition of oesophageal tracings using an oesophageal balloon-tipped catheter,

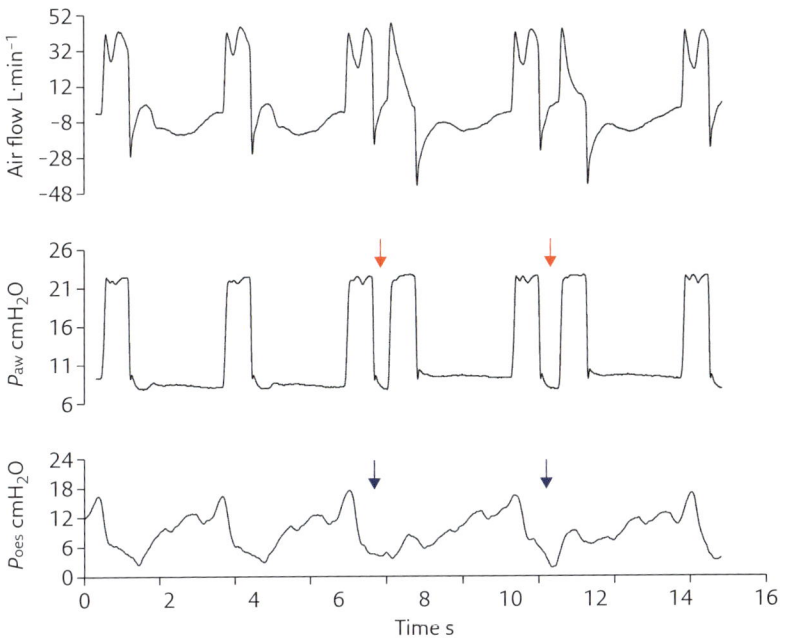

Figure 5. Example of reverse triggering resulting in double cycling in a patient ventilated with pressure assist-controlled mode. The P_{oes} trace shows a decrease in pressure indicating muscular contraction after the time-cycled ventilation insufflations (blue arrows) and is strong enough to trigger a ventilator breath (red arrows). Image courtesy of L. Brochard and T. Pham.

- diaphragmatic electromyography (commercially available in some ventilators), and
- automated algorithms.

The inspection of waveforms from the ventilator screen may provide clues for identifying patient–ventilator dyssynchrony. Recent studies have demonstrated that bedside interpretations of air flow and P_{aw} are helpful for recognising patient–ventilator asynchrony and optimising ventilator settings. It is noteworthy that the ability of clinicians to properly identify these features by visual inspection is partially influenced by their expertise and by the type of dyssynchrony. Moreover, the analysis of breath-to-breath waveforms alone has a very low sensitivity and positive predictive value (22% and 32%, respectively) even among trained physicians, who were able to recognise less than one third of asynchronies. By contrast, a high negative predictive value (close to 90%) is achieved by this method. Additional analysis of P_{oes} traces could help to improve the process and favour better recognition. Unfortunately, it is a minimally invasive manoeuvre that is not routinely used in mechanically ventilated patients that requires experience for proper placing and interpretation.

Electromyographic activity of the diaphragm (EA_{di}), which is commercially available in Servo I ventilators (Maquet, Solna, Sweden) in neurally adjusted ventilator assist

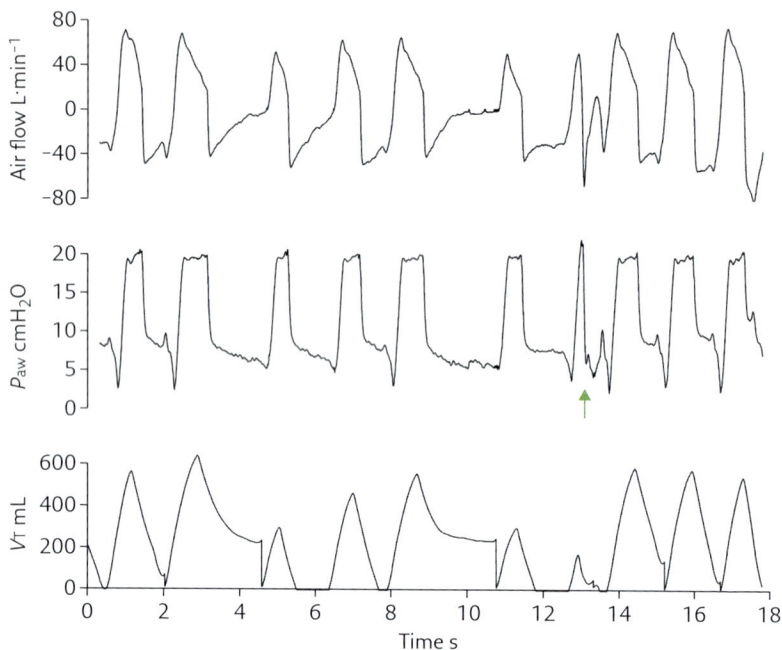

Figure 6. Traces of air flow, Paw and VT in a mechanically ventilated patient on pressure support ventilation. In this mode, each breath is patient triggered and cycling from inspiration to expiration occurs when air flow decreases to a set percentage of peak inspiratory air flow. Short or premature cycling ensues when mechanical insufflation ends before neural inspiration. Therefore, the patient's inspiratory muscles are still active at the beginning of expiration impeding the elastic recoil of the respiratory system. When the inspiratory effort is strong enough, it can trigger a second mechanical breath before complete exhalation resulting in an increase in VT. A short cycle is identified as an inspiratory time less than one-half of the mean inspiratory time (green arrow). Identification of short cycled breaths often requires monitoring Poes or electrical activity of the diaphragm.

(NAVA) mode, provides a reliable insight into patient inspiratory and expiratory time and has been used to detect asynchronies. Supporting ventilation based on EAdi signal should improve the response of the ventilator and synchrony, given that the signal closely reflects the neural time of the control of breathing. Moreover, a direct comparison of asynchronies detection in ICU patients using waveforms analysis or EAdi during the weaning phase has shown that double, premature and late cycling, as well as asynchrony index, were more frequently detected utilising EAdi. Unfortunately, NAVA is only available in Servo I ventilators, and careful adjustments for correct positioning must be made with periodic checks for catheter displacement.

More recently, automated detection algorithms have been developed and validated using the continuous analysis of the flow–time and pressure–time traces to detect asynchronies. There are several available, with different algorithms as well as performances. The BetterCare system (BetterCare, Barcelona, Spain) is one

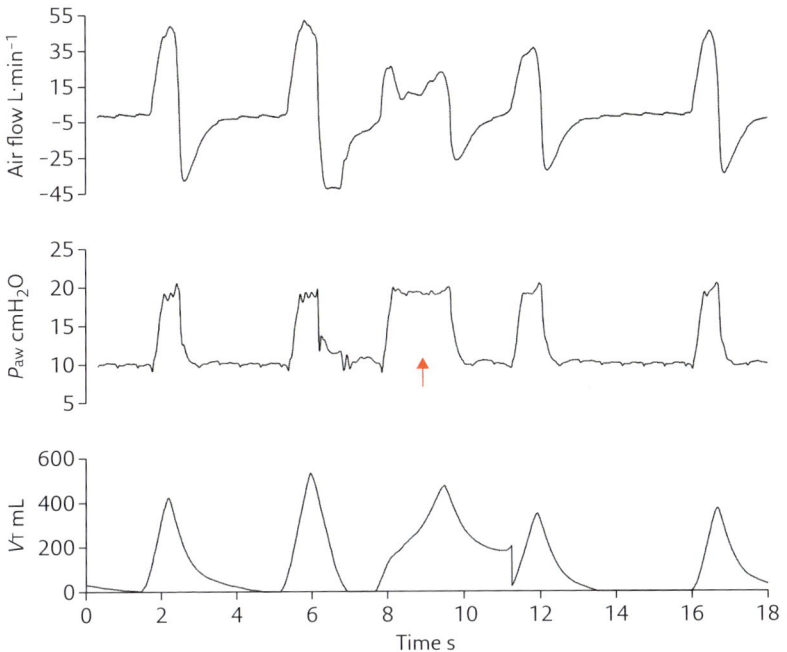

Figure 7. Traces of air flow, Paw and VT in a mechanically ventilated patient on pressure support ventilation. In this mode, each breath is patient triggered and the cycling from inspiration to expiration occurs when air flow decreases to a set percentage of peak inspiratory air flow. Prolonged or delayed cycling (red arrow) occurs when mechanical insufflation continues after neural inspiration has ceased or even during active expiration. High levels of pressure support and increased air flow resistance are predisposing factors. Persistence of mechanical inflation during neural expiration is uncomfortable and patients may exhibit expiratory muscle activity. Identification of prolonged cycled breaths often requires monitoring Poes and gastric pressures.

such algorithm, which could be adapted to any ventilator, that has been validated for the automated detection of ineffective efforts during expiration with a high positive and negative predictive value compared either with expert judgement or physiological measurements obtained by EAdi. There are many other algorithms available (*e.g.* VentMAP platform (University of California Davis, Davis, CA, USA), NeuroSync index (Dr Beck and Dr Sinderby, Toronto, ON, Canada)). We believe that, given the pattern of appearance of patient–ventilator asynchronies over time (these have recently been shown to occur in clusters rather than fixed), automated software for detection and prediction, as well as intelligent alarms, would be more helpful and more accurate in improving patient care during invasive ventilation than visual inspection of the waveforms in a fixed manner, especially given that the latter is time-consuming and the absence of patient–ventilator asynchronies during the observation period does not mean that they would not appear at a later point.

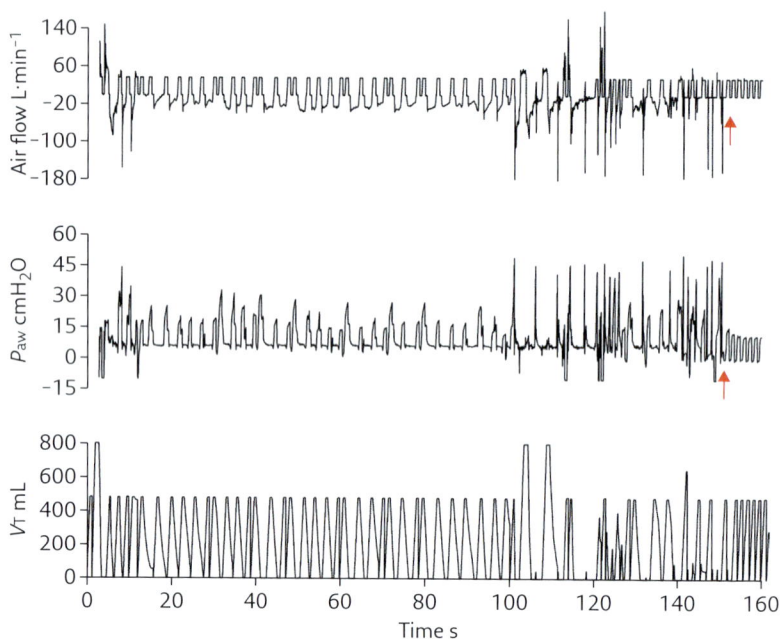

Figure 8. Traces of air flow, Paw and VT in a patient with poor patient–ventilator interaction that ended with an unplanned extubation. The traces show high respiratory rate, repetitive episodes of double and triple cycling with a concomitant deleterious increases in Paw and VT, cough, probably secretions and a final minute of severe fighting with the ventilator. Unplanned extubation and ventilator disconnection is shown when Paw suddenly decreases and no expiratory flow is observed (red arrows).

The figures in this chapter provide a graphical representation and brief explanation of the different types of asynchronies. Although many questions about asynchronies remain unanswered, for example regarding their management and even the effect on outcomes, reducing asynchronies by adapting the ventilator to the patient's demands is feasible and may improve clinical outcomes. Since identification at the bedside can be difficult, technological advances with intelligent algorithms could be a helpful tool in order to identify or predict asynchronies and generate alarms.

Further reading

- Akoumianaki E, *et al.* (2013). Mechanical ventilation-induced reverse-triggered breaths. *Chest*; 143: 927–938.

- Blanch L, *et al.* (2012). Validation of the Better Care® system to detect ineffective efforts during expiration in mechanically ventilated patients: a pilot study. *Intensive Care Med*; 38: 772–780.

- Blanch L, *et al.* (2015). Asynchronies during mechanical ventilation are associated with mortality. *Intensive Care Med*; 41: 633–641.

- Chanques G, *et al.* (2013). Impact of ventilator adjustment and sedation-analgesia practices on severe asynchrony in patients ventilated in assist-control mode. *Crit Care Med*; 41: 2177–2187.

- de Haro C, *et al.* (2018). Double cycling during mechanical ventilation: frequency, mechanisms, and physiologic implications. *Crit Care Med*; 46: 1385–1392.

- de Vries HJ, *et al.* (2019). Respiratory entrainment and reverse triggering in a mechanically ventilated patient. *Ann Am Thorac Soc*; 16: 499–505.

- de Wit M (2011). Monitoring of patient-ventilator interaction at the bedside. *Respir Care*; 56: 61–72.

- Gilstrap D, *et al.* (2013). Patient-ventilator interactions. Implications for clinical management. *Am J Respir Crit Care Med*; 188: 1058–1068.

- Kondili E, *et al.* (2009). Identifying and relieving asynchrony during mechanical ventilation. *Expert Rev Respir Med*; 3: 231–243.

- Marchuk Y, *et al.* (2018). Predicting patient-ventilator asynchronies with hidden Markov models. *Sci Rep*; 8: 17614.

- Marini JJ, *et al.* (1986). The inspiratory workload of patient-initiated mechanical ventilation. *Am Rev Respir Dis*; 134: 902–909.

- Murias G, *et al.* (2016). Does this ventilated patient have asynchronies? Recognizing reverse triggering and entrainment at the bedside. *Intensive Care Med*; 42: 1058–1061.

- Murias G, *et al.* (2016). Patient–ventilator asynchrony. *Curr Opin Crit Care*; 22: 53–59.

- Parthasarathy S, *et al.* (1998). Cycling of inspiratory and expiratory muscle groups with the ventilator in airflow limitation. *Am J Respir Crit Care Med*; 158: 1471–1478.

- Pham T, *et al.* (2018). Asynchrony consequences and management. *Crit Care Clin*; 34: 325–341.

- Schmidt M, *et al.* (2014). Unrecognized suffering in the ICU: addressing dyspnea in mechanically ventilated patients. *Intensive Care Med*; 40: 1–10.

- Sottile PD, *et al.* (2018). The association between ventilator dyssynchrony, delivered tidal volume, and sedation using a novel automated ventilator dyssynchrony detection algorithm. *Crit Care Med*; 46: e151–e157.

- Subirà C, *et al.* (2018). Minimizing asynchronies in mechanical ventilation: current and future trends. *Respir Care*; 63: 464–478.

- Telias I, *et al.* (2018). Is my patient's respiratory drive (too) high? *Intensive Care Med*; 44: 1936–1939.

- Thille AW, *et al.* (2006). Patient-ventilator asynchrony during assisted mechanical ventilation. *Intensive Care Med*; 32: 1515–1522.

- Thille AW, *et al.* (2008). Reduction of patient-ventilator asynchrony by reducing tidal volume during pressure-support ventilation. *Intensive Care Med*; 34: 1477–1486.

- Tobin MJ (2018). Nobel prize symposium Physiologic basis of mechanical ventilation. *Ann Am Thorac Soc*; 15: Suppl. 1, S49–S52.

- Vaporidi K, *et al.* (2017). Clusters of ineffective efforts during mechanical ventilation: impact on outcome. *Intensive Care Med*; 43: 184–191.

- Yoshida T, *et al.* (2017). Fifty years of research in ARDS: spontaneous breathing during mechanical ventilation risks, mechanisms and management. *Am J Respir Crit Care Med*; 195: 985–992.

Extracorporeal lung support

Christoph Fisser and Thomas Bein

In acute severe life-threatening lung failure, the use of ECMO is an "ultima ratio" strategy for the prevention or therapy of severe hypoxaemia. According to the recommendations of the European Branch of the Extracorporeal Life Support Organization (EuroELSO) ECMO is indicated in:

- patients with a high risk of death despite optimisation of conventional treatment,
- with a potentially reversible disease, and
- in the absence of contraindications.

The use of ECMO as a bridging rescue therapy has increased over the past two decades, since ECMO systems have evolved to a more miniaturised form with improved biocompatibility and less complications leading to their widespread use.

In addition, the technique of extracorporeal carbon dioxide removal ($ECCO_2$-R) is of increasing interest for certain indications (*i.e.* exacerbations of COPD, moderate ARDS, "ultra"-protective ventilation, reversal of decompensated hypercapnia/acidosis and hypercapnic weaning failure). $ECCO_2$-R is aimed at removing predominantly carbon dioxide by "medium" ECMO flow. The technique is based on the physiological finding that the diffusion capacity for carbon dioxide is far higher than for oxygen, facilitating effective carbon dioxide removal with lower blood flow rates than those required for oxygenation. However, no large prospective randomised studies in terms of an influence on mortality exist for the use of $ECCO_2$-R systems, and a benefit has only been shown in case reports or (retrospective) observational studies.

Key points

- The technique of extracorporeal oxygenation and carbon dioxide removal substitutes the gas exchange functions of the injured native lung either in part or totally.

- Such a strategy has implications for invasive ventilation: the F_{IO_2} can be reduced, the necessity for recruitment is attenuated, and consequently, the principles of lung protection (low V_T or ΔP, adapted respiratory rate) can be followed.

- Weaning from invasive ventilation and from ECMO requires a specific strategy, including an ECMO withdrawal trial.

In this chapter we discuss the effects of ECMO or $ECCO_2$-R on the capacity and mechanics of the "native" lung and we derive from these findings a strategy for invasive ventilation under extracorporeal support.

The effects of extracorporeal lung support on the native lung

During extracorporeal support the gas exchange functions of the natural (injured) lung may be completely (ECMO) or partly ($ECCO_2$-R) substituted, depending on the extracorporeal blood and sweep gas flow, with the aim of "buying time" for the healing process of the lung. The lung of a patient suffering from ARDS is usually characterised by three compartments:

1) Regions with overdistended and/or normally distended alveoli in the nondependent parenchyma
2) Regions with normal ventilation (V')/perfusion (Q') ratios in the middle part, tending towards a progressive increase in alveoli characterised by a lower than normal V'/Q'
3) In the dependent lung parenchyma most regions are compressed or consolidated

Therefore, invasive ventilation (without extracorporeal lung support) will typically lead to high dead space ventilation in the upper, nondependent parts of the lung, while in the middle and lower parts a high amount of intrapulmonary shunt can be found, and an effective gas exchange can be achieved only partly by recruitment (high PEEP). From this model it is evident that invasive ventilation conducted to correct hypoxaemia and/or hypercapnia combined with a lung protective strategy is difficult to accomplish.

In this scenario ECMO or $ECCO_2$-R will have two main effects, which should have consequences for the ventilation of the native lung:

• An increase of the mixed-venous oxygen saturation and the resolution of critical hypoxaemia
• The removal of the metabolically produced carbon dioxide

How extracorporeal lung support changes the strategy of invasive ventilation

As extracorporeal lung support improves oxygenation and decarboxylation of the blood, the invasiveness of invasive ventilation strategy can be decreased to allow (more) protective ventilation. A "ventilatory rest" of the native lung should enable a reduction of the deleterious effects of invasive ventilation (volutrauma, barotrauma and atelectrauma) to give the lung a better (and faster?) chance to heal. The artificial oxygenation in situations of life-threatening hypoxaemia might enable a reduction in recruitment requirements (high PEEP, which often is associated with overdistention) and a reduction in the F_{IO_2} (high oxygen is associated with negative side-effects). The removal of carbon dioxide through the artificial lung may greatly decrease the harm of invasive ventilation, theoretically up to apnoeic oxygenation. In other words, the application of extracorporeal lung support will change the strategy of invasive ventilation: nearly complete support (ECMO) enhances the reduction of "high oxygen" therapy (high F_{IO_2} and recruitment) and the invasiveness of invasive ventilation; while partial support ($ECCO_2$-R) only promotes lung protection and less invasive mechanical "power" to the lung (without a marked effect on oxygenation). Practical approaches to these aspects are discussed in the following sections.

Invasive ventilation under extracorporeal lung support: oxygenation The correction of hypoxaemia by ECMO makes it possible to reduce the (high) oxygen-associated burden: an adequate reduction in F_{IO_2} should be a first step. Since high PEEP is often followed by hyperinflation of (predominantly ventrally located) lung regions, a moderate reduction in PEEP is suitable, but PEEP levels below 12 cmH$_2$O could promote de-recruitment. However, in studies investigating ARDS patients with dynamic CT it has been shown that PEEP >14 cmH$_2$O were associated with an increasing amount of tidal hyperinflation. Therefore, from a clinical point of view a PEEP level ~12 cmH$_2$O may be a practical compromise between recruitment demand and prevention of hyperinflation. The target blood gases during ECMO treatment are not different from those in non-ECMO patients (figure 1): "normoxia" should be targeted for these patients ($P_{aO_2} = 60-70$ mmHg (8.0–9.3 kPa)) and the negative effects of hypoxaemia (cerebral alterations), as well as hyperoxia (inflammation, radical agents) should be avoided.

In clinical practice the goal of adequate oxygenation in the early phase of ECMO treatment can be achieved by:

- Setting PEEP at a moderate level (~12 cmH$_2$O) as the best empirical way to avoid de-recruitment and hyperinflation
- Reducing F_{IO_2} with the target of "normoxia", avoid hypoxaemia and hyperoxia

Invasive ventilation under extracorporeal lung support: carbon dioxide elimination With artificial lungs sufficient extracorporeal carbon dioxide removal is facilitated to allow the possibility of making several adjustments to reduce ventilator-associated harm to the native lung. The amount of carbon dioxide removal is predominantly controlled by the sweep gas flow through the artificial lung. Practically, a sweep gas flow ≥3 L·min^{-1} should be sufficient for effective carbon dioxide removal, and sweep gas flow rates >8 L·min^{-1} will not further enhance ECCO$_2$-R and might be associated with negative effects.

As a consequence, in most cases a low V_T strategy (V_T=6 mL·kg^{-1} predicted body weight (PBW)) can be applied without the initiation of decompensated hypercapnia/acidosis. A further reduction of V_T to a "ultra-protective" level (V_T<6 mL·kg^{-1} PBW) is advocated by the results of some studies, but robust data regarding an outcome benefit are still lacking and very low V_T might be associated with tidal de-recruitment advancing hypoxaemia. Some working groups promote the monitoring of lung-protective ventilation using ΔP, which represents the ratio between V_T and respiratory system compliance. A lung-protective ΔP level ≤14 mbar is recommended, and ECCO$_2$-R can be used to realise such a goal. Furthermore, ECCO$_2$-R offers the opportunity to balance the RR between 10 and 14 breaths·min^{-1}, since it is hypothesised that even a high RR may contribute to VILI.

In clinical practice the goal of adequate carbon dioxide elimination in the early phase of ECMO treatment can be achieved as follows.

- Set V_T in a lung-protective mode (~6 mL·kg^{-1} PBW). A further reduction of V_T to a "ultra-protective" level is possible, but the aggravation of hypoxia by tidal de-recruitment should be avoided.
- The navigation of lung-protective ventilation by ΔP (≤14 cmH$_2$O) is suggested, to allow a more "flexible" and "situational" application of lung protection.
- Set RR between 10 and 14 breaths·min^{-1}.

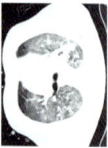

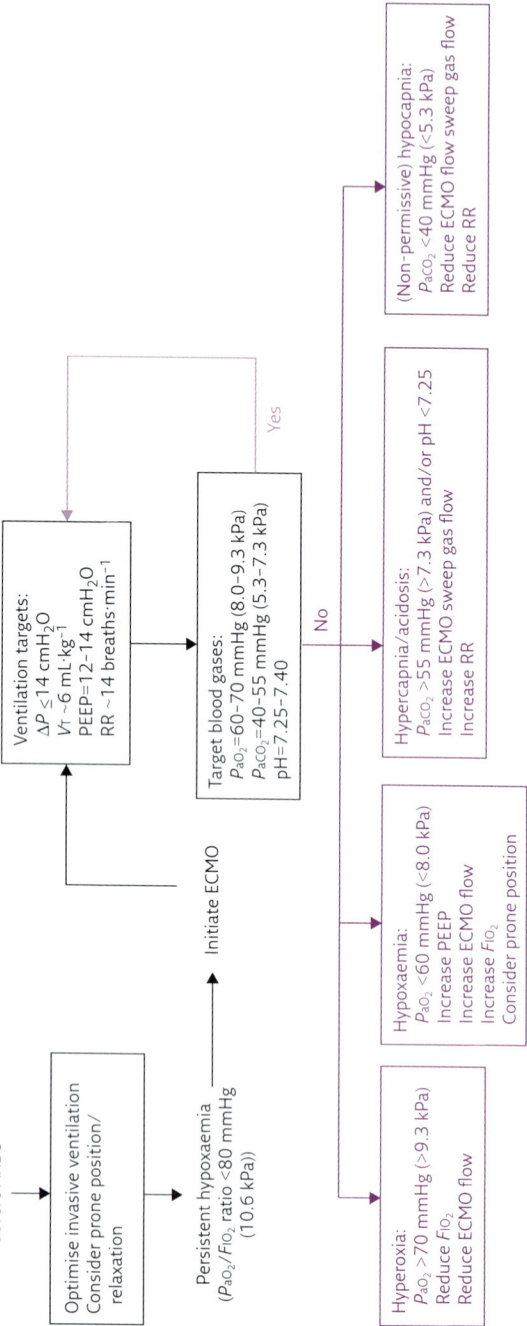

Figure 1. Algorithm for ECMO/ventilator settings based on blood gas analysis. RR: respiratory rate.

Weaning from invasive ventilation in patients on ECMO

Here it is important to distinguish between two different points of interest, *i.e.* the actual process of weaning from invasive ventilation and the correct indication to start the process of weaning from ECMO. In general, weaning is indicated as soon as lung function has recovered sufficiently to allow for adequate gas exchange on moderate positive-pressure ventilator settings without additional ECMO support. An ECMO withdrawal trial, involving switching the sweep gas flow to zero for a certain time (figure 2), is a core measure in these patients.

According to the 2017 ELSO guidelines, <30% of total gas exchange should be provided by the venovenous (V-V) ECMO system before attempting to wean the patient off ECMO. Several parameters are suggested as indicators for the readiness to wean a patient:

- improvement of compromised respiratory mechanics (*i.e.* static compliance in the case of ARDS and airway resistance in the case of asthma),
- improvement of gas exchange, and
- an increased fraction of oxygenation accomplished by the native lungs compared to the oxygenator.

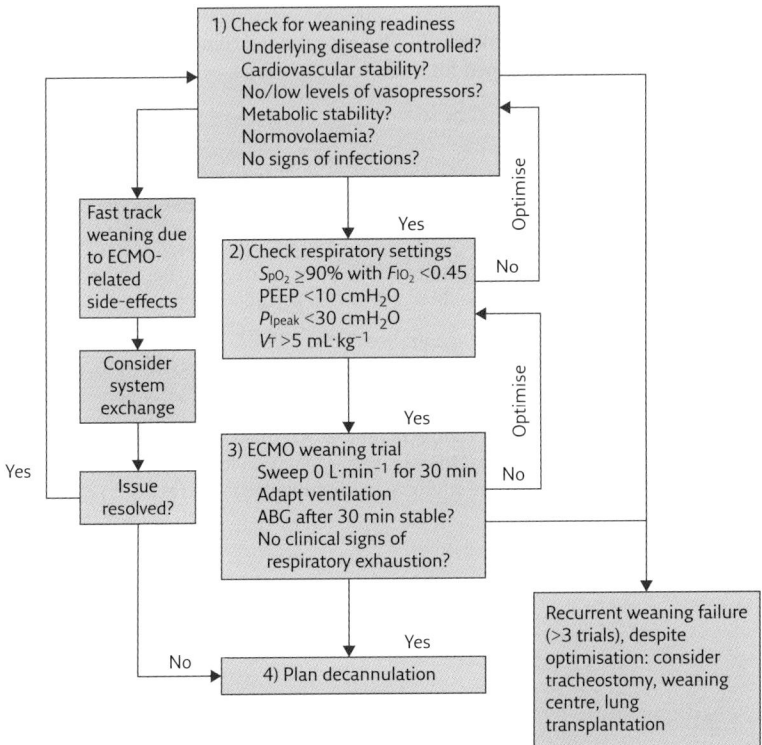

Figure 2. Weaning algorithm for ECMO. ABG: arterial blood gas.

There appears to be a consensus in most publications that the main indicator to start weaning a patient off ECMO is increased lung performance, *i.e.* the native lung being able to provide tolerable gas exchange without further V-V ECMO support. However, a review of existing research shows that in current clinical practice no consensus exists on a set of criteria that indicate a sufficiently recovered native lung. The decision to wean a patient from V-V ECMO is therefore mostly based on a mixture of vaguely determined clinical parameters and the clinician's experience. In addition, the parameters that are currently applied in the decision-making process lack statistical validation, hence requiring more research to satisfy the standards of evidence-based medicine. Some authors advocate the use of ECMO for support of (augmented) spontaneously breathing patients. In this strategy, ECMO should not be discontinued as soon as possible, instead it should stay in place as a part of weaning from invasive ventilation. Although physiologically attractive, such a hypothesis is not yet proven and ECMO use is associated with potentially severe complications (bleeding, clotting and haemodynamic disturbances). Practically, in patients with expected difficult or prolonged weaning the possibility to extubate first and to control the spontaneous breathing capacity under ECMO can be considered. In the second step, ECMO could be weaned by using a stepwise reduction of blood and sweep gas flow in the awake patient. However, ECMO-associated complications might increase with this approach, and a careful decision is mandatory in the individual patient. In any case weaning from invasive ventilation and ECMO should be undertaken in ECMO-experienced centres and integrated into a protocol that can be modified for individual situations.

Further reading

- Boyle AJ, *et al*. (2018). Extracorporeal carbon dioxide removal for lowering the risk of mechanical ventilation: research questions and clinical potential for the future. *Lancet Respir Med*; 6: 874–884.

- Combes A, *et al*. (2018). Extracorporeal membrane oxygenation for severe acute respiratory distress syndrome. *N Engl J Med*; 378: 1965–1975.

- Extracorporeal Life Support Organization (ELSO) (2017). ELSO Guidelines for Adult Respiratory Failure. Ann Arbor, ELSO. https://www.elso.org/Portals/0/ELSO%20 Guidelines%20For%20Adult%20Respiratory%20Failure%201_4.pdf

- Peek GJ, *et al*. (2009). Efficacy and economic assessment of conventional ventilatory support *versus* extracorporeal membrane oxygenation for severe adult respiratory failure (CESAR): a multicentre randomised controlled trial. *Lancet*; 374: 1351–1363.

Prone position in ARDS

Hernán Aguirre-Bermeo and Jordi Mancebo

The first use of prone position in humans was described by Piehl *et al.* (1976). They found that repositioning patients from the supine to the prone position increased P_{aO_2} and facilitated suction of respiratory secretions. Since the publication of that report, several studies have been performed to evaluate the influence of prone position on treatment outcomes. Although previous randomised controlled trials failed to provide evidence for benefit, several variables could have influenced those results, including variations in disease severity, duration of the prone position session, and the time elapsed from the ARDS diagnosis until implementation of prone position. The latest study by Guerin *et al.* (2013) found that the use of early and prolonged prone position sessions in ARDS patients with P_{aO_2}/F_{IO_2} <150 mmHg (20 kPa) was associated with better survival outcomes. Those findings were later confirmed by two meta-analyses. Despite the confirmed benefits of prone position, two recent studies found that prone position was underutilised in severe ARDS (between 16% and 33% of patients). Those two studies clearly indicate that the use of prone position has increased in recent years (and is generally performed in accordance with current recommendations), but it is still underutilised, as evidenced by the low percentage of patients in which prone position is performed.

Key points

- The use of prone position should be considered in patients who fulfil all of the Berlin ARDS criteria with P_{aO_2}/F_{IO_2} <150 mmHg (20 kPa).

- Prone positioning should be initiated in the early stages of ARDS (12–24 h) and the sessions should be relatively long (at least 16 consecutive hours).

- Prone position must be accompanied with invasive ventilation parameters according to the current recommendations (low V_T and moderate PEEP levels to achieve P_{plat} ≤28 cmH$_2$O).

- The use of a protocol and checklist may help to ensure the manoeuvre is performed safely to reduce the likelihood of complications.

Why should we use prone position?

Albert *et al.* (2014) retrospectively analysed the data collected by Guerin *et al.* (2013), showing that the improved survival of severe ARDS patients placed in the prone position does not depend on whether the change in position improves gas exchange. Given this finding, several different mechanisms have been proposed to explain the survival benefit of prone position, as follows:

- Prone position redistributes pleural pressures, thus homogenising transpleural pressures.
- Prone position increases lung volumes, thereby decreasing lung stress and strain.
- The redistribution of lung ventilation in prone position leads to a decrease in mechanical overdistension.
- In the supine position, gravity and shape differences (lungs are cone shaped and chest wall is cylinder) both act in the same direction; as a result, there is a greater expansion of the nondependent regions with less expansion of the dependent parenchyma. However, in prone position, gravitational forces compress the ventral region and thus the gravity and differences in shape act in the opposite direction.
- Other factors, such as the weight of the heart and abdominal pressure, also contribute to differences in density distribution throughout the lung parenchyma.

What are the physiological effects of the prone position?

1) Gas exchange and haemodynamics: the improvement in oxygenation achieved with prone position could be attributable to a decrease in intrapulmonary shunt leading to a decrease in the effect of gravity in the dorsal lung regions, with a redistribution of the aeration resulting in better lung ventilation/lung perfusion ratio matching. As described above, PaO$_2$ increases in prone position (in >85% of patients) but this factor alone does not justify the use of prone position, nor is it associated with improved survival (>80% of patients who do not show PaO$_2$/FIO$_2$ improvement after 1 h of prone ventilation will survive). A decrease in PaCO$_2$ in prone position could indicate lung recruitment, especially if this decrease is accompanied by a decrease in dead space.

2) In severe ARDS, prone position improves right ventricular failure by decreasing right ventricular afterload and increasing right ventricular preload. Systemic venous return increases in prone position due to: 1) transfer of blood volume from the splanchnic compartment; and 2) higher intra-abdominal pressure, which increases mean systemic pressure. Prone position may also increase cardiac output with higher left ventricular afterload, and could improve oxygen transport. However, a slight increase in mean arterial blood pressure due to compression of the abdominal arterial system in prone position could affect left ventricular afterload.

3) Lung volumes and lung strain: lung volumes can be measured at the patient's bedside. Several studies have shown that prone position increases lung volumes. In those studies, the increase in resting lung volumes was primarily related to a redistribution of aeration (a decrease in non-aerated and poorly aerated lung tissue with an increase in well-aerated tissue). Aguirre-Bermeo *et al.* (2018) recently reported that the increase in lung volumes is

accompanied by a decrease in lung strain in the early stages (<72 h) of the ARDS diagnosis. These findings show one mechanism by which prone position improves survival.

4) Respiratory mechanics and transpulmonary pressure: it is well-known that respiratory system elastance depends on chest wall and lung elastance. Chest wall elastance increases in prone position (mainly due to the increase in abdominal pressure) but lung elastance can change depending on the effect of prone position on lung recruitment. For this reason, respiratory system elastance could either increase or decrease in prone position. Mezidi *et al.* (2018) recently evaluated the influence of PEEP and patient positioning on transpulmonary pressure. The authors did not find any variation in transpulmonary pressure due to the position change, regardless of the specific PEEP strategy used (PEEP/F_{IO_2} table *versus* PEEP titrated to reach a $P_{plat} \sim 28$ cmH$_2$O). More studies are needed to confirm these results and to better explore the association between prone position and PEEP titration.

Which patients are eligible for prone position?

Patients must meet all of the Berlin criteria and must have a $P_{aO_2}/F_{IO_2} <150$ mmHg (20 kPa) to be eligible for prone position. In addition, before initiating prone position, invasive ventilation should be optimised (figure 1). The combination of prone position and protective ventilation (low V_T and moderate PEEP levels to achieve $P_{plat} \leq 28$ cmH$_2$O) has shown an improvement in survival in two recent meta-analyses (Beitler *et al.*, 2014, Munshi *et al.*, 2017).

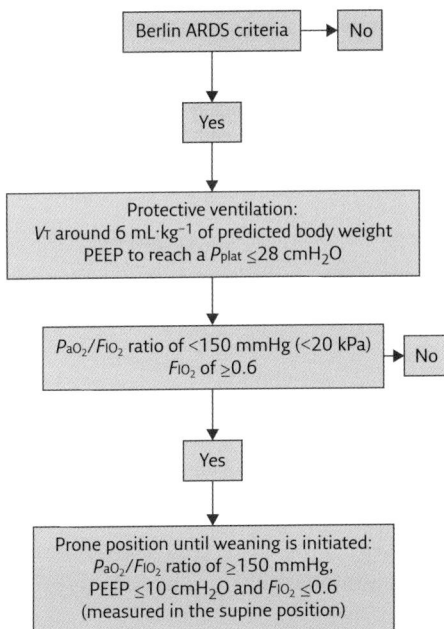

Figure 1. Invasive ventilation and prone position algorithm in severe ARDS patients.

It is important to keep in mind that prone position is not appropriate for all ARDS patients. Guerin *et al.* (2013) found that prone position only improved survival in patients with P_{aO_2}/F_{IO_2} ratio <150 mmHg (20 kPa). In addition, prone position may be contraindicated or difficult in some cases (table 1) and decisions should be individualised according to the patients' clinical characteristics. Note that the experience level of clinical teams (physicians and nurses) with the manoeuvre may affect the likelihood of complications occurring during and after the manoeuvre.

When should prone position be used?

Prone position should be considered in patients who meet the Berlin criteria with P_{aO_2}/F_{IO_2} <150 mmHg (20 kPa) and whose ventilator settings have been optimised according to current recommendations as described above. Guerin *et al.* (2013) demonstrated that the early use of prone position (within 12–24 h after confirming that the patient meets all criteria for ARDS) combined with relatively long prone position sessions (≥16 consecutive hours) improves survival outcomes. A recent meta-analysis by Munshi *et al.* (2017) found that prone position sessions lasting ≥12 consecutive hours significantly improved survival (risk ratio 0.74; 95% CI 0.56–0.99). Aguirre-Bermeo *et al.* (2018) evaluated changes in lung volumes and lung strain in a group of ARDS patients, finding that the application of prone position in the early stages of ARDS (<72 h) increased lung volumes and decreased lung strain. However, when prone position was applied at a later stage (>72 h), those changes were no longer present. The results of the study by Aguirre-Bermeo *et al.* (2018) support the early use of prone position.

How are patients placed in the prone position?

A team of five healthcare professionals is recommended to put patients in the prone position. However, the turn can be done by four professionals, depending of the experience of the team and the clinical context of the patients. The entire process (preparation and turning) typically takes about 10 min. For the turn manoeuvre, one person standing at the head of the bed is responsible for managing the patient's head, the endotracheal tube and the ventilator lines. This same person is also responsible for coordinating the entire procedure, including all of

Table 1. Scenarios to be considered before placing in prone position

---

Conditions that make it difficult to turn patients in the prone position:

External fixators
Multiple pleural tubes
Pericardial drainage
Tracheotomy
Morbid obesity

Clinical conditions that are considered contraindications:

Spinal cord injury with unstable vertebral fractures or pelvic fractures
Open abdominal cavity
Haemodynamic instability
Traumatic brain injury with intracranial hypertension
Pregnancy
Severe burns
Facial lesions

---

the individual steps. The other four people should be placed on each side of the bed (two on each side), near the upper and lower limbs. The two people standing near the upper limbs are responsible for all medical instruments located in this area of the patient's body (*e.g.* electrodes, monitoring cables, pleural drainages, colostomy pouch, *etc.*). The two people standing by the lower limbs are responsible for all medical instruments located in this area (*e.g.* urinary catheter, femoral dialysis catheter, *etc.*). To perform this procedure safely, it is advisable to follow the recommendations provided in box 1.

Box 1. Recommended procedure for placing a patient in the prone position

1) Pre-manoeuvre:
   a. Interrupt enteral nutrition ≥1 h prior to performing the manoeuvre
   b. Pre-oxygenate to reach an S_{aO_2} (pulse oximeter) >95% at least 10 min before the manoeuvre
   c. Check that all necessary materials are available and readily accessible (*e.g.* cushions, electrodes, skin protectors, aspiration equipment, ventilation bag, additional medications, *etc.*)
   d. Evaluate the need to increase analgesia, sedation and curarisation
   e. Perform eye and skin hydration, protect the eyes from erosion and place skin protections
   f. Aspirate the mouth and carefully suction bronchial secretions
2) Performing the manoeuvre:
   a. Ensure that the bed is positioned horizontally
   b. Initiate each step in the manoeuvre only when indicated by the coordinator (the person at the head of the bed). All five people should be in their assigned place and should fully understand their responsibilities (figure 2a)
   c. Move the patient to the side of the bed. While either side can be used, this will depend on the location of the catheters, the mechanical ventilator, the dialysis machine, *etc.* To perform the manoeuvre, the people assigned to the upper and lower limbs should lock their hands together beneath the patient's body. The electrodes should be removed at this time (figure 2b)
   d. The patient should then be placed in the lateral position (figure 2c)
   e. Next, the patient should be turned to the prone position and moved to the centre of the bed. Once this step has been completed, the electrodes and the other monitoring cables and medical instruments should be reconnected (figure 2d)
3) Post-manoeuvre:
   a. Place protective cushions (face, chest, knees, feet) (figure 2d)
   b. Reinsert and confirm the permeability of catheters, drainage tubes, *etc.*
   c. Put the patient in reverse Trendelenburg (30°)
   d. The arms can be placed in two positions: 1) swimmer's position (one arm raised with the head rotated toward the raised arm and the other arm positioned alongside the body) (figure 2d); or 2) the arms can both be positioned alongside the body

---

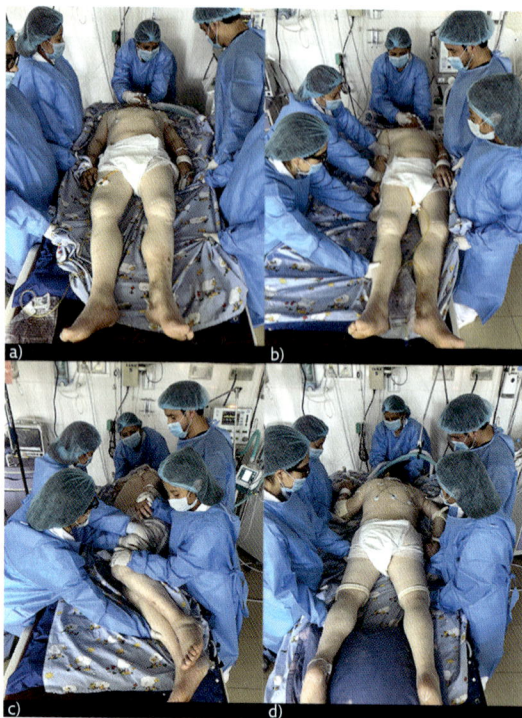

Figure 2. Prone position manoeuvre. a) Patient in supine position and initiation of manoeuvre. b) Patient movement to the side of the bed. c) Patient in lateral position. d) Patient in prone position with monitoring cables and medical instruments reconnected.

After turning the patient, the position (arms, head, neck) should be changed (*i.e.* right to left or left to right) every 2 h. It is important to take special care to monitor pressure points and to monitor the eyes. The enteral nutrition should also be restarted. The patient should be kept in prone position for at least 16 consecutive hours.

The supine position has to be performed with the same steps and with the same precautions and care.

When should prone therapy be stopped?

The main factors to consider when deciding to stop prone position are the improvements in gas exchange and respiratory mechanics that permit continued invasive ventilation in the supine position and then start weaning. Based on the protocol developed by Guerin *et al.* (2013), we recommend stopping prone position when the P_{aO_2}/F_{IO_2} ratio is ≥150 mmHg (20 kPa), with PEEP ≤10 cmH$_2$O and F_{IO_2} ≤0.6 (measured in the supine position 1 h after the last prone position phase).

What are the possible complications of prone position and how can we detect and treat these complications?

Complication rates may be influenced by the team's experience level and the use of institutional protocols. In a recent observational study performed by Guerin *et al.* (2018), 12 out of 101 patients placed in prone position developed at least one complication during the first prone position session.

- Manoeuvre-related complications include the following: unintentional extubation, transient haemodynamic instability, endotracheal tube obstruction, loss of vascular access and transient hypoxaemia. In the study of Guerin *et al.* (2018), four out of 101 patients developed a manoeuvre-related complication in the first session. These complications can be avoided by implementing a specific protocol and by carefully following a checklist.
- Complications caused by skin pressure: the reported rates of pressure ulcers associated with skin necrosis range from 40% to 50%. In the study by Guerin *et al.* (2018), five of the 101 patients developed pressure sores during the first session. The complication rate depends on the duration and number of prone position sessions. However, the incidence of pressure sores can be reduced by implementing a specific protocol with appropriate nursing care and padding.
- Other potential complications include ocular pressure injuries, conjunctival haemorrhage, and elevation of intracranial pressure.

Further reading

- Aguirre-Bermeo H, *et al.* (2018). Lung volumes and lung volume recruitment in ARDS: a comparison between supine and prone position. *Ann Intensive Care*; 8: 25.

- Albert RK, *et al.* (2014). Prone position-induced improvement in gas exchange does not predict improved survival in the acute respiratory distress syndrome. *Am J Respir Crit Care Med*; 189: 494–496.

- Beitler JR, *et al.* (2014). Prone positioning reduces mortality from acute respiratory distress syndrome in the low tidal volume era: a meta-analysis. *Intensive Care Med*; 40: 332–341.

- Blanch L, *et al.* (1997). Short-term effects of prone position in critically ill patients with acute respiratory distress syndrome. *Intensive Care Med*; 23: 1033–1039.

- Gattinoni L, *et al.* (2013). Prone position in acute respiratory distress syndrome. Rationale, indications, and limits. *Am J Respir Crit Care Med*; 188: 1286–1293.

- Guerin C, *et al.* (2013). Prone positioning in severe acute respiratory distress syndrome. *N Engl J Med*; 368: 2159–2168.

- Guerin C, *et al.* (2014). Mechanisms of the effects of prone positioning in acute respiratory distress syndrome. *Intensive Care Med*; 40: 1634–1642.

- Guerin C, *et al.* (2018). A prospective international observational prevalence study on prone positioning of ARDS patients: the APRONET (ARDS Prone Position Network) study. *Intensive Care Med*; 44: 22–37.

- Mancebo J, *et al.* (2006). A multicenter trial of prolonged prone ventilation in severe acute respiratory distress syndrome. *Am J Respir Crit Care Med*; 173: 1233–1239.

- Mezidi M, *et al.* (2018). Effects of positive end-expiratory pressure strategy in supine and prone position on lung and chest wall mechanics in acute respiratory distress syndrome. *Ann Intensive Care*; 8: 86.

- Munshi L, *et al.* (2017). Prone position for acute respiratory distress syndrome. A systematic review and meta-analysis. *Ann Am Thorac Soc*; 14: Suppl. 4, S280–S288.

- Piehl MA, *et al.* (1976). Use of extreme position changes in acute respiratory failure. *Crit Care Med*; 4: 13–14.

- Roche-Campo F, *et al.* (2011). Prone positioning in acute respiratory distress syndrome (ARDS): when and how? *Presse Med*; 40: e585–e594.

Recruitment manoeuvres

Carmen Sílvia Valente Barbas and Gustavo Faissol Janot de Matos

Understanding alveolar or lung recruitment manoeuvres in ARDS patients

ARDS oedematous lung units collapse in the lowermost lung regions leading to pulmonary shunt and increased dead space and decreased lung compliance, and in the most severe cases, leading to critical hypoxaemia and hypercapnia. The patients affected by this syndrome need intubation and invasive ventilation. Lung or alveolar recruitment manoeuvres refer to the re-opening of lung units in ARDS that had previously collapsed due to alveolar instability (figure 1), mainly due to surfactant dysfunction and protein-rich alveolar oedema during the development of ARDS. The recruited alveolar units can re-participate in gas exchange, increasing the P_{aO_2}/F_{IO_2} ratio and making the heterogeneous ARDS lung more homogeneous to allow a more protective PEEP–V_T–respiratory rate interaction.

Gattinoni *et al.* (2006) analysed 68 patients with acute lung injury or ARDS that underwent whole-lung CT during breath-holding sessions at airway pressures of 5, 15 and 45 cmH$_2$O. The percentage of potentially recruitable lung was defined

Key points

- Lung or alveolar recruitment manoeuvres refer to the re-opening of collapsed lung units in ARDS. The recruited alveolar units can then re-participate in gas exchange, increasing the P_{aO_2}/F_{IO_2} ratio.

- It is important to carry out monitored or imaging-guided recruitment manoeuvres in ARDS patients.

- PEEP should be set carefully after a recruitment manoeuvre in ARDS.

- Recruitment manoeuvres in ARDS must be carried out gently, with 5 cmH$_2$O PEEP steps, to avoid stretching the lung tissue too much (which could lead to micro- and macro-barotraumas).

- Monitored recruitment manoeuvres and PEEP titration can be carried out in ARDS patients refractory to the prone position to improve oxygenation and homogenise ventilation.

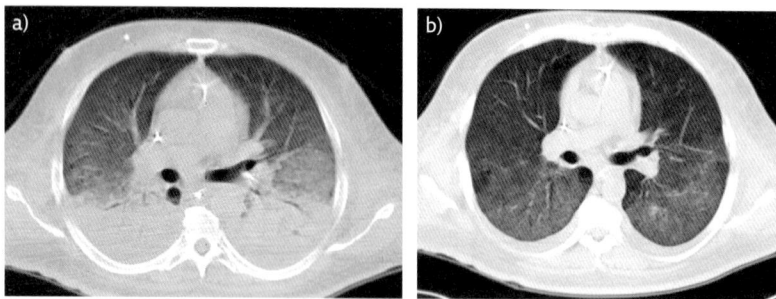

Figure 1. a) ARDS lungs with a huge area of collapse in the lowermost lung regions. b) The same ARDS lungs after an imaging-guided recruitment manoeuvre and PEEP titration.

as the proportion of lung tissue in which aeration was restored at airway pressures between 5 and 45 cmH_2O. The percentage of potentially recruitable lung was shown to vary widely in the population, accounting for a mean±SD of 13±11% of the lung weight, and was highly correlated with the percentage of lung tissue in which aeration was maintained after the application of PEEP ($r^2=0.72$). The study concluded that in ARDS the percentage of potentially recruitable lung is extremely variable and is strongly associated with the response to PEEP.

The importance of undertaking a monitored or imaging-guided recruitment manoeuvre in ARDS patients

Monitored or imaging-guided alveolar recruitment manoeuvres in ARDS patients refer to the re-opening of lung areas that were previously closed guided by pressure–volume curves of the respiratory system, thoracic CT or electrical impedance tomography.

The use of pressure–volume curves of the respiratory system to monitor recruitment manoeuvres and PEEP titration was demonstrated in a prospective controlled trial that analysed 53 patients with ARDS. The trial compared PEEP set 2 cmH_2O above the lower inflection point of the pressure–volume curve of the respiratory system (figure 2) after 40 s of CPAP at 35–40 cmH_2O as a recruitment manoeuvre and V_T of 6 mL·kg^{-1} with patients ventilated with 12 mL·kg^{-1} V_T with the lowest PEEP for acceptable oxygenation without haemodynamic impairment and no recruitment manoeuvres (28-day survival rate of 62% versus 29%, respectively). Another prospective controlled trial, including 103 ARDS patients, compared V_T of 9–11 mL·kg^{-1} predicted body weight and PEEP ≥5 cmH_2O with V_T of 5–8 mL·kg^{-1} predicted body weight and PEEP 2 cmH_2O above the lower inflection point of the pressure–volume curve of the respiratory system (during the performance of the pressure–volume curves, the peak inspiratory pressure achieved was 35–40 cmH_2O, which played the role of a recruitment manoeuvre). This trial demonstrated a significant decrease in both ICU (53.3% versus 32%, respectively) and hospital mortality (55.5% versus 34%, respectively).

Thoracic CT can also be used to guide recruitment manoeuvres and PEEP titration in severe ARDS. Figure 3a shows an ARDS patient with PEEP of 20 cmH_2O and huge collapse at the bottom of the lungs. Increasing PEEP to 25 cmH_2O led to a small decrease in the collapsed lung areas (figure 3b). After a stepwise recruitment

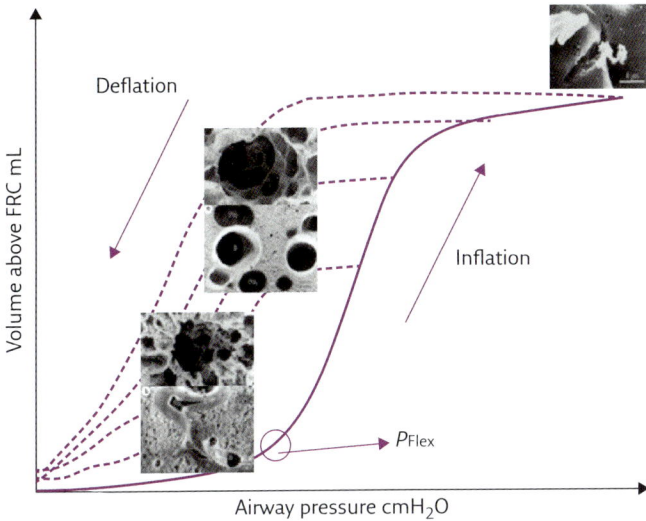

Figure 2. Concept of pressure–volume curve envelopes in ARDS patients to set invasive ventilation to ensure a security window for maintaining an open lung while avoiding overdistension. FRC: functional residual capacity; PFlex: lower inflexion point of the pressure–volume curve of the respiratory system. Reproduced from Barbas et al. (2005), with permission.

manoeuvre with PEEP of 30, 35, 40 and 45 cmH$_2$O and pressure-controlled ventilation of 15 cmH$_2$O and setting 25 cmH$_2$O PEEP after the manoeuvre we can observe an open and homogeneous lung that requires 25 cmH$_2$O PEEP to be kept open (figure 3c). When we decrease PEEP to 20 cmH$_2$O we start to observe collapse of the lower regions of the lung again (figure 3d).

PEEP should be set carefully after a recruitment manoeuvre in ARDS patients

One study demonstrated that most of the collapsed lung tissue observed in early ARDS can be reversed using a monitored recruitment manoeuvre with PEEP titration guided by thoracic CT at an acceptable clinical cost, potentially resulting in better lung protection. The "open-lung hypothesis" would definitely require recruitment manoeuvres in association with individualised, decremental PEEP titration guided by CT.

Another study used a maximal recruitment strategy (MRS) in 51 patients with ARDS. The MRS consisted of 2-min steps of pressure-controlled ventilation with a fixed ΔP of 15 cmH$_2$O, respiratory rate of 10 breaths per min, inspiratory:expiratory ratio of 1:1, and stepwise increments in PEEP levels from 10 to 45 cmH$_2$O (recruitment phase). PEEP was subsequently decreased to 25 cmH$_2$O, and then, from 25 to 10 cmH$_2$O in steps of 5 cmH$_2$O (PEEP titration phase), with each step lasting for 4 min and monitored by CT (figure 4). At each of step CT image sequences from the carina to the diaphragm were acquired during an expiratory pause of 6–10 s. Visual inspection of the images was performed during the tomographic examination to assess the amount of collapse in the lungs bases for an immediate clinical decision, and afterwards offline quantitative analysis was undertaken.

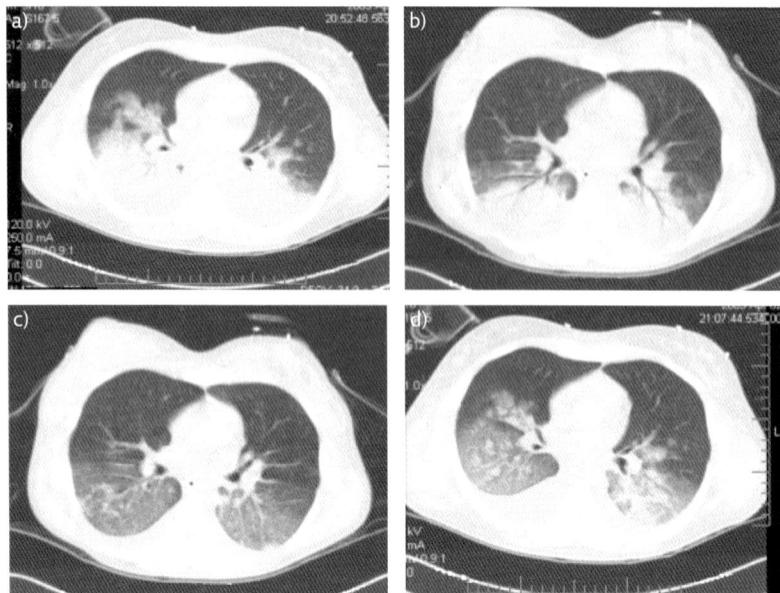

Figure 3. Thoracic CT showing better pulmonary homogenisation and gas distribution after lung recruitment and PEEP titration. a) PEEP of 20 cmH$_2$O before recruitment; b) PEEP of 25 cmH$_2$O before recruitment; c) PEEP of 25 cmH$_2$O after recruitment; d) PEEP of 20 cmH$_2$O after recruitment. Reproduced from Barbas CSV (2017). Ventilation strategies: tidal volume and PEEP. In: Chiumello D, ed. Acute Respiratory Distress Syndrome. Cham, Springer International Publishing, pp. 29–39, with permission.

Non-aerated parenchyma decreased significantly from 53.6% (interquartile range (IQR): 42.5–62.4%) to 12.7% (IQR: 4.9–24.2%) after the MRS. The mean±SD opening Pplat observed during the recruitment protocol was 59.6 ±5.9 cmH$_2$O, and the mean±SD PEEP titrated after MRS was 24.6±2.9 cmH$_2$O. Mean±SD PaO$_2$/FIO$_2$ ratio increased significantly from 125±43 mmHg (16.6±5.7 kPa) to 300±103 mmHg (39.9±13.7 kPa) after MRS and was sustained above 300 mmHg over 7 days. The MRS showed a statistically significant decrease in non-aerated areas of the ARDS lungs, which was accompanied by a significant increase in oxygenation (figure 5). The potentially recruitable lung was estimated to be 45% (IQR: 25–53%). ICU mortality was 28% and hospital mortality was 32%. The independent risk factors associated with mortality were older age and higher ΔP. There were no significant clinical complications or barotrauma with the MRS.

The best way to carry out recruitment manoeuvres in ARDS patients

An analysis of regional lung collapse (across four lung regions) during the recruitment phase and PEEP titration showed that the collapsed lung in the lowermost region of the lungs (region 4) reverted from 100% collapse at a PEEP of 10 cmH$_2$O to 47±30% collapse at PEEP 25 cmH$_2$O (figure 6). These data show that most of the reversal of collapse in the lowermost lung regions occurred at these end-expiratory pressures. This CT analysis suggested that stepwise recruitment manoeuvres in ARDS

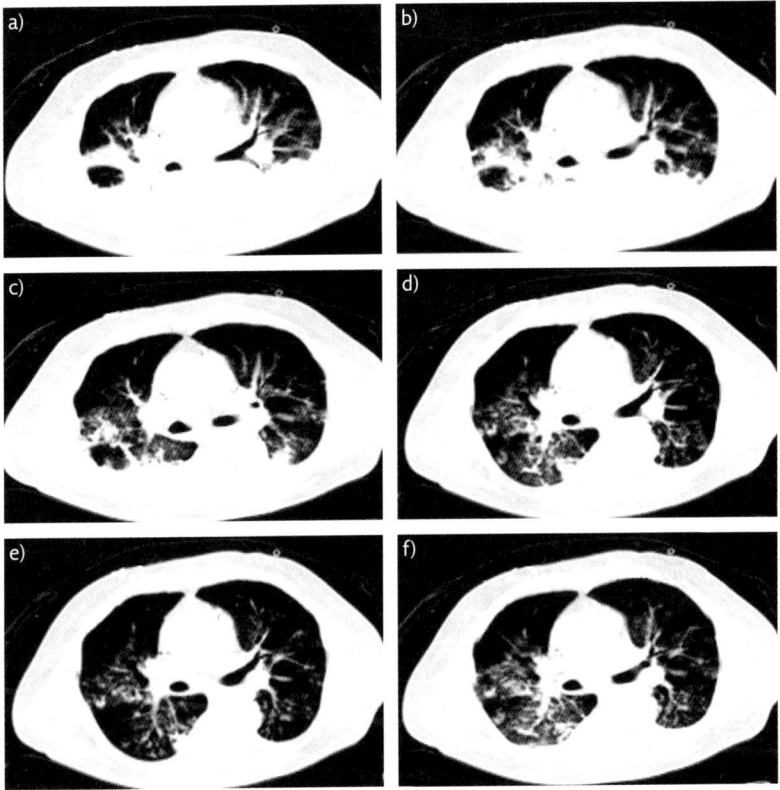

Figure 4. Low-dose radiation CT during the recruitment phase of the MRS (PEEP of a) 10, b) 20, c) 25, d) 35 and e) 45 cmH₂O) and f) at the titrated PEEP of 25 cmH₂O showing less lung collapse in the lowermost ARDS lung and a more homogenised lung with better gas distribution.

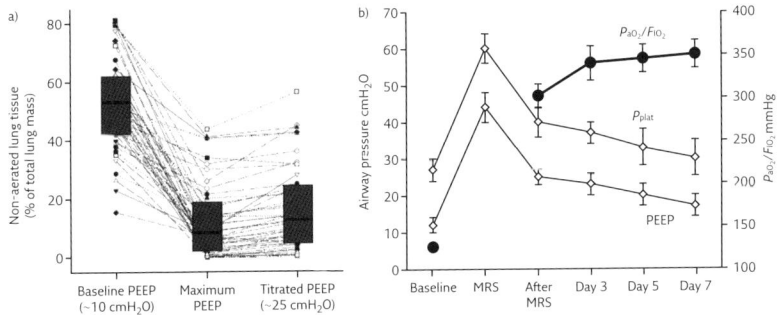

Figure 5. a) A significant decrease in non-aerated lung tissue in 51 ARDS patients following recruitment manoeuvres and b) a significant increase in P_{aO_2}/F_{IO_2} ratio over the 7 days following the MRS. Reproduced from de Matos et al. (2012).

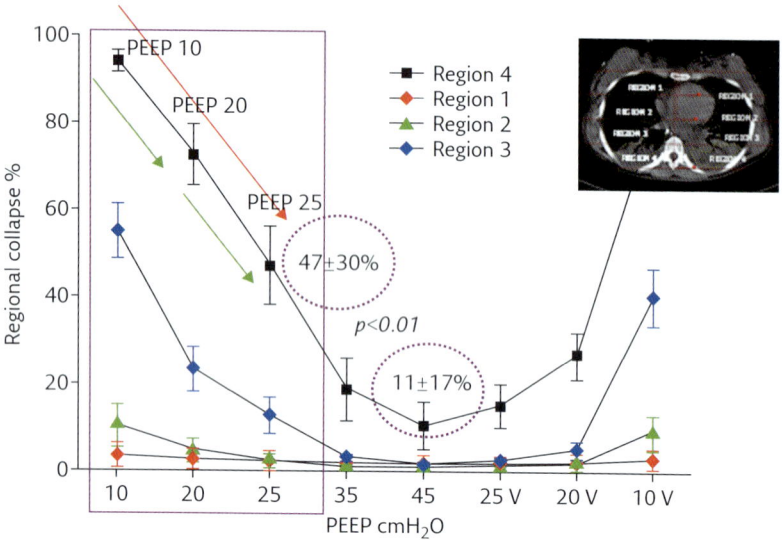

Figure 6. Analysis of percentage regional collapse in 12 ARDS patients during stepwise recruitment manoeuvres and PEEP titration, illustrating that as PEEP increased from 10 to 25 cmH$_2$O there was a 47±30% decrease in non-aerated lung tissue in the lowermost lung regions. PEEP titration should be carried out slowly (green arrows) as stretching the lung tissue too much in a short period of time risks pneumothorax (red arrow). V: measurements made during the decremental phase.

must be carried out gently, with 5 cmH$_2$O PEEP steps, so as not to stretch the lung tissue too much, and thus, to avoid possible micro- and macro-barotraumas.

A recent systematic review and meta-analysis that examined the effects of recruitment manoeuvres for adult patients with ARDS showed an overall pooled effect of a significant decrease in mortality and no associated increase in barotrauma. However, a more recently published, large prospective multicentre RCT (the ART trial) that compared a recruitment manoeuvre and best-compliance PEEP titration in 501 ARDS patients with 509 ARDS patients ventilated with low PEEP showed increased 6-month mortality in both groups, but significantly higher mortality in the recruitment and PEEP titration group (65.3% *versus* 59.9%). However, the recruitment manoeuvre tested in ART trial was abrupt and short: it started at 25 cmH$_2$O PEEP, had a duration of 1 s and was not guided by imaging, which could have contributed to the higher levels of observed barotrauma and mortality. When we combined the results of the systematic review and meta-analysis with the ART trial results, we had a total of 1144 patients undergoing recruitment manoeuvres and PEEP titration and 1179 controls with standard ventilation, with a final result of no significant differences in mortality (relative risk of 0.91, 95% CI 0.74–1.13) (figure 7).

When to apply recruitment manoeuvres in ARDS patients

Clinical, prospective and randomised trials published in the literature have shown that ARDS patients with P_{aO_2}/F_{IO_2} <150 mmHg (<20.0 kPa) and PEEP >5 cmH$_2$O have

	LRM		Control		Risk ratio	RR	95% CI	Weight
Study	Events	Total	Events	Total				
Amato 1998	11	29	17	24		0.54	(0.31-0.91)	11.2%
Meade 2008	145	475	178	508		0.87	(0.73-1.04)	29.8%
Hu 2009	14	30	13	27		0.97	(0.56-1.68)	10.7%
Hodgson 2011	3	10	2	10		1.50	(0.32-7.14)	1.8%
Kackmarek 2016	22	99	27	101		0.83	(0.51-1.36)	12.5%
ART 2017	277	501	251	509		1.12	(1.00-1.26)	34.0%
Random effects model	**1144**		**1179**			**0.91**	**(0.74-1.13)**	**100.0%**

Heterogeneity: I^2=59%, τ^2=0.0307, p=0.03

0.2 0.5 1 2 5
Favours LRMs   Favours no LRMs

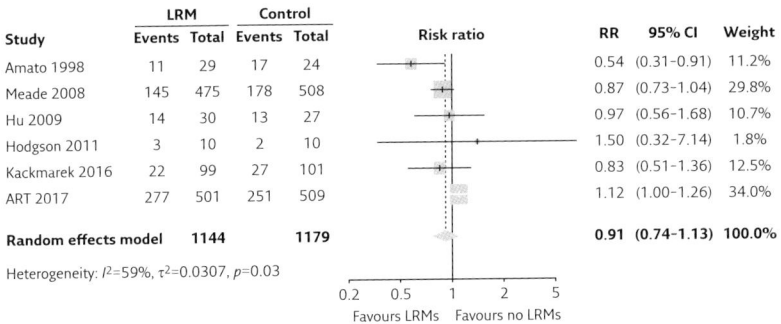

Figure 7. Meta-analysis of the studies included in the meta-analysis by Goligher et al. *(2017) and the ART trial evaluating the mortality risk ratio of lung recruitment manoeuvres (LRMs) in ARDS patients* versus *control. The combined data show no significant difference in mortality. RR: relative risk. Data from Goligher* et al. *(2017) and Writing Group for the Alveolar Recruitment for Acute Respiratory Distress Syndrome Trial (ART) Investigators* et al. *(2017).*

a better survival rate when submitted to the prone position compared with supine position. If a P_{aO_2}/F_{IO_2} <150 mmHg with PEEP >5 cmH$_2$O is identified in an ARDS patient in the supine position, a continuous 16-h period of prone position should be initiated to improve survival rate. If the patient does not improve with prone ventilation or the P_{aO_2}/F_{IO_2} decreases when the patient returns to the supine position monitored recruitment manoeuvres and PEEP titration can be applied in a paralysed patient.

The ART trial showed that unmonitored recruitment manoeuvres with PEEP titration to the best compliance resulted in increased mortality compared with the control group; therefore, we do not recommend carrying out recruitment manoeuvres without respiratory monitoring. If the physician decides to carry out a recruitment manoeuvre as an adjunctive therapy followed by PEEP titration at bedside, they can use the pressure–volume curve of the respiratory system, low radiation thoracic CT or electrical impedance tomography to determine the best personalised and detailed protective PEEP and V_T for ventilation at bedside. Figures 8 and 9 illustrate a recruitment manoeuvre and PEEP titration by electrical impedance tomography in a 47-year-old female patient with an influenza B multiple focal pneumonia aggravated by pneumococcal infection (positive haemoculture). She was intubated and invasive ventilation started with a V_T of 6 mL·kg^{-1} predicted body weight in pressure-controlled ventilation (PCV) mode (ΔPCV of 14 cmH$_2$O), a respiratory rate of 28 breaths per min and PEEP of 8 cmH$_2$O, the S_{pO_2} was 70%. PEEP was increased to 10 cmH$_2$O and S_{pO_2} increased to 85%. Another increment of PEEP to 15 cmH$_2$O increased S_{pO_2} to 90%. She was placed in a prone position for 16 h, keeping PEEP at 10 cmH$_2$O and her P_{aO_2}/F_{IO_2} increased from 60 to 120 mmHg (8.0 to 16.0 kPa). After 16 h, when she was turned supine, with a PEEP of 10 cmH$_2$O, P_{aO_2}/F_{IO_2} decreased from 120 to 80 mmHg (16.0 to 10.6 kPa). Therefore, we decided to prone her again and undertake a monitored recruitment manoeuvre with PEEP titration guided by electrical impedance tomography. We undertook a stepwise recruitment manoeuvre until PEEP was 30 cmH$_2$O with PCV of 15 cmH$_2$O, and then titrated PEEP to obtain the best compromise between collapse/hyperdistension (PEEP of 15 cmH$_2$O) (figure 9).

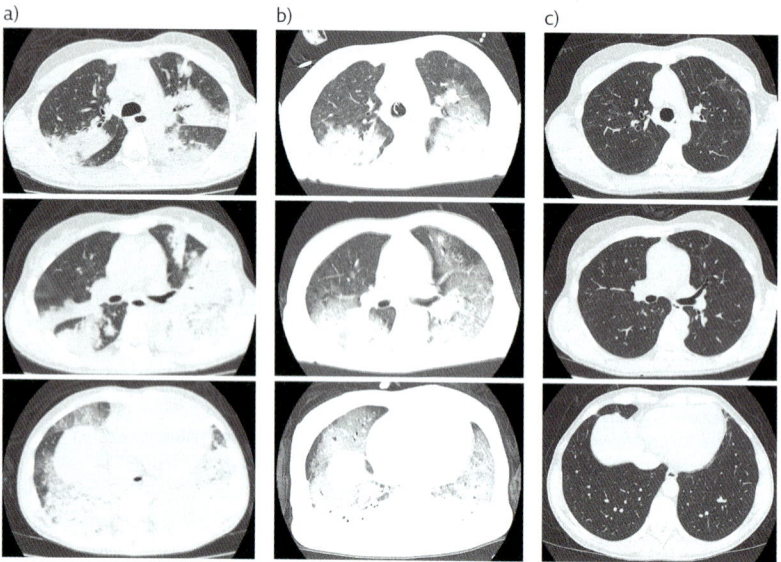

Figure 8. Thoracic CT of a patient with influenza B multifocal pneumonia and ARDS: a) before intubation, b) 6 days after intubation, and c) 10 months after extubation.

After the recruitment manoeuvre and PEEP titration her gas exchange improved to P_{aO_2}/F_{IO_2} of 280 mmHg (37.2 kPa), which was maintained after she turned to supine. After 10 months her thoracic CT was almost normal (figure 8), and S_{pO_2} on room air was 98% without desaturation after exercise. Her pulmonary function tests showed a forced vital capacity of 85%, forced expiratory volume in 1 s of 81%, total lung capacity (TLC) of 99%, residual volume/TLC of 111% and transfer factor of the lung for carbon monoxide of 125% of her predicted value.

In ARDS patients refractory to the prone position, monitored recruitment manoeuvres and PEEP titration can be carried out to improve oxygenation and

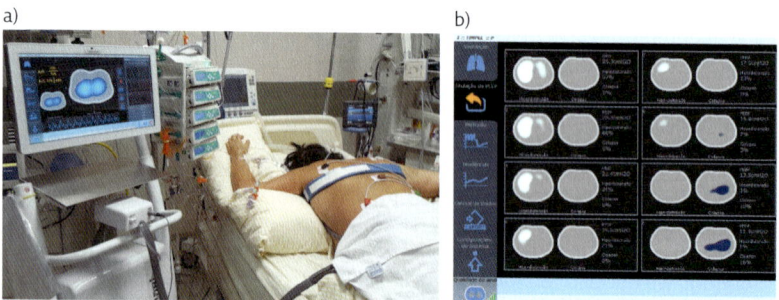

Figure 9. a) Prone position with recruitment manoeuvres and PEEP titration guided by thoracic electrical impedance tomography (b) in the same patient with influenza B multifocal pneumonia and ARDS as in figure 8.

homogenise ventilation. In the most refractory patients, venovenous extracorporeal lung support can be indicated in selected patients and in specialised centres.

Summary

Stepwise monitored recruitment manoeuvres and PEEP titration guided by thoracic tomography have been shown to decrease the amount of collapsed lung tissue and result in better gas distribution and gas exchange in ARDS patients. Monitored lung recruitment manoeuvres and PEEP titration guided by the pressure–volume curve of the respiratory system, thoracic tomography or electrical impedance tomography can be used as an adjunctive therapy to better adjust ventilation and gas exchange in ARDS patients in specialised centres. If physicians decide to apply recruitment manoeuvres in ARDS patients, it is crucial to monitor and perform gentle, stepwise recruitment manoeuvres (increments of 5 cmH$_2$O) and monitor PEEP titration to avoid stretching the lung and possible complications. Aggressive recruitment manoeuvres without adequate monitoring in nonspecialised units are not indicted in ARDS patients because they can increase barotrauma, complications and death. Recruitment manoeuvres in ARDS patients can be used as an adjunctive manoeuvre to improve oxygenation and homogenise ventilation, but the effects of recruitment manoeuvres in clinical outcomes are still unclear. Thoracic electrical impedance tomography with the possibility to undertake ventilation/perfusion analysis of the ARDS patient will allow more detailed and sophisticated protective ventilation in the near future.

Further reading

- Amato MB, *et al.* (1998). Effect of protective ventilation strategy on mortality in the acute respiratory distress syndrome. *N Engl J Med*; 338: 347–354.

- Amato MB, *et al.* (2015). Driving pressure and survival in the acute respiratory distress syndrome. *N Engl J Med*; 372: 747–755.

- Barbas CS, *et al.* (2005). Mechanical ventilation in acute respiratory failure: recruitment and high positive end-expiratory pressure are necessary. *Curr Opin Crit Care*; 11:18–28.

- Barbas CS, *et al.* (2012). Goal-oriented respiratory management for critically ill patients with acute respiratory distress syndrome. *Crit Care Res Pract*; 2012: 952168.

- Barbas CSV, *et al.* (2018). Lung recruitment and positive end-expiratory pressure titration in patients with acute respiratory distress syndrome. *JAMA*; 319: 933.

- Borges JB, *et al.* (2006). Reversibility of lung collapse and hypoxemia in early acute respiratory distress syndrome. *Am J Respir Crit Care Med*; 174: 268–278.

- de Matos GF, *et al.* (2012). How large is the lung recruitability in early acute respiratory distress syndrome: a prospective case series of patients monitored by computed tomography. *Crit Care*; 16: R4.

- Fan E, *et al.* (2018). Acute respiratory distress syndrome: advances in diagnosis and treatment. *JAMA*; 319: 698–710.

- Gattinoni L, *et al.* (2006). Lung recruitment in patients with the acute respiratory distress syndrome. *N Engl J Med*; 354: 1775–1786.

- Goligher EC, *et al.* (2017). Lung recruitment maneuvers for adult patients with acute respiratory distress syndrome. A systematic review and meta-analysis. *Ann Am Thorac Soc*; 14: Suppl. 4, S304–S311.

- Guérin C, *et al.* (2013). Prone positioning in severe acute respiratory distress syndrome. *N Engl J Med*; 368: 2159–2168.

- Kacmarek RM, *et al.* (2016). Open lung approach for the acute respiratory distress syndrome: a pilot, randomized controlled trial. *Crit Care Med*; 44: 32–42.

- Lachmann B (1992). Open up the lung and keep the lung open. *Intensive Care Med*; 18: 319–321.

- Papadakos PJ, *et al.* (2007). The open lung concept of mechanical ventilation: the role of recruitment and stabilization. *Crit Care Clin*; 23: 241–250.

- Writing Group for the Alveolar Recruitment for Acute Respiratory Distress Syndrome Trial (ART) Investigators, *et al.* (2017). Effect of lung recruitment and titrated positive end-expiratory pressure (PEEP) vs low PEEP on mortality in patients with acute respiratory distress syndrome: a randomized clinical trial. *JAMA*; 318: 1335–1345.

Pulmonary vasoactive drugs

Luigi Camporota and Francesco Vasques

Rationale for vasoconstrictors and vasodilators in ARDS: the V'/Q' relationship

The match between alveolar ventilation (V') and perfusion (Q'), *i.e.* an optimal V'/Q' relationship, is crucial to maintain adequate levels of oxygen and carbon dioxide in the arterial blood. In healthy subjects, the average V'/Q' within the whole lung is about 0.8 and tends to be preserved in different physiological conditions (*e.g.* exercise) by the balanced variation in ventilation and perfusion. The V'/Q', however, may range from 0 (in nonventilated, perfused lung units) to infinity (in ventilated, nonperfused alveoli). The spectrum within these extremes identifies all the possible combinations of alveolar ventilation and perfusion.

Functionally, however, it is possible to identify a three-compartment model:

1) Nonventilated, perfused alveoli (intrapulmonary shunt), where $V'/Q'=0$
2) Ventilated, nonperfused alveoli (alveolar dead space), where $V'/Q'=$infinity
3) Ventilated and perfused alveoli, where V'/Q' has intermediate values with various degrees of V'/Q' mismatch

Gas exchange can occur exclusively in perfused and ventilated lung units. The proportion of pulmonary units with extremes of the V'/Q' spectrum is negligible in

Key points

- Nitric oxide is a selective vasodilator of the pulmonary vasculature that may be administered by inhalation to improve oxygenation and decrease pulmonary artery pressure in patients with refractory hypoxaemia.

- Almitrine is a peripheral respiratory stimulant that can increase minute ventilation in conditions of hypoxaemia or hypercarbia.

- Almitrine can potentiate hypoxic pulmonary vasocontriction and therefore improve gas exchange by restoring ventilation/perfusion ratio.

- Although both inhaled nitric oxide and almitrine improve systemic oxygenation in ARDS patients, neither is associated with improved survival in this population.

young healthy humans but tends to increase with age and in lung disease, when V'/Q' mismatch (dead space or shunt) determines the severity of the impairment of gas exchange abnormalities. In particular, intrapulmonary shunt is the mechanism of hypoxaemia in patients with ARDS. In these patients, the hypoxic vasoconstriction plays a major role in diverting the blood flow from poorly aerated and non-aerated lung units to better aerated regions, hence limiting the shunt. This compensation is nonetheless limited and for shunt >30% the increasing F_{IO_2} alone is insufficient at reversing hypoxaemic respiratory failure.

Drugs, either inhaled or administered intravenously, can affect regional lung perfusion (through vasoconstriction or vasodilation), restore V'/Q' relationship and therefore improve systemic oxygenation (*i.e.* reduce the intrapulmonary shunt) in ARDS patients. This can be achieved by maximising vasodilation and perfusion of ventilated pulmonary units and/or inducing vasoconstriction of perfused but hypoventilated pulmonary units.

In this chapter we will discuss the use of inhaled nitric oxide and intravenous almitrine as pharmacological strategies to improve V'/Q' matching and therefore improve pulmonary gas exchange.

Inhaled nitric oxide

Nitric oxide is a free-radical gas generated by nitric oxide synthetase from L-arginine and rapidly inactivated to nitrosyl haemoglobin. Nitric oxide produced by endothelial cells is the main determinant of the vascular tone. Therefore, it is a key component of the vascular autoregulation and tissue perfusion and, as such, plays an essential role in the local regulation of tissue oxygen delivery and utilisation. By activating the soluble guanylate cyclase in the vascular smooth muscle, an increase in nitric oxide production by enzymatic or non-enzymatic mechanisms produces a local decrease in vascular resistance, with a proportional increase in blood flow. At the same time, it controls mitochondrial oxygen consumption by inhibiting cytochrome c oxidase.

Mechanism of action The exogenous administration of nitric oxide through inhalation exerts a relaxing effect on the smooth musculature of both the vascular and bronchial trees. After vaporisation in the ventilator circuit, inhaled nitric oxide will reach primarily the well-ventilated lung units, reducing the pulmonary vascular resistance and therefore increasing regional pulmonary blood flow. In other words, inhaled nitric oxide improves the V'/Q' relationship by diverting the pulmonary blood flow from poorly aerated and non-aerated to well-aerated lung units, hence reducing the intrapulmonary shunt. As a consequence of the decreased resistance induced in the pulmonary vascular tree, the administration of inhaled nitric oxide decreases the pressures in the pulmonary arteries and the afterload of the right ventricle.

Evidence Studies in patients with ARDS and pulmonary hypertension show that the effects of inhaled nitric oxide on the pulmonary vasculature of ventilated lung units result in improved oxygenation and haemodynamics. A recent systematic review showed that in a mixed cohort of patients with acute hypoxaemic respiratory failure included in 11 trials, inhaled nitric oxide was associated with a significant improvement in P_{aO_2}/F_{IO_2} and oxygenation index at 24 h. However, despite the clear improvement in oxygenation, clinical studies have so far failed to show a survival benefit in ARDS patients treated with inhaled nitric oxide or an improvement in ventilation-free days. Although the routine use of inhaled nitric oxide in ARDS is not supported by current evidence, it is frequently used in many institutions. Epidemiological studies show that inhaled pulmonary vasodilators are used in ~8% of patients with ARDS and in 13% of patients with severe ARDS. However, use can increase substantially (up to 80%) in studies that have enrolled a very severe cohort of ARDS patients.

Clinical use The two main indications for pulmonary vasodilators in the critically ill are ARDS and pulmonary arterial hypertension. A summary of potential uses is given in table 1. Clinical use of nitric oxide must consider the following points:

- Inhaled nitric oxide is considered a salvage therapy in patients with severe ARDS and refractory hypoxaemia, as an adjunctive treatment to high PEEP, muscle relaxation, prone position or extracorporeal support. It is also indicated in the presence of pulmonary hypertension and right ventricular impairment, in order to reduce right ventricular afterload and therefore improve cardiac output.
- The administration of inhaled nitric oxide requires a specific nebulisation system that must be added to the mechanical ventilator, and a dedicated scavenging system.
- Monitoring of the clinical response to inhaled nitric oxide includes S_{aO_2}, P_{aO_2}/F_{IO_2} ratio and pulmonary artery pressure. Although the risk for systemic complications is low, the invasive monitoring of systemic arterial pressure is recommended and usually already in use in this group of patients.
- The dose required to produce a reduction in pulmonary artery pressure is higher than that needed to improve P_{aO_2}. Inhaled nitric oxide is commonly used at doses of 10–20 ppm to improve systemic oxygenation. Higher doses do not add therapeutic benefit and may increase the risk of adverse effects. However, higher concentrations can be effective to reduce pulmonary arterial pressure (20–40 ppm). The administration of inhaled nitric oxide is initiated at low dose and titrated up (*e.g.* doubling the dose every 60 min), on the basis of the clinical response and improvement in oxygenation.
- The administration of inhaled nitric oxide should not be suspended abruptly. In fact, a slow weaning is indicated to avoid a rebound effect. There is no optimal weaning protocol. A possible approach could be reducing inhaled nitric oxide by 2 ppm every 2 h down to 1 ppm, and then by 0.2 ppm every 2 h down to 0 ppm.

Table 1. Potential uses of inhaled nitric oxide (NO) and almitrine

	Hypoxaemia	Right ventricular failure	Pulmonary hypertension	ARDS
Inhaled NO, lower dose	++	++	++	++
Inhaled NO, higher dose	++	+++	+++	++
Almitrine	++	−	−	+
Inhaled NO plus almitrine	+++	+/−	+/−	+

−: not useful; +: somewhat useful; ++: useful; +++: especially useful.

Adverse effects

- Effects on the systemic circulation. When entering the circulation, inhaled nitric oxide is rapidly taken up by the red blood cells and deactivated by haemoglobin binding. As a consequence, the benefits of low doses of inhaled nitric oxide (commonly between 10 and 20 ppm) on the pulmonary vasculature are associated with very limited effects on the systemic circulation (*i.e.* systemic arterial hypotension).
- Adverse effects on intrapulmonary shunt and oxygenation. At low doses (<20 ppm), inhaled nitric oxide determines the selective vasodilation in ventilated areas of the pulmonary vasculature. Conversely, at higher doses (80–100 ppm), the diffusion of inhaled nitric oxide (a very lipophilic substance) may easily extend to non-aerated areas, increasing the intrapulmonary shunt and reversing the positive effect on oxygenation. However, these doses are not used clinically and are associated with significant pulmonary and systemic toxicity.
- Methaemoglobinaemia. This may be induced by inhaled nitric oxide, but is clinically more important in neonates than it is in adults, due to the lower level of the enzyme methaemoglobin reductase. The concentration of inhaled nitric oxide used in clinical practice is associated with a very low risk of toxicity. However, intermittent measurement of methaemoglobin is recommended with more prolonged use.
- Platelet effects. Dose-dependent inhibition of platelet adhesion and aggregation by interference with molecular signalling may increase the risk of bleeding in patients given inhaled nitric oxide.
- Inhibition of endogenous nitric oxide production. This is particularly relevant during prolonged administration of inhaled nitric oxide and mandates the slow weaning from exogenous inhaled nitric oxide in order to prevent possible rebound phenomena with impaired systemic oxygenation and pulmonary hypertension and possible acute right heart failure.
- Nephrotoxicity. Inhaled nitric oxide has been associated with increased nephrotoxicity, and several studies, systematic reviews and recent cohort studies have reported an association between the use of inhaled nitric oxide and a statistically significant increase in renal failure.

Almitrine

Almitrine bismesylate is a piperazine derivative developed in the 1970s as a respiratory stimulant for patients with COPD. Almitrine is not licensed in the USA and in Europe it is only licensed in France, Portugal and Poland.

Mechanism of action

- Effects on ventilation. Almitrine increases minute ventilation by selectively stimulating peripheral chemoreceptors (in the carotid body). At lower, sub-stimulatory doses, almitrine can increase ventilation in response to hypoxaemia and hypercapnia but has no effect in normoxic or normocapnic conditions.
- Effects on V'/Q'. When infused intravenously, almitrine exerts a dose-dependent effect on the pulmonary vasculature. At doses <10 $\mu g \cdot kg^{-1} \cdot min^{-1}$ it determines selective pulmonary vasoconstriction, enhancing hypoxic pulmonary vasoconstriction and improving the V'/Q' relationship. At doses

>10 µg·kg^{-1}·min^{-1}, almitrine may have no additional effect or may induce vasodilation. Almitrine has no effect on systemic vascular resistance. The pharmacological potentiation of hypoxic pulmonary vasoconstriction can be advantageous in clinical conditions that result in blunting or abolition of the normal hypoxic pulmonary vasoconstriction (*e.g.* in the post-operative period or in ARDS). The effect of almitrine on the vascular tone, however, comes at the cost of increased pulmonary vascular resistance.

Evidence The intravenous infusion of almitrine may increase systemic oxygenation by improving the V'/Q' relationship *via* the direct vasoconstriction of the pulmonary vasculature, reinforcing the hypoxic vasoconstriction. The clinical effect is frequently already evident at infusion rates <10 µg·kg^{-1}·min^{-1}. In a recent small observational study carried out in patients with severe ARDS requiring ECMO, it was reported that ~70% of the patients demonstrated a significant (35%) improvement in P_{aO_2}/F_{IO_2} post almitrine infusion. However, 22% of patients had side-effects probably related to almitrine (*i.e.* acute cor pulmonale, hepatic dysfunction and hyperlactatemia), which were reversed after stopping the infusion. There is evidence that combined use of almitrine and inhaled nitric oxide allows control of the pulmonary pressure elevation induced by almitrine and significantly increases systemic oxygenation in ARDS patients. However, neither almitrine bismesylate alone nor its combination with inhaled nitric oxide have been associated with a greater survival in ARDS patients, despite the improvement in oxygenation and the synergic effect.

Clinical use Despite the initial enthusiasm accompanying its introduction in ARDS in the late 1990s, at present almitrine bismesylate is infrequently used in clinical practice. A summary of potential uses is given in table 1. Clinical use of almitrine must consider the following points:

- Almitrine was initially introduced for the management of patients with COPD. Its use in these patients is discouraged due to the incidence of long-lasting peripheral neuropathy and weight loss. However, almitrine is still occasionally used a respiratory stimulant in patients with reduced respiratory drive post-operatively and in COPD.
- The use of almitrine has been recently proposed in severe ARDS patients with persisting refractory hypoxaemia despite treatment with ECMO.
- The use of intravenous almitrine alone in ARDS patients with refractory hypoxaemia is limited by the risk of increase in pulmonary vascular resistance, with potential repercussions on the right ventricular function. The combined use of almitrine and inhaled nitric oxide limits the deterioration of the right ventricular function induced by almitrine and may have synergistic effects on the V'/Q' matching, maximising the positive effects on systemic oxygenation.
- The recommended dose of almitrine is <10 µg·kg^{-1}·min^{-1} infusion, and is frequently 4 µg·kg^{-1}·min^{-1}. Low-dose almitrine infusion (4 µg·kg^{-1}·min^{-1}) may be considered to increase pulmonary hypoxic vasoconstriction in the treatment of hypoxaemia during one-lung ventilation in surgical patients with no significant repercussions on the right ventricular function. Higher doses of almitrine (*e.g.* 16 µg·kg^{-1}·min^{-1} has been tested *versus* 4 µg·kg^{-1}·min^{-1}) further improves systemic oxygenation but exposes the patient to significant risks of right ventricular dysfunction.

Adverse effects

- Increased pulmonary arterial pressure. Acute and short-term use of almitrine is generally well tolerated, and increases in pulmonary arterial pressure are generally modest. However, in conditions of pulmonary hypertension and with higher doses of continuous infusion, there is potential to induce secondary right ventricular dysfunction.
- Weight loss and peripheral neuropathy are also potential adverse effects of almitrine. These are more frequent in patients receiving prolonged treatment with almitrine bismesylate (*e.g.* for COPD). Neuropathy seems to be due to the toxic effects of active metabolites, causing axonal degradation and large myelinated fibres.

Further reading

- Adhikari NK, *et al.* (2007). Effect of nitric oxide on oxygenation and mortality in acute lung injury: systematic review and meta-analysis. *BMJ*; 334: 779.

- Afshari A, *et al.* (2010). Inhaled nitric oxide for acute respiratory distress syndrome (ARDS) and acute lung injury in children and adults. *Cochrane Database Syst Rev*; 7: CD002787.

- Esnault P, *et al.* (2019). Evaluation of almitrine infusion during veno-venous extracorporeal membrane oxygenation for severe acute respiratory distress syndrome in adults. *Anesth Analg*; 129: e48–e51.

- Gallart L, *et al.* (1998). Intravenous almitrine combined with inhaled nitric oxide for acute respiratory distress syndrome. The NO Almitrine Study Group. *Am J Respir Crit Care Med*; 158: 1770–1777.

- Golder FJ, *et al.* (2013). Respiratory stimulant drugs in the post-operative setting. *Respir Physiol Neurobiol*; 189: 395–402.

- Taylor RW, *et al.* (2004). Low-dose inhaled nitric oxide in patients with acute lung injury: a randomized controlled trial. *JAMA*; 291: 1603–1609.

Inhalation therapy in ventilated patients

Federico Longhini and Paolo Navalesi

Today, bronchodilators are administered *via* the inhalational route in spontaneously breathing patients with airflow obstruction. When acute respiratory failure (ARF) ensues and invasive ventilation is necessary, bronchodilators are still required in these patients. The inhalational route of administration is generally preferred, offering significant advantages, such as selective treatment of the target sites, *i.e.* the airways and lung parenchyma, with higher drug concentration, rapid onset and fewer systemic adverse effects. The administration of aerosolised medications for treatment of spontaneously breathing patients with asthma, COPD and cystic fibrosis was introduced and standardised decades ago. In patients undergoing invasive ventilation, inhalational therapy is hampered by several technical limitations that need to be overcome to guarantee proper drug availability.

An international survey conducted in 611 departments across 70 countries in 2011 and published in 2013 reported that 99% of ICUs used inhalational therapies, with the most commonly used drugs being bronchodilators, steroids, aminoglycosides and colistin. Surprisingly, however, the optimal implementation of inhalation therapies was infrequently applied, suggesting the need for better education and knowledge dissemination.

Key points

- Inhalation therapy can be administered in patients receiving invasive ventilation by means of both metered dose inhalers (MDIs) and nebulisers.

- Inhaled β_2-agonists are effective to treat acute airway obstruction in mechanically ventilated patients.

- Short-acting β_2-agonists (SABAs) are the most frequently used and studied inhalational drugs during invasive ventilation.

- Nebulised aminoglycosides and colistin, in association with systemic administration, are increasingly used, despite limited evidence, to treat ventilator-associated pneumonia due to multidrug-resistant (MDR) bacteria.

In this chapter we will provide a brief practical guide on the use of inhalation therapy in intubated patients undergoing invasive ventilation.

Devices for inhalation therapy

Metered dose inhalers   Aerosol therapy can be delivered by means of either MDIs or nebulisers. Both techniques have been shown to be effective, without clear evidence in favour of one technique or the other. Although drug delivery is affected by air humidification with both MDIs and nebulisers, when adopting proper modes of administration, the quota of the nominal dose actually delivered to the lower respiratory tract during invasive ventilation slightly exceeds 10% with MDIs, and ranges between 5% and 10% with continuous and inhalation actuated nebulisation, respectively. It should be noted that dry-powder inhalers and soft-mist inhalers are not applicable during invasive ventilation.

According to the aforementioned survey of 611 ICU departments across 70 countries, MDIs are the most widely prescribed device for inhalation therapy in mechanically ventilated patients. Originally, MDIs contained chlorofluorocarbon (CFC) as the propellant associated with small amounts of excipients, such as valve lubricants. Because of stratospheric ozone depletion, CFC inhalers were completely phased-out of production in 2013 in the USA and in 2016 in Europe. CFC inhalers were also affected by the so-called cold freon effect, limiting patient compliance to therapy. The CFC propellant was replaced by hydrofluoroalkane (HFA), which guarantees a slower and warmer release of the drug in the airways, further enhanced by the presence of small amount of ethanol. Unfortunately, in mechanically ventilated patients HFA-propelled MDIs, as opposed to CFC-propelled MDIs, lessen MDI delivery.

Lack of actuation–inhalation coordination, failure to exhale to residual volume before inhaling and the impossibility of taking a deep breath soon after drug administration are the major drawbacks of MDI use during invasive ventilation. The use of large volume chamber spacers limits these drawbacks, to some extent, but could diminish drug availability because of accumulation of electrostatic charge on the plastic surface of the chamber. Coating spacers with ionic detergent reduces the electrostatic charge on the chamber surface. Recently, antistatic spacers have become commercially available. However, while it is well recognised that the

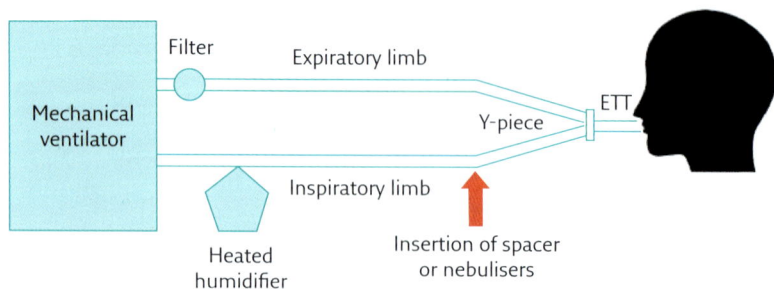

Figure 1. Schematic representation of the ventilator circuit during aerosol therapy with MDIs and nebulisers, which are both located between the distal end of the inspiratory limb of the circuit and the Y-piece. ETT: endotracheal tube.

electrostatic charge reduces MDI aerosol drug delivery, it remains unclear whether or not this truly affects aerosol clinical outcome.

The chamber spacer needs to be inserted on the inspiratory limb side of the ventilator circuit, approximately 15 cm from the endotracheal tube (figures 1 and 2). To optimise drug delivery, one single dose should be actuated into the spacer after shaking the canister prior to ventilator insufflation. Furthermore, the V_T should be no lower than 0.5 L. Repeated shaking of the canister between actuations should be avoided, while the duration of the intervals between puffs does not affect aerosol delivery.

It has been observed *in vitro* and then confirmed in mechanically ventilated COPD patients that the amount of β_2-agonist delivery by MDI is no different with total or partial forms of mechanical ventilatory assistance. Based on *in vitro* studies, the ventilator settings have been proposed as important determinants of the amount of drug actually delivered to the lung. However, a series of studies performed on mechanically ventilated COPD patients showed that end-inspiratory pause, inspiratory duty cycle, inspiratory flow pattern and flow rate had little or no impact on MDI efficacy. Two studies evaluated the consequence of the application of PEEP with controversial results.

Nebulisers Nebulisers convert a drug solution into small droplets. Three types of nebulisers are available for mechanically ventilated patients: jet, ultrasonic and vibrating mesh (figure 2).

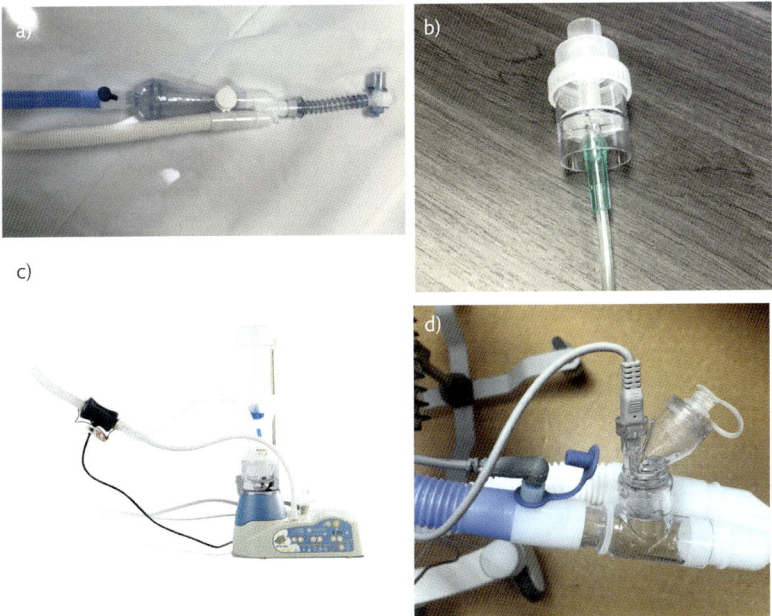

Figure 2. a) A chamber spacer for metered-dose delivery. Examples of b) jet, c) ultrasonic (DP100+ Ultrasonic nebuliser and humidifier, image reproduced with permission from Syst'am, Villeneuve sur Lot, France) and d) vibrating mesh nebulisers.

Jet nebulisers are the most commonly used type of nebuliser, because of ease of use and low costs. However, they are affected during invasive ventilation by drawbacks such as entrainment of external gas into the ventilator circuit, which may significantly add to the preset V_T and alter triggering performance. In addition, these nebulisers necessitate equipment preparation and cleaning, and increase the risk of contamination of the ventilator circuit and ventilator-acquired pneumonia. A recent meta-analysis did not find significant differences in clinical outcome between MDIs and jet nebulisers in mechanically ventilated patients.

There are remarkable differences in the performance of different jet nebulisers, which makes crucial to know the efficiency of a specific device before its use in mechanically ventilated patients. Ventilator mode, pulmonary mechanics, inspiratory flow rate and the distance of the nebuliser from the endotracheal tube affect drug delivery, while PEEP does not remarkably affect aerosol efficiency. Furthermore, the additional flow from the compressed gases required to nebulise drugs increases the V_T actually delivered to the patient and affects triggering performance during partial ventilatory support.

Ultrasonic nebulisers aerosolise drugs through high frequency waves generated by vibration of a piezoelectric crystal on the surface of the drug solution. The vibration nebulises the drug into small droplets more quickly than a jet nebuliser; aerosol particle size and drug output are affected by the amplitude and frequency of the vibration. Ultrasonic nebulisers do not add gas to the ventilator circuit, but they can heat the solution and inactivate some molecules.

Vibrating mesh nebulisers vibrate a piezo that moves the solution through a fine mesh to generate aerosols. There are single use devices with a vibrating aperture plate designed to deliver aerosolised medications to mechanically ventilated patients. Vibrating mesh nebulisers offer some advantages, including:

- smaller residual volume,
- no gas added to the ventilator circuit,
- higher available solution fraction, and
- unaltered temperature of the solution.

This makes it possible to reduce the dose of drugs administered for achieving a clinical response, when compared with jet or ultrasonic nebulisers. This is particularly important when delivering drugs with narrow therapeutic indices and is the reason why these nebulisers are increasingly used for delivery of aerosolised antibiotics in mechanically ventilated patients.

Drugs

β_2-agonists An acute airway obstruction consequent to a COPD exacerbation or an acute asthma attack is the commonest indication for inhaled β_2-agonists in patients receiving invasive ventilation. The administration of β_2-agonists reduces airway resistance (R_{aw}) and auto or intrinsic PEEP (PEEPi). β_2-agonists available for aerosol therapy (with both MDIs and nebulisers) are either short-acting (SABAs), *i.e.* salbutamol, or long-acting (LABAs), *i.e.* formoterol and salmeterol. SABAs are preferred in mechanically ventilated patients with ARF and acute airway obstruction, while the use of LABAs, although not contraindicated *per se*, is not currently supported by data.

The administration, with appropriate technique, of aerosolised salbutamol at a dose of four puffs (400 µg) with an MDI or 2.5 mg with a nebuliser in mechanically ventilated patients with airflow obstruction has significant bronchodilator effects, reducing R_{aw} and PEEPi. Higher doses produce a negligible additional therapeutic advantage, while exposing the patient to increased risk of side-effects, such as hypokalaemia, tachycardia and arrhythmias. In critically ill patients, salbutamol should be repeated every 3–4 h to sustain a bronchodilator response, as it has been shown that, in mechanically ventilated COPD, the bronchodilator effect is sustained for 2–4 h.

Nebulised fenoterol at a dose of 0.4 mg was also found effective in reducing R_{aw}, PEEPi and end-expiratory lung volume (EELV) in intubated COPD patients; increasing the dose up to 1.2 mg did not produce further significant improvement.

In patients with severe asthma, continuous or repetitive nebulisation of salbutamol should be preferred because SABAs duration of activity and effectiveness are inversely related to the severity of airways obstruction. Furthermore, continuous nebulisation of 10 mg salbutamol nebulised in 70 mL over 2 h decreases the hospital admission rate and improves the peak expiratory flow when compared with intermittent therapy with 2.5 mg nebulised salbutamol at 30, 60, 90 and 120 min after the initial treatment.

Anticholinergics Ipratropium bromide is currently available only as solution for nebulisation. The combination of ipratropium bromide and fenoterol delivered by nebuliser (0.5 mg and 1.25 mg, respectively) was shown to reduce R_{aw}, PEEPi and EELV in mechanically ventilated patients with COPD.

Corticosteroids Inhaled corticosteroids are the first-line treatment for outpatients with asthma and are used in stable COPD with a high blood eosinophil count and recurrent exacerbations, while in severe acute asthma and COPD with ARF systemic corticosteroids are indicated, regardless of the need for invasive ventilation. Inhalational therapy with corticosteroids in mechanically ventilated patients has not been specifically studied.

Antibiotics Ventilator-associated pneumonia, due to MDR Gram-negative bacteria, is considered one of the most challenging infections in intubated patients. Inhaled aminoglycosides and colistin have been introduced to clinical use to achieve high drug concentrations in the lung, while reducing drug-related complications and side-effects. Delivery of antibiotics in the lung requires efficient nebulisation; vibrating mesh nebulisers greatly enable antibiotic aerosol therapy when compared with other devices. It should be noted that a viscous solution of antibiotics for inhalation may result in obstruction of the filter at the distal end of the expiratory limb of the circuit, causing hyperinflation.

Although increasingly used over the past decade, true evidence in favour of this treatment is currently lacking, and recent guidelines provide only a weak recommendation for use in patients with ventilator-associated pneumonia due to Gram-negative bacteria susceptible to aminoglycosides or colistin only, in association with systemic drug administration.

Other drugs Mucolytic agents, surfactant and prostaglandins can also be delivered to mechanically ventilated patients by means of nebulisers.

Summary

The primary indication for aerosol therapy during invasive ventilation is treatment of acute airflow obstruction, which can be effectively achieved by means of MDIs and nebulisers. However, both techniques, have specific features that, if ignored, may lead to frustrating results. SABAs are still the most commonly investigated and used drugs in these patients. Aerosolised antibiotics are a promising form of treatment; however, well designed clinical trials are necessary to confirm their clinical efficacy.

Further reading

- Ari A (2012). Aerosol therapy for mechanically ventilated patients: devices, issues, selection and technique. *Clinical Foundations*; 14: 1-12. http://clinicalfoundations.org/assets/cf_14.pdf

- Dhand R (2017). How should aerosols be delivered during invasive mechanical ventilation? *Respir Care*; 62: 1343-1367.

- Dhand R, *et al.* (2008). How best to deliver aerosol medications to mechanically ventilated patients. *Clin Chest Med*; 29: 277-296.

- Fink JB, *et al.* (1999). Reconciling *in vitro* and *in vivo* measurements of aerosol delivery from a metered-dose inhaler during mechanical ventilation and defining efficiency-enhancing factors. *Am J Respir Crit Care Med*; 159: 63-68.

- Holland A, *et al.* (2013). Metered dose inhalers *versus* nebulizers for aerosol bronchodilator delivery for adult patients receiving mechanical ventilation in critical care units. *Cochrane Database Syst Rev*; 6: CD008863.

- Laube BL, *et al.* (2011). What the pulmonary specialist should know about the new inhalation therapies. *Eur Respir J*; 37: 1308-1331.

- Levy SD, *et al.* (2016). High-flow oxygen therapy and other inhaled therapies in intensive care units. *Lancet*; 387: 1867-1878.

- Palmer LB, *et al.* (2017). Is there a role for inhaled antibiotics in the treatment of ventilator-associated infections? *Semin Respir Crit Care Med*; 38: 359-370.

- Russell CJ, *et al.* (2016). The use of inhaled antibiotic therapy in the treatment of ventilator-associated pneumonia and tracheobronchitis: a systematic review. *BMC Pulm Med*; 16: 40.

Weaning definition and outcome

Laurent Brochard, Michael Sklar and Martin Dres

The separation of patients from invasive ventilation, referred to as the weaning process, concerns all ventilated patients and is therefore essential. It is sometimes a long and complex process when faced with various difficulties but is simple for a majority of patients. This simplicity, however, does not imply that it is conducted in an optimal way in such cases. Indeed, discontinuation of ventilatory support and extubation should occur as expeditiously as possible to minimise the iatrogenic consequences of intubation and invasive ventilation, including infectious complications, complications of bed rest and, importantly, ventilator-induced diaphragm dysfunction. Therefore, the weaning process aims at identifying patients early to separate them from invasive ventilation. Overall, three groups of patients have been identified from observational studies. A majority of patients are separated easily at the first attempt. Because this group

Key points

- The majority of patients are separated at first attempt.

- The first reason for delayed extubation is a lack of systematic screening to determine if the patient is ready to be extubated.

- Weaning and extubation can be delayed by sedation practices, since drugs often accumulate and delay the time of full awakening.

- A small group of patients (~10–15%) will become ventilator dependent, even after 1 week of weaning attempts. In these patients, a global approach including mobilisation, nutrition and therapies focusing on psychological factors is essential.

- When doing a test for separation from invasive ventilation, a key aspect is to consider pre-test probability of success in order to interpret the result of the test.

- A T-piece or a test on a ventilator without support best simulate the ventilation conditions after extubation.

is large (the majority of invasively ventilated patients), small benefits in this group can turn into large reductions in ICU days. Most weaning or liberation protocols target this group by proposing systematic approaches and tests, but an important aspect is to consider pre-test probability of success when interpreting any test, as will be discussed later. The other groups are referred to as difficult or prolonged weaning (taking <1 week or >1 week) and are explained by specific causes of weaning difficulties, including volume overload and weaning-induced pulmonary oedema, respiratory muscle weakness, and inadvertently prolonged sedation. The third group (prolonged weaning) represents patients entering the general definition of ventilator-dependent patients, who are usually tracheostomised and may benefit from specialised weaning centres. The advantages of early discontinuation must also be balanced against the detrimental consequences of reintubation. Patients who fail extubation and require reintubation (around 15%) have a high mortality, which to some degree may be precipitated by the extubation failure itself.

Understanding these three groups is essential to applying weaning strategies and tests based on the pre-test probability of successful separation. As an example, for simple weaning, short spontaneous breathing trials (SBTs) and, in some cases, no SBT when pre-test probability of success is very high, are sufficient. At the other extreme, for ventilator-dependent tracheostomised patients, periods of several days disconnected from the ventilator are necessary before deciding on decannulation.

General approach

From the moment that invasive ventilation is introduced, it is important that clinicians start planning for eventual discontinuation of ventilatory support. The reason for emphasising the need for a systematic screening and SBT are two-fold:

1) clinicians naturally tend to wait until a natural improvement in the patient's condition before extubation, which may keep patients unduly intubated;
2) several studies have suggested that there are no other ways to "test" a patient than to watch them breathe spontaneously.

Predicting accurately when a patient is ready to breathe without support has been repeatedly proven to be inaccurate under mechanical assistance. A key aspect of weaning recommendations is serial evaluation, together with aggressive treatment of the factors contributing to the patient's ventilatory dependence. The first reason for delayed extubation is, therefore, a lack of systematic screening to determine if the patient is ready to be extubated. This can be performed by routine SBTs as soon as the patient meets a number of simple criteria. These criteria include: oxygenation criteria ($P_{a}O_2/F_{I}O_2$ >200 mmHg (>26.6 kPa)), PEEP level (not higher than 5 cmH_2O, sometimes 8 cmH_2O), interruption of sedation (except for pain or agitation), and no need for vasopressors (some people ask for very low doses). We will discuss later the role of the rapid shallow breathing index, which is essential in the weaning process and we will spend time describing how to use it and which test should be performed.

The majority of patients (60–75%) will be successfully separated from the ventilator and eventually extubated on the first attempt. Several studies have demonstrated that protocols implemented by non-physician healthcare professionals improved care and were associated with substantial cost savings compared with standard management approaches, even though the specifics of the protocols were different. A landmark trial describing a systematic approach aimed at finding simple criteria for performing a test has shown interest in significantly shortening the duration of invasive ventilation and reducing associated complications. In this study, Ely *et al.* (1996) developed predefined criteria that, when met, led clinicians to initiate a SBT. The criteria were variables that were easily obtained at the patient's bedside and that showed the level of oxygenation, haemodynamic stability, the presence of a cough and the measurement of the respiratory rate/V_T ratio. Using this approach significantly reduced the duration of invasive ventilation without any additional complications such as reintubation. More recently, a strategy that paired spontaneous awakening, based on the interruption of sedatives, with SBTs improved extubation rates, reduced ICU length of stay and decreased mortality by 32%. Therefore, bundles have been proposed to facilitate separation form invasive ventilation. On the contrary, one study reported a high rate of reintubation (37%) in a population of patients ventilated on average for 9 days and separated from the ventilator based on clinical criteria without a SBT. The usual rates of reintubation are ~10–15%.

The global approach to weaning is therefore based on the following:

- Screening for readiness should be performed daily, using relatively simple criteria of stability (*e.g.* patient has shown some improvement in the underlying process); the patient should be haemodynamically stable with no or minimal need for vasopressors; the patient has met reasonable oxygen requirements that can be met by a face mask once the patient is extubated (*e.g.* $F_{IO_2} < 50\%$ and/or P_{aO_2}/F_{IO_2} ratio >200 mmHg (>26.6 kPa) and PEEP <8 or 10 cmH$_2$O).
- A specific screening test that allows the continuation and practice of a SBT to be determined is the rapid shallow breathing index, which is measured over 2 or 3 min without assistance. The cut-off value is 105 and has been simplified as 100 breaths·min^{-1}·L^{-1}. Below this value a trial of spontaneous breathing should be attempted. This test is very useful for screening, *i.e.* when the pre-test probability of success is close to complete uncertainty. It is probably not necessary when the pre-test probability is >80%.
- If the patient meets these general criteria (and has a reasonably low value of the rapid shallow breathing index), a SBT is recommended; if the patient passes the trial, the next question is whether the patient can be extubated.
- Gradual weaning is not necessary, instead, patients should be assessed on a daily basis regarding their suitability for removal from ventilatory support, and if they are not ready, a comfortable, non-fatiguing form of invasive ventilation should be used between the assessments, allowing the patient to use the respiratory muscles. Modes optimising patient-ventilator synchrony may be of major interest. Evidence suggests that after extubation, NIV may be beneficial in hypercapnic or elderly high-risk patients. Among extubated patients at low risk for reintubation, some data suggest that high-flow nasal cannula oxygen reduces the risk of reintubation within 72 h compared with conventional oxygen therapy and is as good as NIV for high-risk patients.
- Despite repeated attempts, there will still be a small group of patients (~10–15%) who will continue to be ventilator dependent, even after 1 week of weaning attempts. In these patients, a global approach including mobilisation,

nutrition and therapies focused on psychological factors may be important; specialised weaning centres may be useful. It is possible that respiratory muscle rehabilitation may help but the evidence is weak, and simple trach mask trials may be the preferred approach for weaning.

A central component: the SBT

The central question is to predict, as much as possible and more precisely, the future of patients after extubation. The clinician navigates between two risks: separating ventilation of patients who still need it too early, or keeping patients ventilated for too long and exposing them to increased risks. Several modalities of SBT are available for clinicians (T-piece, minimal pressure support with/without PEEP, no pressure support, no PEEP). The SBT is a test that is supposed to reproduce ventilation conditions after extubation (table 1). From a physiological point of view, T-piece better reflects spontaneous breathing without assistance compared to other methods; breathing without support on the ventilator seems equivalent. All forms of support (CPAP and low pressure support ventilation) provided by modern ventilators reduce the work of breathing and do not accurately reflect patient capability of being extubated. When the probability of weaning success is high, the SBT should quickly reassure that the patient is ready and the type of test may not be critical (in fact some patients are even extubated without SBTs, such as after cardiac surgery). In a population selected by the failure of a first or further separation attempts, it is logical to use accurate tests such as T-piece (or

Table 1. Comparison of the main modalities of spontaneous breathing trials

	T-piece	Low pressure support	Unsupported on the ventilator
Method	Disconnection of the endotracheal tube Oxygen can be administered	Pressure support alone (usually 7 cmH$_2$O) Pressure support + PEEP PEEP alone (CPAP)	Pressure support 0, PEEP 0
Rationale	Mimic "post extubation" respiratory conditions	Compensate breathing through a ventilator circuit	Mimic "post extubation" respiratory conditions
Advantages	Standardisation	Simplicity Monitoring	Standardisation Monitoring
Disadvantages	Clinical monitoring only Uncertainty of F_{IO_2}	Major practice heterogeneity (pressure support and PEEP combinations, depend on ventilator brand) Deliver efficient ventilator support reducing the test function (not "spontaneous" any more)	Less clinical results Minimal support may still be delivered (may vary with ventilator brands)

on the ventilator without ventilatory support) in order to avoid underestimation of a potential next failure.

Physiological and clinical consequences of a SBT

The physiological effects of the SBT performed with a T-piece or with low levels of PEEP and/or pressure support ventilation in patients who were difficult to wean have been well described. The inspiratory effort was lower with any form of ventilatory assistance compared to the T-piece and decreased when PEEP increased. The conclusion suggested that respiratory work could be largely underestimated by the addition of ventilatory support in patients with heart failure. A recent meta-analysis confirmed the findings that a SBT without support best predicts the post extubation situation. It contradicts the widespread belief that the T-piece test is more physiologically demanding for patients. More "demanding" than other tests, yes, but not more "demanding" than extubation itself.

Clinical studies comparing the two techniques did not show a clear superiority, however, and recent meta-analyses suggest a possible small advantage of low pressure support levels. A possible clinical advantage (which remains to be confirmed) of a low level of inspiratory support, is possibly explained by the inclusion of patients who are mostly easy to wean. Indeed no test is perfect, always exposed to the risks of false negatives or false positives. As we said previously, the performance of a test (its predictive value) is not absolute but very strongly depends on the pre-test probability and therefore on the population tested.

Artificial intelligence has also been used in the weaning process. The SmartCare system (Dräger, Lübeck, Germany) has been shown to either be equivalent to best practices or to significantly reduce the duration of ventilation until the first SBT and extubation. This system is based on a gradual but mostly automatic reduction of ventilatory assistance, automatically guided by the ventilator from simple signals (mainly respiratory rate). Upon detection of predefined thresholds, the system undertakes a SBT (minimal help) and, if necessary, indicates on the screen that the patient is ready to be extubated. The effectiveness of this system has been confirmed in a meta-analysis of all studies. The main reason for these results is the inclusion of easy to wean patients where an automated system can outperform what can be done in a busy ICU.

How to integrate these data into a decision-making process

As discussed above, the majority of patients can and should be extubated easily and quickly. Paradoxically, the implementation of complex predictive indices that cannot claim a perfect specificity could delay the extubation of patients who are "easily weanable". Thus, the essential prerequisite is to identify these patients as soon as possible. This step can be enhanced by setting up systematic protocols for stopping sedation and identifying criteria for separation. Therefore, if the patient meets these criteria (without waiting for a full correction of various clinical or laboratory abnormalities), a SBT must be performed. At this stage, the use of the rapid shallow breathing index is helpful in case of indeterminate pre-test probability and to avoid exposing patients to a SBT if the patient fails immediately. With the two modalities (T-piece and low pressure support without PEEP) being equivalent for an unselected population, there is no reason to recommend one over the other at this stage, except according to the habits and tendencies of the clinician. After failure of spontaneous ventilation or extubation failure, a T-piece or a test on a ventilator without support best simulates the ventilation conditions after extubation.

Weaning and extubation can be delayed by sedation practices, since drugs often accumulate and delay the time of full awakening. In practice, the failure of the first SBT selects a group of patients that justifies a rigorous and systematic diagnostic and therapeutic approach to the weaning process. As this is a common and easily treatable cause, the hypothesis of weaning-induced pulmonary oedema must be evoked, sought and possibly treated. Fluid overload is usually a major component of this "cardiac" failure and giving diuretics titrated on biomarkers of fluid overload has been proven to reduce the duration of weaning. The presence of respiratory muscle weakness should also be assessed since it is highly associated with weaning difficulties. Specific rehabilitation methods may be helpful and special attention should be devoted to sleep quality, prevention of delirium, mobilisation and treatment of depression.

Further reading

- Beduneau G, *et al.* (2017). Epidemiology of weaning outcome according to a new definition. The WIND Study. *Am J Respir Crit Care Med*; 195: 772–783.

- Boles JM, *et al.* (2007). Weaning from mechanical ventilation. *Eur Respir J*; 29: 1033–1056.

- Burns KE, *et al.* (2008). Automating the weaning process with advanced closed-loop systems. *Intensive Care Med*; 34: 1757–1765.

- Burns KEA, *et al.* (2017). Trials directly comparing alternative spontaneous breathing trial techniques: a systematic review and meta-analysis. *Crit Care*; 21: 127.

- Dres M, *et al.* (2017). Coexistence and impact of limb muscle and diaphragm weakness at time of liberation from mechanical ventilation in medical intensive care unit patients. *Am J Respir Crit Care Med*; 195: 57–66.

- Ely EW, *et al.* (1996). Effect on the duration of mechanical ventilation of identifying patients capable of breathing spontaneously. *N Engl J Med*; 335: 1864–1869.

- Girard TD, *et al.* (2008). Efficacy and safety of a paired sedation and ventilator weaning protocol for mechanically ventilated patients in intensive care (Awakening and Breathing Controlled trial): a randomised controlled trial. *Lancet*; 371: 126–134.

- Goligher EC, *et al.* (2018). Mechanical ventilation-induced diaphragm atrophy strongly impacts clinical outcomes. *Am J Respir Crit Care Med*; 197: 204–213.

- Goligher EC, *et al.* (2019). Diaphragmatic myotrauma: a mediator of prolonged ventilation and poor patient outcomes in acute respiratory failure. *Lancet Respir Med*; 7: 90–98.

- Jubran A, *et al.* (2019). Long-term outcome after prolonged mechanical ventilation: a long-term acute-care hospital study. *Am J Respir Crit Care Med*; 199: 1508–1516.

- Klompas M (2015). Potential strategies to prevent ventilator-associated events. *Am J Respir Crit Care Med*; 192: 1420–1430.

- Mancebo J (1996). Weaning from mechanical ventilation. *Eur Respir J*; 9: 1923–1931.

- Mekontso-Dessap A, *et al.* (2006). B-type natriuretic peptide and weaning from mechanical ventilation. *Intensive Care Med*; 32: 1529–1536.

- Rochwerg B, *et al.* (2017). Official ERS/ATS clinical practice guidelines: noninvasive ventilation for acute respiratory failure. *Eur Respir J*; 50: 1602426.

- Sklar MC, *et al.* (2017). Effort to breathe with various spontaneous breathing trial techniques. A physiologic meta-analysis. *Am J Respir Crit Care Med*; 195: 1477–1485.

- Straus C, *et al.* (1998). Contribution of the endotracheal tube and the upper airway to breathing workload. *Am J Respir Crit Care Med*; 157: 23–30.

- Strøm T, *et al.* (2010). A protocol of no sedation for critically ill patients receiving mechanical ventilation: a prospective randomised trial. *Lancet*; 375: 475–480.

- Thille AW, *et al.* (2011). Outcomes of extubation failure in medical intensive care unit patients. *Crit Care Med*; 39: 2612–2618.

- Thille AW, *et al.* (2013). The decision to extubate in the intensive care unit. *Am J Respir Crit Care Med*; 187: 1294–1302.

- Yang KL, *et al.* (1991). A prospective study of indexes predicting the outcome of trials of weaning from mechanical ventilation. *N Engl J Med*; 324: 1445–1450.

Weaning protocols and automatic modes

Louise Rose

Thorough standardisation of weaning processes, weaning protocols and automated weaning modes may facilitate systematic and timely recognition of spontaneous breathing ability and the potential for discontinuation of invasive ventilation. Weaning protocols empower the ICU interprofessional team to initiate and progress weaning, which may reduce practice variation and improve efficiency by enabling timely and objective decision making. Automated weaning modes use continuous monitoring and closed-loop control based on decision rules that adapt the level of ventilatory support to patient need. Automated weaning modes can be viewed as a computerised version of a written weaning protocol.

This chapter will discuss the definition and content of weaning protocols, the reasons for their use, and will briefly outline how to develop and implement a weaning protocol. In addition, this chapter will describe types of automated weaning modes and reasons for their use.

Weaning protocols

Definition Weaning protocols are step-by-step guides to clinical decision making that provide clinicians with direction in terms of:

- When to initiate the weaning process, *i.e.* recognition of readiness to wean
- How to conduct the weaning process, *i.e.* reduction of support provided by the ventilator
- When to extubate, *i.e.* recognition of readiness for extubation

Key points

- Weaning protocols are step-by-step guides as to when to initiate weaning, how to conduct weaning, and when to extubate.

- Weaning protocols can reduce the duration of invasive ventilation, weaning and ICU length of stay without increasing complications.

- Automated weaning modes can be viewed as a computerised version of a written weaning protocol. Both automated and non-automated protocols facilitate systematic and timely recognition of spontaneous breathing ability and the potential for ventilation discontinuation.

> *Box 1. Common criteria used in weaning protocols to recognise readiness to wean*
>
> 1) Initiating spontaneous breaths >6 breaths·min^{-1}
> 2) Respiratory rate ≤35 breaths·min^{-1}
> 3) S_{pO_2} >90% on F_{IO_2} of 0.4 or P_{aO_2}/F_{IO_2} ratio ≥200 mmHg (≥26.6 kPa)
> 4) No significant respiratory acidosis
> 5) PEEP ≤10 cmH$_2$O
> 6) Clinical stability indicated by heart rate ≤140 beats·min^{-1}; systolic blood pressure 90–160 mmHg, and no or minimal vasopressors
> 7) Ratio of respiratory frequency (fR) to V_T (fR/V_T) <105 breaths·min^{-1}·L^{-1}
> 8) Cooperative and pain free
> 9) Adequate cough and absence of excessive secretions

Recognition of readiness to wean This weaning protocol component comprises criteria that indicate if a patient is ready for a reduction in ventilator support. Common criteria are listed in box 1.

How to conduct the weaning process Weaning protocols usually recommend a decremental reduction in ventilator support, daily (or more frequent) spontaneous breathing trials (SBTs), or a combination of both. A SBT is a focused assessment of a patient's capacity to breathe with either substantially reduced or no ventilatory support (figure 1).

Weaning protocols that recommend a decremental approach generally suggest reduction in pressure support, *i.e.* reduction by 2–4 cmH$_2$O, with a period of review of patient response prior to further reduction. This review period can vary from as little as 30 min to a day. For optimal decision-making regarding progression to extubation, weaning protocols should advocate for the length of this review period to be adjusted to the individual patient response to the decrement in support. Box 2 lists common criteria used in weaning protocols to indicate weaning failure, and therefore, the need to discontinue or reverse the decrement of ventilatory support.

Weaning protocols that recommend SBTs include recommendations on the type, duration and frequency of SBT. The type of SBT refers to use of reduced pressure support, CPAP *via* the ventilator, or a T-piece attached to the distal end of the endotracheal tube. Duration typically ranges from 30 min to 2 h. Frequency typically ranges from once to twice daily. Weaning protocols that contain guidance for patients experiencing difficult (*i.e.* patients that fail the initial weaning attempt and take up to 7 days to wean) or prolonged (*i.e.* patients that fail the initial weaning attempt and take >7 days to wean) weaning generally recommend SBTs of a longer duration. For patients with a tracheostomy *in situ*, the weaning protocol may include use of tracheostomy mask trials of progressively lengthening duration.

Weaning protocols that recommend both a decremental and SBT approach generally start with the decremental approach and culminate with a SBT to determine readiness for extubation.

Recognition of readiness for extubation Weaning protocols provide guidance on minimal levels of ventilatory support prior to an extubation attempt, as well as criteria for extubation readiness. If a SBT is recommended in the weaning protocol and is

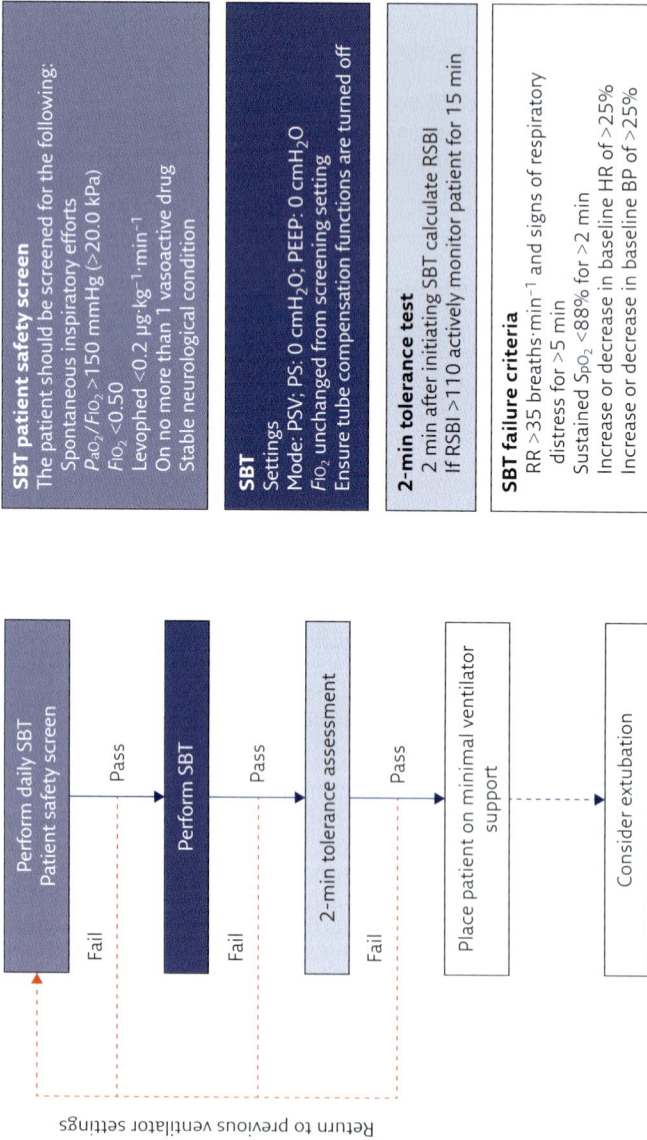

SBT patient safety screen

The patient should be screened for the following:

Spontaneous inspiratory efforts

P_{aO_2}/F_{IO_2} >150 mmHg (>20.0 kPa)

F_{IO_2} <0.50

Levophed <0.2 µg·kg^{-1}·min^{-1}

On no more than 1 vasoactive drug

Stable neurological condition

SBT

Settings

Mode: PSV; PS: 0 cmH$_2$O; PEEP: 0 cmH$_2$O

F_{IO_2} unchanged from screening setting

Ensure tube compensation functions are turned off

2-min tolerance test

2 min after initiating SBT calculate RSBI

If RSBI >110 actively monitor patient for 15 min

SBT failure criteria

RR >35 breaths·min^{-1} and signs of respiratory distress for >5 min

Sustained S_{pO_2} <88% for >2 min

Increase or decrease in baseline HR of >25%

Increase or decrease in baseline BP of >25%

Perform daily SBT Patient safety screen

Pass

Fail

Perform SBT

Pass

Fail

2-min tolerance assessment

Pass

Fail

Place patient on minimal ventilator support

Consider extubation

Return to previous ventilator settings

Figure 1. Toronto city-wide SBT policy (reproduced courtesy of the Interdepartmental Division of Critical Care Medicine, University of Toronto, with permission). If a patient has failed three consecutive SBTs consider reassessing the weaning care plan. PSV: pressure support ventilation; PS: pressure support; RSBI: rapid shallow breathing index; RR: respiratory rate; HR: heart rate; BP: blood pressure.

Box 2. *Common criteria used in weaning protocols to identify weaning failure*

1) Respiratory rate >35 breaths·min^{-1}
2) f_R/V_T ratio >105 breaths·min^{-1}·L^{-1}
3) $P_{aO_2} \leq 60$ mmHg (≤ 8.0 kPa) on $F_{IO_2} \geq 0.5$ or $S_{aO_2} < 90\%$
4) $P_{aCO_2} > 50$ mmHg (>6.7 kPa), pH <7.32
5) Clinical instability indicated by heart rate >140 beats·min^{-1}; systolic blood pressure <90 mmHg or >160 mmHg, or >20% change
6) Arrhythmia
7) Increased work of breathing indicated by increased accessory muscle activity
8) Dyspnoea, anxiety, agitation, distress

passed successfully, the weaning protocol may provide additional guidance as to other considerations (*i.e.* airway considerations) before extubation occurs. Currently a SBT is advocated as the best method to ascertain readiness for extubation.

Why use a weaning protocol?

Use of a weaning protocol has been demonstrated in numerous studies and several systematic reviews to reduce the duration of invasive ventilation, weaning and ICU length of stay with no increase in complications. However, their effect will be moderated by usual weaning practices and the context in which they are introduced. For example, weaning protocols may have less of an effect in units with frequent assessment of weaning readiness and relative autonomy of the ICU professional team regarding weaning decision making.

Weaning protocols are generally considered to empower members of the ICU interprofessional team in terms of weaning decision making and are particularly useful to junior clinicians with less experience in ventilator weaning. Due to the heterogeneity of the ICU patient population requiring weaning from invasive ventilation, a single weaning protocol may not be applicable to all patients. Therefore, individualisation of a weaning plan with input from the interprofessional team, and whenever possible the patient and family, within the framework of a weaning protocol is recommended. This is particularly important for those patients experiencing difficult or prolonged weaning.

How to develop and implement a weaning protocol

As with any ICU protocol, its development should be informed by the current evidence base. The protocol should be simple, clearly laid out and easy to follow. Engagement of the ICU interprofessional team in protocol development will result in more consistent implementation into practice.

Automated weaning modes

Automated weaning modes may improve adaptation of ventilatory support to a patient's individual ventilatory needs. Automated weaning modes facilitate systematic and early recognition of the ability to breathe spontaneously and the potential for ventilation discontinuation.

Early automated modes focused on controlled reduction of the mandatory breath rate based on monitoring the spontaneous breath rate to maintain a predetermined minute ventilation. More recent automated modes, such as INTELLiVENT-ASV (adaptive support ventilation (ASV)), monitor and automate multiple parameters throughout the trajectory of invasive ventilation. See table 1 for descriptions of automated modes that enable reductions in ventilatory support that support weaning.

SmartCarePS is an automated mode specifically designed for weaning, which monitors:

- spontaneous breath frequency
- V_T
- end-tidal carbon dioxide tension (P_{ETCO_2})

Monitoring occurs every 2 or 5 min, with adaptation of pressure support to maintain the patient in a "respiratory zone of comfort". Once a minimal level

Table 1. Automated weaning modes

Mode	Brief description
ASV	Weaning occurs through automated switching to PSV and adaption of pressure support based on RR and V_T.
Automode	Weaning occurs through switching from a controlled mode to PSV based on detection of the patient triggering two consecutive breaths.
INTELLiVENT-ASV Quick Wean	Weaning occurs through pressure support reduction based on end-tidal carbon dioxide, oxygenation and RR. Option to include a SBT.
Mandatory minute ventilation (MMV)	Weaning occurs through closed-loop control of the mandatory breath rate while monitoring the spontaneous breath rate using a clinician predetermined minute ventilation.
Mandatory rate ventilation (MRV)	Weaning occurs through closed-loop control to adjust pressure support based on a target RR.
Proportional assist ventilation (PAV)+	Weaning occurs through changes in pressure support in accordance with changes in patient demand *via* continuous monitoring of flow and volume.
Proportional pressure support (PPS)	Weaning occurs through provision of pressure support proportional to changes in airway resistance and lung compliance.
Neurally adjusted ventilator assist (NAVA)	Weaning occurs through reductions in ventilatory support proportional to inspiratory diaphragmatic electrical activity measured *via* an oesophageal catheter.
SmartCarePS	Weaning occurs through a reduction in pressure support based on monitoring of RR, V_T and P_{ETCO_2}. A 1-h SBT determines readiness for extubation.

of pressure support is reached, the SmartCarePS mode conducts a 1-h SBT on minimal pressure support and then recommends whether to "consider separation", *i.e.* extubation.

Effort adapted automated proportional modes include PAV and NAVA (discussed further in the chapter "Proportional modes"). Unlike PSV, which provides the same level of preset pressure during inspiration regardless of inspiratory effort, these modes adjust the level of ventilatory assistance using continuous measurement of inspiratory effort. As the patient recovers respiratory function, ventilatory support is automatically decreased until a minimal level is reached. Unlike SmartCarePS, these proportional modes do not conduct a SBT or provide any recommendation for separation from the ventilator.

The automated mode INTELLiVENT-ASV (discussed further in the chapter "Automated modes") also includes an optional automated weaning protocol with the proprietary name of Quick Wean. This is an operator configurable weaning protocol and comprises three phases:

1) screening and reduction
2) observation
3) an optional SBT

In the screening and reduction phase, the protocol reduces pressure support based on monitoring of S_{pO_2}, P_{ETCO_2} and RR parameters. If these parameters remain stable, Quick Wean then enters the observation phase continuing to monitor to ensure these parameters remain within the acceptable range with no further reduction in support. If enabled, the observation phase is followed by a SBT on low levels of pressure support.

Why use an automated weaning mode?

As with weaning protocols, the use of an automated weaning mode has been demonstrated in numerous studies and several systematic reviews to reduce the duration of invasive ventilation, weaning and ICU length of stay with no increase in complications. Automated weaning modes can be used in simple weaning, such as in short-term postoperative ventilatory failure, as well as in those patients experiencing difficult and prolonged weaning. As discussed in the chapter "Proportional modes", effort adapted automated proportional modes also improve patient–ventilator synchrony thereby increasing patient comfort during weaning.

Further reading

- Epstein SK, *et al.* (2019). Methods of weaning from mechanical ventilation. UpToDate. https://www.uptodate.com/contents/methods-of-weaning-from-mechanical-ventilation

- Holets SR, *et al.* (2016). Is automated weaning superior to manual spontaneous breathing trials? *Respir Care*; 61: 749–760.

- Peñuelas Ó, *et al.* (2015). Discontinuation of ventilatory support: new solutions to old dilemmas. *Curr Opin Crit Care*; 21: 74–81.

- Rose L (2015). Strategies for weaning from mechanical ventilation: a state of the art review. *Intensive Crit Care Nurs*; 31: 189–195.

- Wallet F, *et al.* (2016). Automated weaning modes. *In:* Esquinas A, eds. Noninvasive Mechanical Ventilation and Difficult Weaning in Critical Care. Cham, Springer; pp. 21–28.

Failure to wean and causes for difficult weaning

Alexandra Beurton and Martin Dres

Weaning from invasive ventilation is the process of reducing ventilatory support, ultimately resulting in a patient breathing spontaneously and being extubated. This process can be achieved easily in 60% of patients when the original cause of the respiratory failure has been improved. The remaining cases will require a longer duration of weaning from invasive ventilation, which is associated with a longer stay in the ICU and a high morbidity and mortality rate. Difficult weaning is an important ICU challenge and it is important to find the key factors causing it. Critical causes seem to be cardiac dysfunction and fluid overload. In this chapter, we will define weaning failure and difficult weaning along with the pathophysiology of weaning failure. Diagnostic and therapeutic approaches will also be briefly discussed.

Definitions

What is weaning failure? The weaning process starts when the original cause of the respiratory failure has improved. A spontaneous breathing trial (SBT) assesses the patient's ability to breathe while receiving minimal or no ventilator support. Weaning guidelines suggest performing the SBT without or with the lowest level of ventilator assistance (T-tube with oxygen or CPAP set to zero). The SBT is currently the best diagnostic tool used to determine whether a patient can breathe without the ventilator, but it is important to emphasise that it doesn't evaluate whether the patient still requires the endotracheal tube. A patient could very well tolerate the SBT and fail the extubation because of inability to cope with abundant secretions,

Key points

- Weaning failure is defined as the inability to pass a spontaneous breathing trial and/or the need for reintubation within 48 h to 7 days following extubation.

- Difficult weaning occurs in a minority (<20%) of patients but it is associated with a high morbidity rate, which in turn causes a heavy burden on healthcare resources.

- The main causes of difficult weaning are cardiac dysfunction, fluid overload and diaphragm dysfunction.

swallowing disorders or laryngeal oedema. Therefore, generally speaking, weaning failure refers to SBT failure and extubation failure. In this chapter, only the causes for SBT failure will be discussed.

What is the definition of weaning failure? An international classification published by Boles *et al.* (2007) recommended that patients should be categorised into three groups based on the difficulty and duration of the weaning process: simple, difficult and prolonged weaning. "Simple weaning" refers to patients who can be successfully extubated after the first SBT and "difficult weaning" refers to patients who require up to three SBTs (or as long as 7 days) to be successfully extubated. "Prolonged weaning", which includes patients who fail three SBTs or are still on invasive ventilation more than 7 days after the first SBT, affects a relatively small proportion of ICU patients but these, however, require disproportionate resources. The management of the difficult weaning group is particularly challenging. All efforts have to be taken to understand the reasons for failure and to implement proper interventions. Otherwise, patients will fall into the prolonged weaning group and this is associated with a longer ICU stay, increased utilisation of ICU resources, and a worse outcome than the two other groups.

Pathophysiology of weaning failure

The pathophysiology of weaning failure is complex and multifactorial. Several circumstances may lead to an imbalance between the respiratory capacity and the respiratory load during the SBT (figure 1). On the one hand, a respiratory muscle dysfunction and/or a decreased respiratory drive can impair the respiratory capacity; on the other hand, cardiac dysfunction, lung or chest wall diseases may increase the load on the respiratory system.

What loads applied to the respiratory system may lead to weaning failure? Airway resistance is the resistance of the respiratory tract to airflow during inhalation and expiration. Increased airway resistance and cardiac dysfunction during the SBT increase the work of breathing and thus contribute to weaning failure.

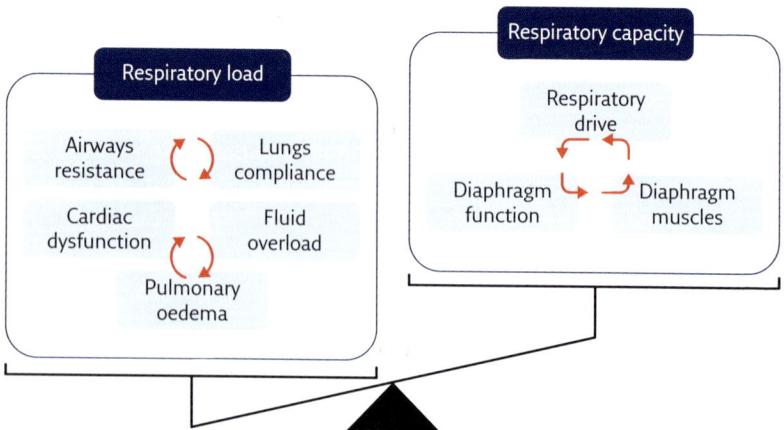

Figure 1. Schematic representation of the load/capacity balance of the respiratory system.

Increased airway resistance is frequent in patients with COPD, which explains the high prevalence of weaning failure in COPD patients. Increased airway resistance leads to intrinsic PEEP, in particular with a reduced expiratory time when a patient develops a rapid breathing pattern. For the respiratory system, intrinsic PEEP acts as a supplementary load to overcome before inspiratory flow will start. Observation of the ventilator waveforms may facilitate the identification of this phenomenon and might lead to prompt changes in the cycling settings to reduce intrinsic PEEP and the work of breathing. In this context, the easiest setting to implement is to decrease the level of pressure support (to decrease the duration of inspiration and increase the duration of expiration) and to set the expiratory trigger to allow the longest expiratory time. In practice, setting the expiratory trigger at 30% of the expiratory peak seems appropriate in most patients, although occasionally higher values of the expiratory trigger (*e.g.* 50–60%) are necessary to limit hyperinflation. In the case of patients with COPD, bronchodilators should also be administered to decrease the work of breathing.

A SBT can be considered a form of physical exercise; therefore, haemodynamic compromise can occur during the weaning process in critically ill patients. Figure 2 displays the main physiological mechanisms potentially leading to cardiac dysfunction and pulmonary oedema during a SBT. Given the close interactions between the cardiovascular function and the respiratory system, all these mechanisms may be exacerbated in a patient with COPD. The main trigger is the decrease in intrathoracic pressure induced by the switch from invasive ventilation (positive intrathoracic pressure) toward spontaneous breathing (negative intrathoracic pressure). The consequence is an increase in venous return that could lead to right ventricle dilation and interventricular interdependence. The decrease in intrathoracic pressure also generates an increase in left ventricle afterload (the

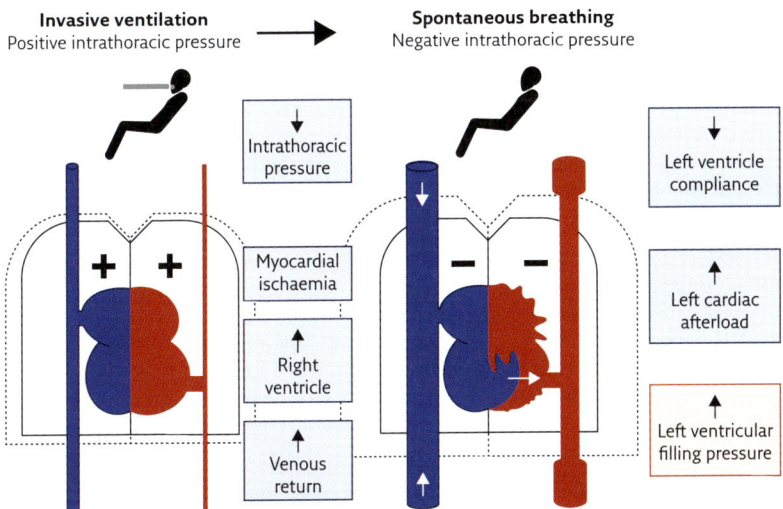

Figure 2. Main mechanisms potentially leading to cardiac dysfunction and pulmonary oedema during the SBT.

left ventricle has to overcome the decrease in intrathoracic pressure before ejecting the blood outside the thorax). In addition, myocardial ischaemia can occur and may worsen the left ventricle function. All these mechanisms are likely to lead to a weaning-induced cardiac dysfunction and subsequently to pulmonary oedema and SBT failure.

Echocardiography is probably the best tool to diagnose weaning-induced cardiac dysfunction as it is noninvasive and highly available at the bedside. Weaning-induced cardiac dysfunction may be suspected in cases of SBT failure when the left ventricle filling pressure is elevated. A normal left ventricle ejection fraction does not prevent weaning-induced cardiac dysfunction as left ventricle diastolic function plays a major role. The left ventricle filling pressure is estimated by assessing the profile of the mitral inflow recorded by the pulse wave Doppler (PWD) and tissue Doppler imaging (TDI). PWD measures the E wave corresponding to the early diastole and the A wave corresponding to the late diastole, and both depend on left ventricle diastolic function and filling pressure. TDI of the mitral annulus evaluates the left ventricle relaxation (e' wave at early diastole) and left ventricle filling pressure (E/e' ratio). In cases of clinical intolerance during the SBT, the combination of E/A >0.95 and E/e' >8.5 indicates failure from cardiac origin.

The diagnosis of weaning-induced cardiac dysfunction can also be made by measuring indirect signs of pulmonary oedema, namely the filtration of fluid from the vascular compartment toward the alveoli and the interstitium. This transfer of fluid induces a plasma volume contraction that can be evidenced by an increase in plasma protein concentration (or haematocrit) >5% between the beginning and the end of the SBT.

The treatment of weaning-induced cardiac dysfunction (and pulmonary oedema) mainly relies on fluid removal and antihypertensive agents. Considering the cardiovascular disturbances occurring during weaning-induced cardiac dysfunction, administration of inotropes does not appear as a logical therapeutic option. Any clear suspicion of myocardial ischaemia should lead to a coronary angiogram.

Changes in lung and/or chest wall compliance induced by pleural effusion may also be involved during weaning failure but data are conflicting on this question. The principle of *primum non nocere* (first, do no harm) should apply and a decision of pleural drainage will have to be wisely considered before proceeding.

What can decrease the capacity of the respiratory system? The capacity of the respiratory system may be reduced in cases of decreased respiratory muscle force and/or decreased respiratory drive. Impaired respiratory drive is an obvious cause of weaning failure, frequently observed in patients with stroke, central hypoventilation and metabolic alkalosis. Low respiratory drive should be suspected in a patient with hypercapnic acidosis and low breathing effort after a failed SBT. Another frequent reason for a decreased respiratory drive is simply the use of sedatives that are not always (or are insufficiently) interrupted at the time of weaning.

Critical illness, polyneuropathy and myopathy are frequently observed in patients who fail the SBT and cause respiratory muscle weakness. Among the respiratory muscles, the diaphragm plays a crucial role in the respiratory system capacity. Thus, diaphragm dysfunction has been associated with SBT failure. The prevalence of diaphragm dysfunction is high at the time of weaning (two-thirds of the patients); thus, such dysfunction may be frequently involved in weaning failure (SBT and extubation). The diaphragm is particularly sensitive to the physiological derangements of critical illness. Among them, some are present before and during the ICU stay (sepsis, shock) while others develop during the stay. In particular, the negative impact of prolonged invasive ventilation on the diaphragm function has been highlighted in several studies. Nevertheless, it is important to keep in mind that, despite the presence of diaphragm dysfunction, some patients successfully pass the SBT and the extubation. Therefore, the implication of the diaphragm dysfunction in cases of weaning failure needs to be made after having ruled out other reasons of failure, particularly weaning-induced cardiac dysfunction.

Diaphragm dysfunction can be detected by several methods. The physiological method for assessing diaphragm dysfunction aims to evaluate its capacity to generate a pressure. In practice, this method can be performed only in expert centres, since it requires sophisticated and dedicated resources. A simplified method is to measure the maximal inspiratory pressure (P_{Imax}), which provides a global assessment of the respiratory muscle function (not specifically the diaphragm). Measuring the P_{Imax} is easy to do with a one-way valve that is adapted on the external tip of the endotracheal tube and measured during a 30-s manoeuvre. During the measurement, the patient can only breathe out and can not breathe in. This results in the inspiratory efforts generating a maximal drop in the airway pressure, indicating the P_{Imax}. Patients who cannot generate a P_{Imax} more negative than -30 cmH$_2$O are considered to have respiratory muscle weakness. Unfortunately, the accuracy of the P_{Imax} in predicting weaning outcome varies widely. Recently, the use of ultrasound has gained interest in the evaluation of diaphragm function. Ultrasound is largely available in the ICU and it is totally noninvasive. As with every other muscle, the diaphragm contracts and thickens. The thickening of the diaphragm can be measured by ultrasound to evaluate the diaphragm function. With this method, the diaphragm is examined on its zone of apposition to the rib cage or through the subcostal approach. While promising, the use of ultrasound to evaluate the diaphragm function still remains in the field of research. Further advances are needed to improve the feasibility and reproducibility of the technique before generalising its routine use.

Other causes of weaning failure There are many other conditions that could explain weaning failure (SBT and extubation). Acute brain dysfunction, delirium and sleep deprivation are frequent in patients at the time of weaning and may be involved in weaning failure. Specific measures (reducing noise and light, sedative sparing) have to be initiated to ensure the best management at the time of weaning. Anaemia is a relevant question in the context of difficult weaning but no haemoglobin level targets have been proposed. Lastly, metabolic disturbances such as hypokalaemia, hypophosphataemia, hypomagnesaemia, myxoedema and malnutrition can cause global muscle weakness and could contribute to weaning failure.

Summary

Management of SBT failure requires a holistic approach where determinants of the respiratory load/capacity balance have to be evaluated clinically and possibly through dedicated investigations. Cardiac dysfunction with or without fluid overload are the most frequent causes of weaning failure for patients with difficult weaning. Echocardiography is the best option in this context. Diaphragm dysfunction may be suspected when initial investigations fail to demonstrate an obvious cause of weaning failure. Diaphragm dysfunction is frequent at the time of weaning but its presence should not discourage caregivers from undertaking weaning and eventually extubating patients.

Further reading

- Boles JM, *et al.* (2007). Weaning from mechanical ventilation. *Eur Respir J*; 29: 1033–1056.

- Dres M, *et al.* (2014). Weaning the cardiac patient from mechanical ventilation. *Curr Opin Crit Care*; 20: 493–498.

- Dres M, *et al.* (2018). Diaphragm dysfunction during weaning from mechanical ventilation: an underestimated phenomenon with clinical implications. *Crit Care*; 22: 73.

- McConville JF, *et al.* (2012). Weaning patients from the ventilator. *N Engl J Med*; 367: 2233–2239.

- Tobin MJ, ed. (2013). Principles and Practice of Mechanical Ventilation. 3rd Edn. New York, McGraw-Hill Medical.

Weaning: a practical approach

Rebecca F. D'Cruz, Nicholas Hart and Georgios Kaltsakas

Weaning must be considered at initiation of invasive ventilation. For this chapter, weaning is defined as the initiation of pressure support ventilation (PSV), proceeding to spontaneous breathing trials (SBTs), with successful weaning defined as liberation from all forms of invasive ventilation for more than 48 h. Longer duration of invasive ventilation is associated with substantial mortality and complications including ventilator-associated pneumonia, airway trauma and extubation failure. The majority (>75%) of patients undergo a simple weaning process, with successful weaning achieved following the first weaning attempt. A smaller proportion of patients require prolonged weaning. Such patients use a significant proportion of critical care resources and have poorer clinical outcomes. In this chapter, we provide a practical approach to weaning from invasive ventilation.

Weaning stages

1) Treatment of the underlying cause of acute respiratory failure
2) Assessment of readiness to wean
3) Weaning (reduction in PSV, T-piece trial)
4) Liberation from invasive ventilation

Assessment of readiness to wean

It is essential to assess readiness to wean early in critical illness. This involves clinical assessment (review cough strength, airway secretions and progress in

Key points

- Patients' readiness to wean must be assessed early in the critical care admission.

- Spontaneous breathing trials are used to determine the likelihood of successful extubation.

- NIV and oxygen delivered through humidified high-flow nasal cannula may be implemented as bridges to liberation from ventilation in selected patients at high risk of post-extubation respiratory failure.

- Patients undergoing prolonged weaning should be managed in specialist weaning units.

Table 1. Physiological parameters that determine readiness to wean

---

Clinical stability

    Cardiovascular: heart rate ≤140 beats·min⁻¹, systolic blood pressure 90–160 mmHg, no/minimal vasopressors

    Metabolic: replacement of electrolytes, where appropriate

Adequate oxygenation

    Oxygen saturation >90% on F_{IO_2} of ≤0.4 (or P_{aO_2}/F_{IO_2} ≥150 mmHg (≥20.0 kPa))

    PEEP ≤8 cmH₂O

Respiratory function

    Respiratory rate ≤35 breaths per min

    Maximal inspiratory pressure ≤–20 to –25 cmH₂O

    V_T >5 mL·kg⁻¹ predicted body weight

    Vital capacity >10 mL·kg⁻¹ predicted body weight

    Rapid shallow breathing index <100–105 breaths·min⁻¹·L⁻¹

    No significant respiratory acidosis

Neurological status

    No sedation, or

    Adequate mentation on sedation, or

    Stable neurological patient

Adapted from Boles *et al.* (2007).

the treatment of the underlying illness precipitating acute respiratory failure) and review of physiological parameters that may be used to determine readiness for the first SBT (table 1). Predictors of weaning failure may be considered, although both single physiological measurements (*e.g.* respiratory rate, V_T, vital capacity, minute ventilation, maximal inspiratory pressure, airway occlusion pressure) and composite indices (*e.g.* rapid shallow breathing index) have limited value in predicting weaning success.

Spontaneous breathing trial (PSV or T-piece)

The SBT is a diagnostic tool to predict the likelihood of successful extubation through a reduction in ventilator support for a short period (30–120 min). The SBT simulates the load on the respiratory muscle pump that will be experienced by patients following extubation and enables clinical review of patients' ability to breathe spontaneously. A SBT should be performed as soon as the patient is assessed as ready to wean. Different techniques for SBT have been applied, including use of a T-piece (where the patient is disconnected from the ventilator and breathes through a T-piece connected to supplementary oxygen), CPAP and low pressure support (5–8 cmH₂O) with or without low PEEP (5 cmH₂O). There is no advantage of one method over another, with each having similar rates of SBT and weaning success, re-intubation, duration of invasive ventilation, pneumonia, ICU mortality, and ICU and hospital length of stay. SBT duration of

Table 2. Weaning methods

Recommended	
T-piece	Patient is disconnected from the ventilator and connected to a T-piece, through which they breathe spontaneously.
PSV	Patient remains connected to the ventilator on pressure support mode. Pressure support is reduced gradually to 5–8 cmH$_2$O ±5 cmH$_2$O PEEP.
Emerging	
Automated tube compensation	A closed-loop system that compensates for the additional work of breathing imposed by the endotracheal tube. It does not account for resistance caused by airway inflammation so may underestimate post-extubation work of breathing. Preliminary evidence suggests that it is noninferior to T-piece and PSV SBT.
Mandatory minute ventilation	An advanced closed-loop system that considers patient effort and delivers mandatory breaths and PSV to augment spontaneous breaths.
Adaptive support ventilation	Automatic selection of target ventilation based on data input by the clinician (predicted body weight, minimum minute volume, pressure limit). Automatic adaption of pressure support, respiratory rate and inspiratory time of ventilator-delivered breaths.
Proportional assist ventilation	Ventilator delivered pressure is based on patient effort to amplify inspiratory effort. No pre-set target volume or pressure.
Neurally adjusted ventilator assist	Automatic adjustment of ventilator setting based on invasive measurement of diaphragm electromyography using a multipair electrode oesophageal catheter.

30 min is recommended. Alternative SBT methods are emerging; however, there are insufficient data to recommend their use at present. Ventilator modes that can be used for weaning are listed in table 2.

SBT success is defined using patients' respiratory pattern, comfort, gas exchange and haemodynamic stability. Following SBT success, a clinical review of neurological status, secretion burden and cough strength, and risk of upper airway obstruction should be undertaken. The latter may involve performing a cuff leak test: if air leaks around the endotracheal tube following cuff deflation, extubation can be considered. Systemic steroids may be administered to patients at risk of stridor.

Liberation from invasive ventilation

Extubation should be performed following a successful SBT and subsequent clinical review. 75% of patients will be successfully liberated from ventilation within 10 days of weaning initiation. Up to 20% of patients considered ready to wean require re-intubation, as indicated by agitation, respiratory distress, tachycardia, hyper/hypotension, impaired gas exchange or acidosis. Predictors of extubation failure include duration of ventilation of >72 h, a prior failed weaning attempt, upper airway pathology or stridor at extubation, excessive secretions, weak cough, post-extubation $P_{a}CO_2$ >45 mmHg (>6.0 kPa) and severe left ventricular dysfunction.

40% of patients are difficult to wean. These patients should be rested on PSV and possible causes of SBT failure should be addressed. Examples of causes of SBT failure include an imbalance in the load–capacity–drive relationship of the respiratory muscle pump (see the chapter "Respiratory mechanics"), cardiac dysfunction, psychological issues, inappropriate nutrition and ventilator circuit issues (dead space, secretion retention or asynchrony). Patient posture and secretion management must also be optimised. Weaning should be resumed using PSV or a T-piece SBT of longer duration (30–120 min), terminating early if the patient fatigues.

Post-extubation, NIV or humidified high-flow nasal cannula oxygen (HFNC) may be used as bridges to liberation from invasive ventilation to reduce the risk of post-extubation respiratory failure.

Noninvasive ventilation NIV has been evaluated in early extubation and post-extubation and is most effective in patients with COPD. Early extubation of hypercapnic and difficult-to-wean patients onto NIV following a successful SBT reduces the risk of post-extubation respiratory failure and re-intubation, and shortens the duration of invasive ventilation and ICU length of stay compared with invasive PSV weaning. It does not appear to confer long-term benefits, with recent data demonstrating no difference in time to weaning success, 30- and 180-day survival or 3- and 6-month health-related quality of life compared with invasive PSV weaning.

Patients at high risk of extubation failure, those who are difficult-to-wean and patients with COPD should be considered for extubation onto NIV for 24–48 h post-extubation. This reduces the incidence of post-extubation respiratory failure and pneumonia, and may reduce the re-intubation rate compared with supplementary oxygen in this patient cohort. Post-extubation NIV also improves 90-day survival in patients with chronic respiratory failure and those who develop hypercapnia during a SBT.

Humidified high-flow nasal cannula oxygen HFNC delivers warmed, humidified gas at up to 60 L·min^{-1} and may improve oxygenation and secretion clearance and reduce upper airways obstruction. It is superior to conventional oxygen in reducing the risk of post-extubation respiratory failure and reintubation in low-risk patients, and noninferior to NIV in preventing post-extubation respiratory failure and reintubation within 72 h of extubation in patients at high-risk of reintubation. HFNC is well tolerated by patients and may facilitate NIV breaks for administration of nutrition and medications, or be implemented in those who cannot tolerate NIV.

Prolonged weaning

25% of patients require invasive ventilation beyond 10 days from weaning initiation, or undergo >3 SBTs or >7 days of weaning following the first weaning attempt. Such patients should undergo early tracheostomy and be referred to a specialist weaning unit (SWU), where a personalised weaning plan involving multidisciplinary input from specialist physicians, nurses, therapists and physiologists can be implemented (figure 1). 34–60% of SWU patients are weaned successfully, which may take several months. A proportion of patients are unweanable, 25% of SWU patients remain ventilator-dependent 1 year after index hospitalisation with acute respiratory failure and are managed either at home with trained carers or in long-term care facilities. Given the limited evidence in this small patient cohort, prolonged weaning methods are typically based on local experience and preferences. We recommend the following holistic approach to prolonged weaning.

Ventilation and tracheostomy strategy

1) Downsize the tracheostomy tube (7.0–8.0 mm cuffed tubes recommended) and use PSV.
2) Cuff deflation trials with introduction of a one-way speaking valve in the ventilator circuit. Trials should be increased in duration and frequency as tolerated (figure 1). Assess inspiratory and expiratory muscle function by reviewing thoracoabdominal movements and cough strength during cuff deflation trials. Target a P_{aCO_2} of 52–56 mmHg (6.9–7.5 kPa), particularly if bicarbonate is >40 mmol·L^{-1}.
3) Change to a cuffless tracheostomy tube.
4) Daytime self-ventilation with a "capped" tracheostomy tube and overnight PSV.
5) Daytime self-ventilation with daytime and nightime "capped" tracheostomy tube and NIV applied overnight with higher pressure support than delivered invasively.
6) Consideration of mini-tracheostomy insertion for secretion management and review vocal cord function.
7) Decannulation and continuation of nocturnal NIV.

If patients are unable to tolerate NIV due to interface issues, HFNC can be implemented as an alternative.

Secretion clearance A personalised secretions management plan addressing upper and lower airway secretions should be implemented. This should include the following:

• Pharmacotherapy: transdermal anti-muscarinics reduce saliva production, nebulised antibiotics may be considered in patients at risk of *Pseudomonas* colonisation.
• Physiotherapy: tracheobronchial suctioning, percussion and vibration, lung volume recruitment with manual inflation, postural drainage.
• Mechanical insufflation–exsufflation (MIE): improves cough function and effectively clears airways secretions in patients with neuromuscular disease.

Rehabilitation Passive and active movements and exercise are used to improve muscle power and endurance. Early mobilisation reduces duration of invasive ventilation and is associated with a higher proportion of patients who are able to walk at hospital discharge. It should therefore be introduced as early as possible.

Ventilator weaning

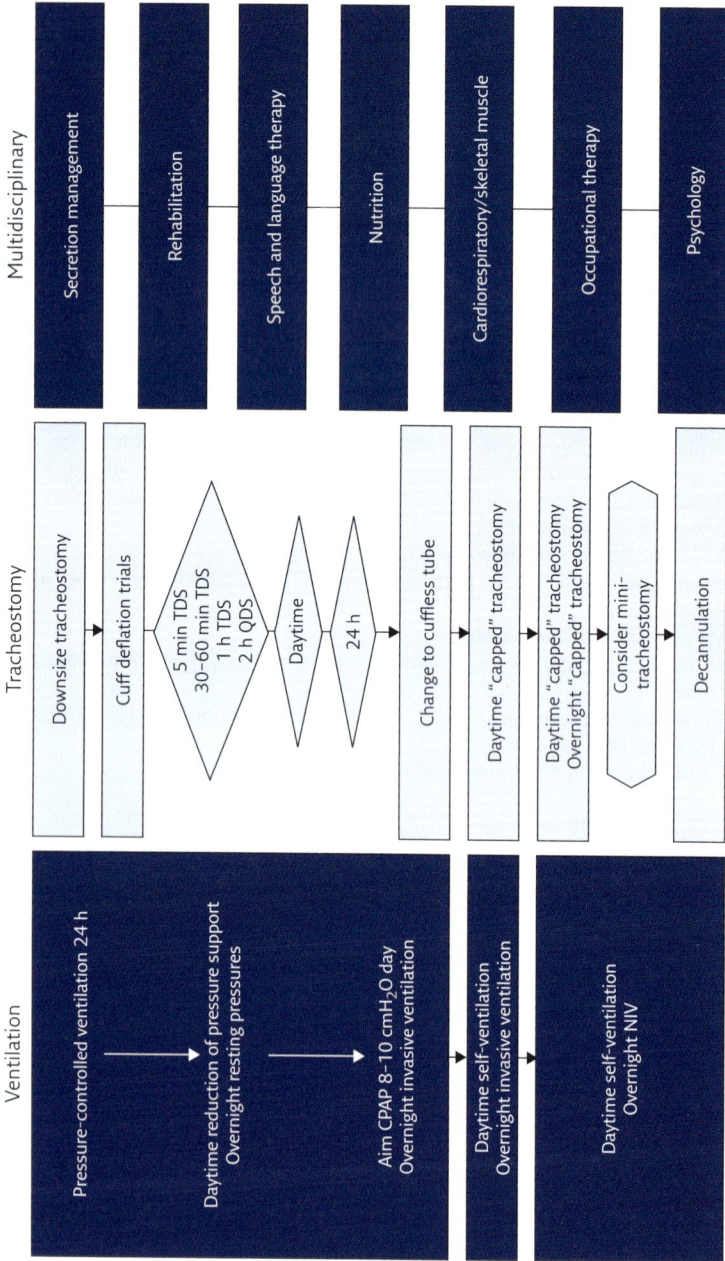

Figure 1. Practical approach to prolonged weaning following transfer to the SWU. The depicted stepwise ventilation and tracheostomy strategies should be conducted in parallel, with concurrent multidisciplinary management throughout the prolonged weaning process. TDS: three times daily; QDS: four times daily.

Nutrition Nasogastric tube size should be downsized where possible to improve comfort and swallow function. Subject to clinical progress, the feed should be reduced from 24 to 20 h. Consider oral intake if cuff down trials are successful and bulbar function is intact.

Cardiorespiratory status Monitor cardiorespiratory status and maintain a neutral fluid balance. Investigations to identify cardiac insufficiency (echocardiography), causes of chronic respiratory failure (high-resolution thoracic imaging) or sleep disordered breathing (polysomnography or respiratory polygraphy) should be considered.

Skeletal muscle ICU-associated weakness (ICUAW) is common and its severity should be assessed and monitored. Neurological investigations, including electromyography, nerve conduction studies, brain and spinal magnetic resonance imaging, should be performed if neurological signs are inconsistent with ICUAW, such as fasciculations, brisk reflexes or a sensory level.

Psychological Among patients undergoing prolonged weaning, depression and anxiety are common, health-related quality of life is lower and post-traumatic stress disorder following critical illness is increasingly recognised. Perform mental health assessments regularly and consider patients' premorbid level of function and patients' and relatives' expectations of recovery. Patients with capacity may request withdrawal of invasive ventilation or decline recommencement of invasive ventilation in the event of deterioration. In these circumstances, shared decision-making with patients, relatives and a multidisciplinary team of specialist palliative care physicians, nurses and therapists is crucial.

Summary

The practical approach to weaning involves: 1) treatment of the underlying clinical condition resulting in acute respiratory failure; 2) assessment of readiness to wean; 3) weaning; and 4) liberation from invasive ventilation. Assessment of readiness to wean should be performed at an early stage of critical illness. Most patients wean successfully following their first SBT. In difficult-to-wean patients, identify and treat possible causes of weaning failure and perform regular, prolonged SBTs if tolerated. Prolonged weaning should be undertaken in specialist weaning, rehabilitation and home ventilation centres where patients receive personalised, holistic management.

Further reading

- Boles JM, *et al.* (2007). Weaning from mechanical ventilation. *Eur Respir J*; 29: 1033–1056.

- Creagh-Brown B, *et al.* (2014). Prolonged weaning. *In:* Stevens R, *et al.*, eds. The Legacy of Critical Care: A Textbook of Post ICU Medicine. Oxford, Oxford University Press.

- Girard TD, *et al.* (2017). An official American Thoracic Society/American College of Chest Physicians clinical practice guideline: liberation from mechanical ventilation in critically ill adults. Rehabilitation protocols, ventilator liberation protocols, and cuff leak tests. *Am J Respir Crit Care Med*; 195: 120–133.

- Hart N (2010). Weaning from mechanical ventilation. *In:* McLuckie A, ed. Respiratory Disease and its Management: Competency-Based Critical Care. London, Springer, pp. 157–165.

- Ouellette DR, *et al.* (2017). Liberation from mechanical ventilation in critically ill adults: an official American College of Chest Physicians/American Thoracic Society clinical practice guideline: inspiratory pressure augmentation during spontaneous breathing trials, protocols minimizing sedation, and noninvasive ventilation immediately after extubation. *Chest*; 151: 166–180.

- Thille AW, *et al.* (2013). The decision to extubate in the intensive care unit. *Am J Respir Crit Care Med*; 187: 1294–1302.

Tracheostomy

Elise Morawiec, Bernard Fikkers and Alexandre Demoule

Tracheostomy is often considered a means to facilitate the weaning process when the need for invasive ventilation is expected to be prolonged. The other indications of tracheostomy, such as airway protection or upper airway obstruction, are beyond the scope of this chapter. This chapter will discuss the following points: benefits and risks of tracheostomy, patient and technique selection, daily management of a tracheostomised patient and decannulation.

Benefits and risks

Tracheostomy improves respiratory mechanics as it reduces airway resistance and work of breathing, reduces the level of intrinsic PEEP, and improves patient–ventilator synchrony. It is unclear whether or not it reduces the incidence of ventilation-acquired pneumonia. It improves patient comfort (which translates into a reduction in sedative drugs) and can allow the patient to eat, drink and talk. It facilitates nursing care and physiotherapy. Patients can be detached from the ventilator for increasing periods of time with the security of a fast and easy reconnection to the ventilator.

Key points

- In appropriately selected patients, tracheostomy is a great tool to achieve gradual weaning and has several advantages over the endotracheal tube.

- However, as with any invasive device, complications can occur and these are sometimes severe. ICU physicians and nurses should know how to avoid and/or recognise and treat such complications.

- Tracheostomy should come with a weaning protocol (*e.g.* daily sessions of unassisted breathing) that should be implemented as soon as possible, along with other measures that promote weaning and global rehabilitation (physiotherapy, *etc.*).

- It is advised to refer to decision trees, algorithms and written protocols and procedures for matters regarding tracheostomy (indication, realisation, daily management and decannulation).

Complications can occur during the tracheostomy procedure (bleeding, misplacement or accidental extubation), or later on (asphyxia following accidental tube obstruction, tracheal stenosis, bleeding or impaired swallowing). Careful patient and technique selection and proper team training can reduce the occurrence of complications.

Patient and technique selection

The question of tracheostomy usually arises when difficult weaning from invasive ventilation is observed or expected. Tracheostomy is a complex ethical issue in patients with chronic respiratory failure or degenerative neuromuscular disease. The decision to perform a tracheostomy in these patients should be thoroughly discussed.

Tracheostomy in the context of weaning is not an emergency, and therefore should only be performed on a clinically stable patient (figure 1). The percutaneous dilatational technique (PDT) is the method of choice, except for patients with

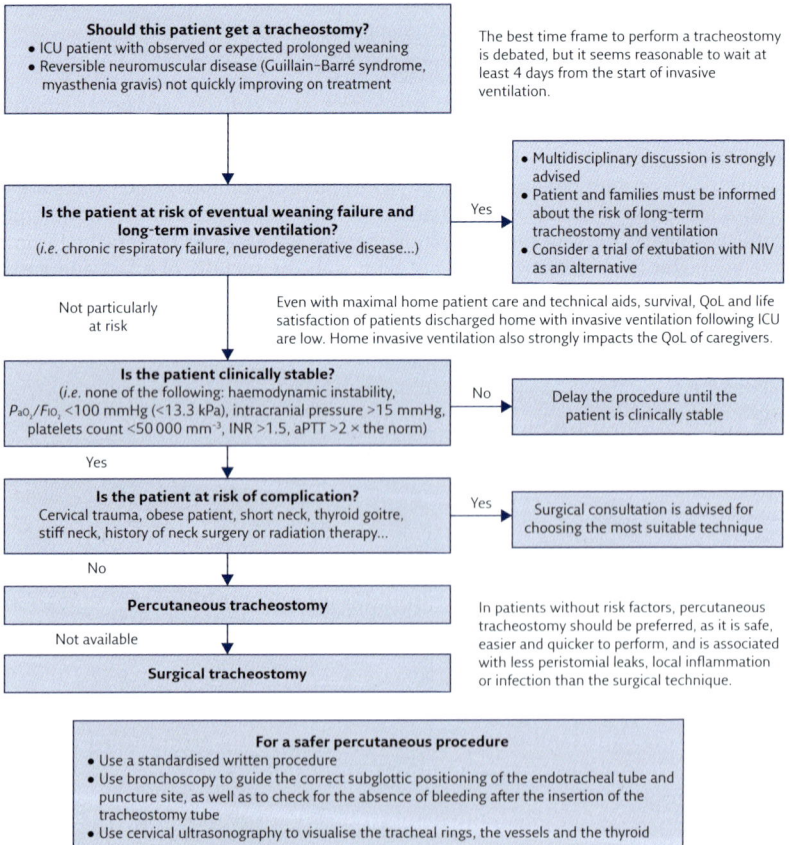

Figure 1. Tracheostomy decision tree. QoL: quality of life; INR: international normalised ratio; aPTT: activated partial thromboplastin time.

cervical abnormalities (figure 1). In such patients, surgical consultation is advised to select the most suitable technique. To limit the potential risks of the procedure, it is advised to use a standardised written procedure, bronchoscopy and cervical ultrasonography. Figure 1 presents the different questions that should be answered for optimal patient, timing and technique selection.

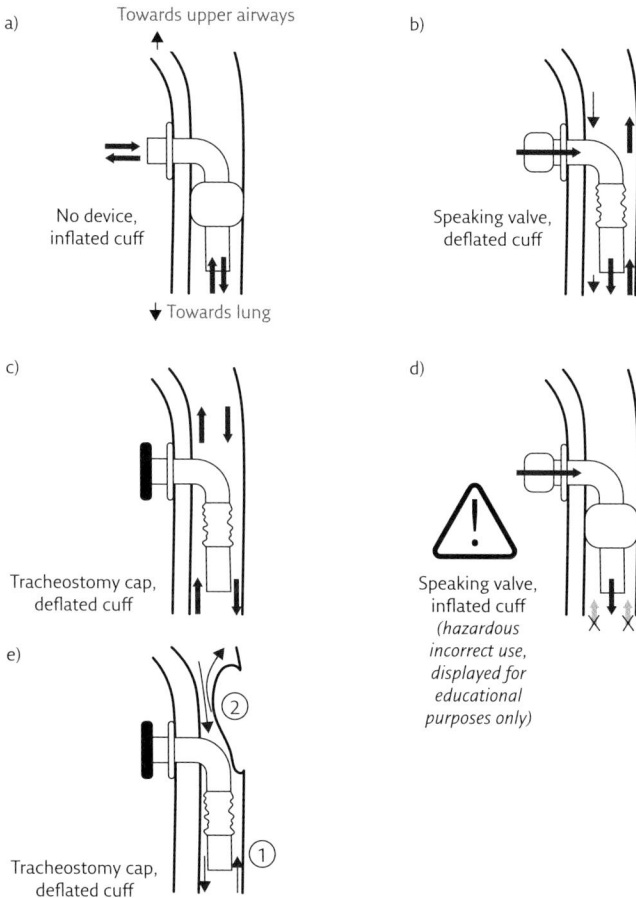

Figure 2. Inspiratory and expiratory flow patterns in a spontaneously breathing tracheostomised patient. a) No speaking device, inflated cuff: air flows in and out through the tracheostomy tube (TT). b) Speaking valve, deflated cuff: air flows in through the TT, but flows out through the upper airways. c) Tracheostomy cap, deflated cuff: air flows in and out through the upper airways. d) Speaking valve, inflated cuff (incorrect use): expiratory flow is blocked. A few inspiratory breaths are possible before asphyxiation occurs, often with a tension pneumothorax. e) Tracheostomy cap, deflated cuff. This example shows two possible causes of airflow limitation: a high tube-to-trachea ratio (1) and an upper tracheal granuloma (2). Symptoms depend on the severity of the limitation and range from mild dyspnoea to asphyxia.

Daily management of a tracheostomised patient

Nursing care

- In most cases, simple peristomal care with saline solution is sufficient. The peristomal zone should be kept as dry as possible. A slightly inflammatory aspect is frequent with surgical tracheostomies. Complications to look for are cervical cellulitis, pressure ulcers and peristomal granulomas that can be treated with silver nitrate.
- When the cuff is inflated, cuff pressure should be monitored every 4–8 h and should be between 20 and 25 mmHg (or 25–30 cmH$_2$O).
- Humidification systems should be used during invasive ventilation and spontaneous breathing. Thick or sticky secretions can indicate a lack of humidification that can lead to accidental tube obstruction.
- Most tracheostomy tubes used in the ICU have an inner cannula, which can be removed and cleaned daily or as needed (including in cases of an obstructive plug).
- Systematic regular tube changes (*i.e.* every week) are not recommended.
- Readiness to perform an unassisted breathing session must be assessed every day.

Weaning protocol Weaning time is reduced when a systematic weaning protocol is applied. A protocol using daily sessions of unassisted breathing is more efficient that a protocol based on a progressive decrease in the pressure support level. Applying a nurse-led systematic weaning protocol also appears to reduce weaning time.

Box 1. How to use a speaking valve or a tracheostomy cap safely

Use only on a thoroughly deflated cuff.

Using a speaking valve or tracheostomy cap on a patient with complete tracheal or upper airways obstruction (*e.g.* inflated cuff, obstructive granuloma or glottic oedema) can lead to asphyxia, barotrauma and cardiac arrest.

Patients with partial obstruction can display symptoms ranging from severe dyspnoea, expiratory noise and/or stridor, delayed respiratory fatigue or poor exercise tolerance.

If this occurs:

- immediately remove the device in case of asphyxia or severe respiratory distress;
- check for proper cuff deflation;
- consider changing the tracheostomy tube for a smaller or thinner one (a high tube-to-trachea diameter ratio is a cause of increased airway resistance); and
- if the problem persists, consider fibrescopy to look for a cause of airway obstruction.

Speaking valves do not provide any humidification of inspired gases. Consider alternating with a humidification filter or using a tracheostomy cap instead.

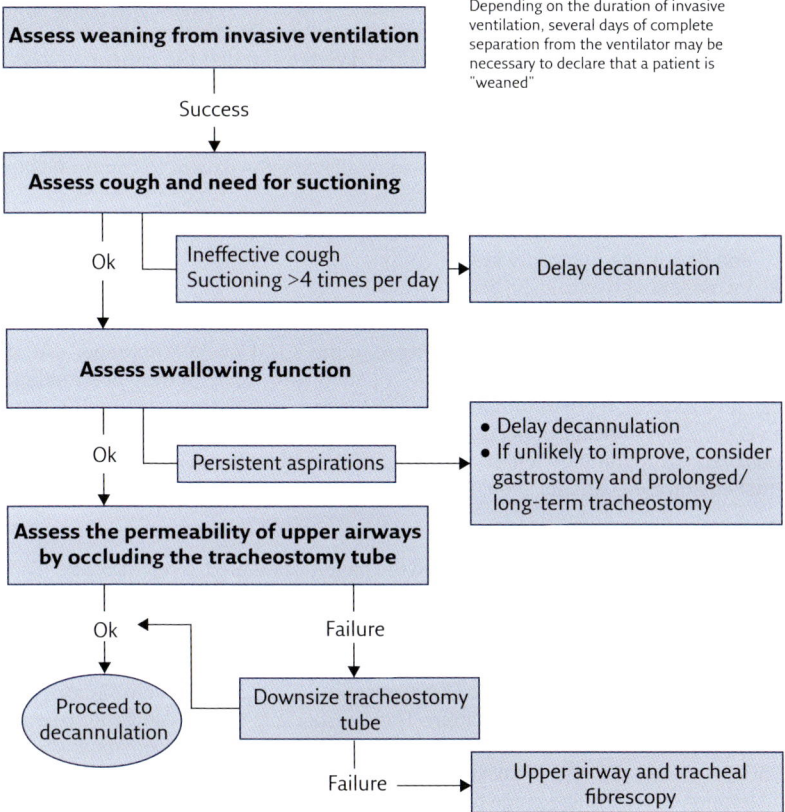

Depending on the duration of invasive ventilation, several days of complete separation from the ventilator may be necessary to declare that a patient is "weaned"

Figure 3. Decannulation decision tree.

Cuff management During spontaneous breathing, cuff deflation:

- decreases airway resistances and work of breathing;
- is safer (in case of accidental tube obstruction);
- relieves the tracheal mucosa from cuff pressure, thereby preventing the occurrence of tracheal stenosis;
- is associated with a decreased weaning time and infection rate while improving swallowing function; and
- allows the use of phonation devices.

Cuff deflation should therefore be the default procedure. The cuff should remain inflated in patients with profuse salivary aspiration, but this should be reassessed regularly, as it usually improves over time. Caution should be used in patients at high risk of aspiration (neurological patients, and patients with a history of neck surgery or radiation therapy).

Speaking valves and tracheostomy caps A speaking valve is a one-way valve that allows the air to flow through the tracheostomy during inspiration, but not during expiration. The expiratory flow is therefore diverted through the patient airways, around the tracheostomy tube (and/or through fenestrations in cases where a fenestrated cannula is used), and through the vocal cords and upper airways, thus allowing speech. A tracheostomy cap is a plug that completely occludes the tracheostomy tube (figure 2a–c). Aside from allowing the patient to communicate more effectively, these devices:

- improve swallowing and reduce aspirations through the restoration of pressure and flow in the upper airways;
- increase cough efficiency; and
- increase lung recruitment.

Their use should therefore be encouraged in the ICU. However, improper use of these devices (on an inflated cuff or in a patient with upper airway obstruction) can lead to tension pneumothoraces, asphyxia and cardiac arrest (figure 2d). Poor tolerance can indicate upper airways complications such as glottic oedema or upper tracheal granuloma (box 1 and figure 2e). All staff involved in the care of tracheostomised patients should be adequately trained (box 1).

Decannulation

Decannulation can be considered when the patient is weaned, is not dependent on suctioning, is not at high risk of aspiration, and has unobstructed upper airways. A 24–48 h capping trial allows the assessment of most of these aspects and can help predict a successful decannulation (figure 3).

NIV can be considered to facilitate decannulation and/or consolidate the weaning process after decannulation. This is especially the case in patients with underlying respiratory conditions or in patients who remain hypercapnic ($P_{a}CO_2$ >50–55 mmHg (6.7–7.3 kPa)). Of note, if tracheostomy capping is well tolerated, adaptation to NIV can be made before the decannulation in fragile patients.

Further reading

- Alansari M, *et al.* (2015). Use of ultrasound guidance to improve the safety of percutaneous dilatational tracheostomy: a literature review. *Crit Care*; 19: 229.

- Diehl J-L, *et al.* (1999). Changes in the work of breathing induced by tracheotomy in ventilator-dependent patients. *Am J Respir Crit Care Med*; 159: 383–388.

- Hernandez G, *et al.* (2013). The effects of increasing effective airway diameter on weaning from mechanical ventilation in tracheostomized patients: a randomized controlled trial. *Intensive Care Med*; 39: 1063–1070.

- Huttmann SE, *et al.* (2018). Quality of life and life satisfaction are severely impaired in patients with long-term invasive ventilation following ICU treatment and unsuccessful weaning. *Ann Intensive Care*; 8: 38.

- Jubran A, *et al.* (2013). Effect of pressure support *vs* unassisted breathing through a tracheostomy collar on weaning duration in patients requiring prolonged mechanical ventilation: a randomized trial. *JAMA*; 309: 671–677.

- Jubran A, *et al.* (2019). Long-term outcome after prolonged mechanical ventilation: a long-term acute-care hospital study. *Am J Respir Crit Care Med*; 199: 1508–1516.

- O'Connor LR, *et al.* (2018). Physiological and clinical outcomes associated with use of one-way speaking valves on tracheostomised patients: a systematic review. *Heart Lung*; 48: 356–364.

- Singh J, *et al.* (2019). Performance, long-term management, and coding for percutaneous dilational tracheostomy. *Chest*; 155: 639–644.

- Trouillet J-L, *et al.* (2018). Tracheotomy in the intensive care unit: guidelines from a French expert panel: the French Intensive Care Society and the French Society of Anaesthesia and Intensive Care Medicine. *Anaesth Crit Care Pain Med*; 37: 281–294.

- Yarmus L. Percutaneous tracheotomy. *In*: Ernst A, *et al.*, eds. (2012). Principles and Practice Of Interventional Pulmonology. New York, Springer Science and Business Media, pp. 683–696.

Physiotherapy and speech therapy in ventilated patients

Rik Gosselink and Christina Iezzi

23-30% of patients fail discharge from invasive ventilation and require a disproportionate amount of resources. Several factors contribute to weaning failure including inadequate ventilatory drive, respiratory muscle weakness, increased work of breathing, excessive airway secretions, ineffective cough, lung dysfunction, brain dysfunction and cardiac failure, as well as endocrine and metabolic dysfunctions. Tracheostomy is one of the most common procedures performed in intensive care for prolonged invasive ventilation or difficult-to-wean patients and is also associated with impaired communication and swallowing. This, along with the growing critical care population means there is an increasing demand for a collaborative multi- and interdisciplinary approach to weaning. Physiotherapists and speech and language therapists are involved in both assessment and treatment of patients with weaning failure. The specific aims of physiotherapy are to:

- initiate and guide early mobilisation and physical activity
- improve lung inflation
- clear airway secretions
- enhance inspiratory muscle function

Key points

- To understand the assessment of physiotherapists and speech and language therapists in patients with difficult weaning.

- To understand the different modalities of physiotherapy and speech and language therapy in the treatment of patients with difficult weaning.

- Weaning from invasive ventilation needs to be bespoke/ individualised for each patient, including assessment and treatment by speech and language therapists and physical therapists.

- Multi- and interdisciplinary multi-modal approaches including both speech and language therapy and physical therapy approaches are warranted.

Speech and language therapists aim to:

- optimise communication
- provide assessment and management of secretions and swallowing
- assist in the evaluation of laryngeal function

Early mobilisation and physical activity

Early mobilisation and physical activity during ICU admission has been shown to be safe and feasible, while improving functional status and mobility level during ICU stay and hospital discharge, as well as decreasing duration of invasive ventilation, and ICU and hospital length of stay. A standardised multidisciplinary protocol, "Start To Move As Soon As Possible" (figure 1), was developed to facilitate safe and early mobilisation in critically ill patients. The protocol consists of an objective diagnostic assessment, which is subsequently linked to different treatment levels consisting of gradually progressing early mobilisation exercises adapted to the physical and mental conditions of patients. In a first step, patients are ranked into one of six different mobility levels according to their medical condition (cardiorespiratory and neurological status), level of cooperation and functional status (muscle strength and level of mobility). Each of the six levels are subsequently linked to a number of specific physiotherapy treatment options and mobilisation exercises that gradually increase in intensity and difficulty from level 0 to 5. Patients in the ICU are evaluated on a daily basis and classified into one of the six "start to move" levels which determine the daily physiotherapy treatment options.

Assessment of suitability for extubation

A spontaneous breathing trial can be used to assess readiness for extubation with the performance of serial measurements. Early detection by the interdisciplinary team of worsening clinical signs such as distress, rapid shallow breathing, paradoxical chest wall motion, abdominal contraction during expiration, airway obstruction and impaired secretion clearance contribute to the prevention of serious problems.

Secretion clearance and cough efficacy

The ability to effectively eliminate secretions from the central airways is dependent on the expiratory flow rate. Patients who are difficult to wean are often suffering from ineffective cough due to either insufficient inspiratory volume, expiratory muscle weakness, poor bulbar and glottis function or upper airway instability. Airway patency and protection (*i.e.* an effective cough mechanism) should be assessed prior to commencement of weaning. Vital capacity and cough peak expiratory flow can be assessed on the ventilator or spirometer connected to the artificial airway. Cut-off scores of cough peak expiratory flow ranging from <35–70 L·min^{-1} were proposed to identify extubation failure or the use of prophylactic NIV to prevent extubation failure.

Oropharyngeal dysphagia and swallowing

Oropharyngeal dysphagia is common in critical care patients. It has been identified in specific clinical subgroups including ARDS, cardiac surgery, sepsis and critical illness polyneuropathy. Additionally, the impact of interventions in ICU such as endotracheal intubation and tracheostomy contributes to the complexity of dysphagia in this patient cohort. There is increasing evidence around the incidence

Multidisciplinary approach

	Level 0	Level 1	Level 2	Level 3	Level 4	Level 5
	No cooperation SSQ1=0-5	Variable cooperation SSQ1=0-5	Variable cooperation SSQ1=0-5	Close-full cooperation SSQ1≥4/5	Full cooperation SSQ1=5	Full cooperation SSQ1=5
Clinical investigation	Fails basic assessment[2]	Passes basic assessment[3]	Passes basic assessment[3]	Passes basic assessment[3]	Passes basic assessment[3]	Passes basic assessment[3]
		Transfer to chair not allowed because of neurological or surgical trauma condition	Active transfer to chair not allowed because of obesity or neurological or surgical or trauma condition	MRCsum ≥36 (MRCsumʟ ≥18) BBS Sit to stand=0 BBS Standing=0 BBS Sitting ≥1	MRCsum ≥48 (MRCsumʟ ≥24) BBS Sit to stand ≥0 BBS Standing >0 BBS Sitting ≥2	MRCsum ≥48 BBS Sit to stand ≥1 BBS Standing ≥2 BBS Sitting ≥3
Rehabilitation	Body positioning[4] 2 h turning Splinting Positioning	Body positioning[4] 2 h turning Splinting Fowler's position	Body positioning[4] 2 h turning Splinting Upright sitting position in bed Passive transfer bed to chair	Body positioning[4] 2 h turning Passive transfer bed to chair Sitting out of bed Standing with assistance (≥2 persons)	Body positioning[4] Active transfer bed to chair Sitting out of bed Standing with assistance (≥1 person)	Body positioning[4] Active transfer bed to chair Sitting out of bed Standing
	Physiotherapy No treatment	Physiotherapy[4] Passive/active ROM Passive/active leg and/or arm cycling in bed NMES ADL	Physiotherapy[4] Passive/active ROM Resistance training arms and legs Passive/active leg and/or arm cycling in bed or chair NMES ADL	Physiotherapy[4] Passive/active ROM Resistance training arms and legs Active leg and/or arm cycling in bed or chair Standing (with assistance/frame) NMES ADL	Physiotherapy[4] Passive/active ROM Resistance training arms and legs Active leg and/or arm cycling in bed or chair Walking (with assistance/frame) NMES ADL	Physiotherapy[4] Passive/active ROM Resistance training arms and legs Active leg and/or arm cycling in bed or chair Walking (with assistance) NMES ADL

Figure 1. Continued on the facing page.

1: Score 5 questions: adequate response to 5 standardised orders
2: Fails: at least 1 risk factor present
3: If basic assessment failed, decrease to level 0
4: Safety and feasibility: each activity should be deferred if severe adverse events (cv., resp., internal and subject intolerance) occur during the intervention

ADEQUACY SCORE
A. Open and close your eyes
B. Look at me
C. Open your mouth and put out your tongue
D. Nod your head
E. Raise your eyebrows when I have counted up to five

BASIC ASSESSMENT
Cardiorespiratory unstable
MAP <60 mmHg **or**
F_{IO_2} >60% **or**
P_{aO_2}/F_{IO_2} <200 mmHg **or**
RR >30 beats·min^{-1}
Neurologically unstable
Acute surgery
Temperature >40°C

Sitting with back unsupported but feet supported on floor or on a stool
4 able to sit safely and securely for 2 min
3 able to sit 2 min under supervision
2 able to sit 30 s
1 able to sit 10 s
0 unable to sit 10 s unsupported

BERG BALANCE SCORE
Sitting to standing
4 able to stand without using hands and stabilise independently
3 able to stand independently using hands
2 able to stand using hands after several tries
1 needs minimal aid to stand or stabilise
0 needs moderate or maximal assist to stand

Standing unsupported
4 able to stand safely for 2 min
3 able to stand 2 min with supervision
2 able to stand 30 s unsupported
1 needs several tries to stand 30 s unsupported
0 unable to stand 30 s unsupported

MRC-SUMSCORE Pre-existing NMD: ☐ No ☐ Yes: ____

MRC-SCALE
0 = no visible contraction
1 = visible contraction without movements of the limbs
2 = movements of the limbs but not against gravity
3 = movement against gravity over (almost) the full range
4 = movement against gravity and resistance
5 = normal

	Right	Reason	EP	Left	Reason	EP
MS: Abduction of the arm						
MS: Flexion of the arm						
MS: Extension of the wrist						
MS: Flexion of the leg						
MS: Extension of the knee						
MS: Dorsal flexion of the foot						

Dominance

STRENGTH SUBTOTAL VALUE	STRENGTH TOTAL=
EP SUBTOTAL VALUE	EP TOTAL=
MRC TOTAL SUMSCORE	

Figure 1. UZ Leuven "Start To Move As Soon As Possible" protocol levels from day 2 with an expected prolonged ICU stay of ≥5 days. S5Q: adequacy score; MRC: Medical Research Council; MRCsumLL: MRCsum of the lower limbs; BBS: Berg Balance Scale; ROM: range of motion; NMES: neuromuscular electrical stimulation; ADL: activities of daily living; MAP: mean arterial pressure; RR: respiratory rate; NMD: neuromuscular disease; MS: muscle strength; EP: extrapolation; cv: cardiovascular; resp: respiratory.

of laryngeal injury and post-extubation dysphagia following endotracheal intubation. Dysphagia prevalence following extubation has been reported in 20–83% of patients intubated for >48 h and the loss of both motor and sensory laryngeal function can occur. Consequently, there is a high prevalence of undetected silent aspiration in ICU patients and aspiration is a leading cause of pneumonia in the ICU environment, contributing significantly to morbidity and mortality. Prolonged invasive ventilation is independently associated with post-extubation dysphagia, which is independently associated with tracheostomy requirement, increased length of stay and poor patient outcomes. There is an absence of validated swallowing screening tools for ICU patients and current screening methods are unreliable and insufficient in identifying silent aspiration. The gold standard for early and accurate assessment for oropharyngeal dysphagia in tracheostomised patients is evaluation by an appropriately skilled speech and language therapist who would employ instrumental assessments as indicated. Videofluoroscopy or fibreoptic endoscopic evaluation of swallowing (FEES) can provide comprehensive evaluation of swallowing function, including identifying and quantifying (silent) aspiration risk. Both instrumental swallow assessments can be employed to develop dysphagia and weaning management plans; however, FEES is more accessible for this patient population and can be performed at the patient bedside *via* video-nasendoscope. Considering laryngeal susceptibility to injury following intubation, access to FEES or flexible nasendoscopy is essential for effective evaluation of laryngeal function. This requires both direct visualisation of laryngeal structures and dynamic assessment of laryngeal function and competence. Additionally, FEES provides assessment of secretions which can assist decision making around suitability for cuff deflation plus evaluation of swallow function and aspiration risk, which provides invaluable information for tracheostomy weaning decisions. This may include establishing appropriateness for use of one-way/speaking valves to restore voice and cough function and decannulation decisions. It can also be utilised to establish candidacy for above cuff vocalisation in patients who are not able to tolerate cuff deflation in the early stages of weaning. Speech and language therapists input should be ideally sought as soon as the decision to wean from the ventilator has been made and sedation hold has commenced.

In the absence of access to appropriately skilled speech and language therapists and instrumental swallow assessments, a water swallow test (WST) can offer sufficient utility in screening for swallowing difficulties and overt aspiration in non-tracheostomised or ventilated patients. Systematic review and meta-analysis for screening accuracy for aspiration using WST highlighted 71% sensitivity and 90% specificity for single sip volumes (1–5 mL), and 91% sensitivity and 53% specificity for consecutive sips of water (90–100 mL). The authors suggested that WSTs adopt a combination of both single sips and consecutive sips with large volumes in patients to improve screening accuracy. There is a paucity of research evaluating screening accuracy of WST in the ICU population, particularly in tracheostomised patients. This, in combination with the high prevalence of silent aspiration in ICU patients, does warrant caution and WSTs should be avoided in tracheostomised and ventilated patients. As screening tests are reliant on symptoms such as changes to vocal quality and coughing post swallowing, caution should also be exercised in the dysphonic or aphonic patient and the use of WST is contraindicated in cuff inflated tracheostomy patients. This highlights the invaluable contribution of instrumental assessments in the evaluation of dysphagia in a complex patient group.

Respiratory muscle function

The inability to breathe spontaneously relates to an imbalance between load on the respiratory muscles and the capacity of the respiratory muscles. A high rate of respiratory muscle effort (ratio of load and muscle capacity (P_I/P_{Imax})) is a major cause of ventilator dependency and predicts the outcome of successful weaning. Clinical signs of the high respiratory effort are the rapid shallow breathing index (V_T/respiratory rate >105), accessory inspiratory muscle contractions, paradoxical (inward) abdominal motion, and expiratory abdominal muscle contraction. A more objective assessment of the capacity of the respiratory muscles include the measurement of the maximal inspiratory and expiratory airway pressures (P_{Imax} and P_{Emax}, respectively) at the tracheostomy or endotracheal tube opening during temporary occlusion of the airway. The procedure for inspiratory pressure measurement involves a unidirectional valve to allow the patient to expire while inspiration is occluded. Optimal length of occlusion time is considered to be 25–30 s in adults. The presence of inspiratory weakness is accepted when P_{Imax} is <50% of the predicted value. Recently, ultrasound assessment of the diaphragm thickness, thickening index and excursion has been proposed as a reliable and useful noninvasive method to assess diaphragm dysfunction and contribute to the prediction of weaning success. Expiratory airway pressures will be measured during a Vasalva manoeuvre from total lung capacity and will be informative to assess cough effectiveness. Normal values are available.

Treatment

Environmental influences, such as ambulating with a portable ventilator, have been shown to benefit attitudes and outlooks in long-term ventilator-dependent patients. In addition, exercise training (ambulation, cycling, walking) will activate respiratory muscles, increase minute ventilation and enhance airway clearance. Early mobilisation has been shown to shorten the duration of invasive ventilation. However, the amount of rehabilitation performed in ICUs is often inadequate. Different (modifiable) barriers were identified by nurses, physiotherapists and physicians, *i.e.* limited (experienced) staff and supporting equipment, no protocol, no mobility culture, lack of planning and coordination, no "champion" in the team or "standing bed rest" order. However, the risk of moving a critically ill patient (*i.e.* endotracheal tube displacement, cardiovascular instability) should be weighed against the risk of immobility and recumbency and when employed, it requires stringent monitoring to ensure that the mobilisation is instituted appropriately and safely. A variety of programmes to guide a (interdisciplinary) step-up approach of progressive mobilisation and physical activity are available.

Airway clearance and lung recruitment

In intubated or cannulated patients several modalities are available to assist in secretion clearance: manual hyperinflation or ventilator hyperinflation, postural drainage, spontaneous coughing, cough-assist devices, expiratory chest wall compression and airway suctioning. Manual hyperinflation is applied in uncooperative patients to prevent pulmonary atelectasis, re-expand collapsed alveoli, improve lung compliance and oxygenation, and enhance secretion removal. Manual hyperinflation involves a slow deep inspiration with a manual resuscitator bag, an inspiratory hold of 2–3 s, followed by a quick release of the bag to enhance expiratory flow and mimic a forced expiration. Manual hyperinflation might have important negative side-effects. A pressure of 40 cmH$_2$O has been recommended as an upper limit. Alternatively, in more cooperative intubated or cannulated patients with an ineffective cough due to impaired inspiratory volume, expiratory force or glottis dysfunction, the mechanical insufflator-exsufflator can be applied. The mechanical insufflator-exsufflator device delivers adjustable positive inspiratory pressures (+30–60 cmH$_2$O) and negative expiratory pressures (−3–60 cmH$_2$O) to enhance lung inflation and increase expiratory flow rate to mobilise bronchial secretions. The effectiveness of the mechanical insufflator-exsufflator has been shown specifically in patients with neuromuscular disease and its application has become more popular. However, in the ICU population the mechanical insufflator-exsufflator did not improve secretion removal and respiratory mechanics, but increased extubation success significantly.

In patients with ineffective cough and an inability to clear secretions, airway suctioning *via* the artificial airway (endotracheal tube or tracheostomy) or nasotracheal suctioning is needed. Airway suctioning may have detrimental side-effects (bronchial lesions and hypoxaemia), but reassurance, sedation and pre-oxygenation of the patient may minimise these effects. Suctioning can be performed *via* an in-line closed suctioning system or an open system. Although frequently used, the in-line system does not appear to decrease the incidence of ventilator-associated pneumonia or the duration of invasive ventilation, length of ICU stay or mortality. Personal practices and established practice in the ICU seems to be the most important factors in suctioning practice. The routine instillation of normal saline before airway suctioning has potential adverse effects on oxygen saturation and cardiovascular stability, and variable results in terms of increasing sputum yield. Chest wall compression prior to endotracheal suctioning did not improve airway secretion removal, oxygenation or ventilation after endotracheal suctioning in an unselected population of invasively ventilated patients.

Communication

One-way/speaking valves The prevalence of communication difficulties in this population is reported to be between 16% and 24%. The loss of speech and the inability to express basic needs as a result of invasive ventilation can adversely affect patients' mood, cause anxiety, lead to difficulty participating in treatment decisions and lead to disengagement with subsequent nonadherence to necessary rehabilitation. Restoring or facilitating verbal communication enables the patient to actively participate in their treatment and can improve the intensive care experience for patients. Early introduction of one-way speaking valves in ventilated dependent patients has a dynamic role beyond the immediate and obvious benefits of restoring verbal communication. There is also an emerging role for early introduction of one-way valves in line with ventilator dependent patients to facilitate weaning. Once patients have commenced laryngeal weaning and are able to tolerate full cuff deflation, one-way valves can be utilised in line with positive pressure ventilation. This allows exhaled air to pass through the larynx instead of the ventilator circuit.

Early cuff deflation and insertion of one-way valves during invasive ventilation has been shown to restore speech sooner for ventilated patients when compared to patients only using one-way valves during spontaneous breathing trials and without an increase in complications. Furthermore, despite a deflated tracheostomy cuff, speaking valves have also been shown to improve lung recruitment. For example, the Passy Muir speaking valve (Passy Muir Inc., Irvine, CA, USA) can be used in line with invasive ventilation and should be considered for use as part of standard care in prolonged weaning patients.

Above cuff vocalisation If cuff deflation is not tolerated, above cuff vocalisation can be utilised in the short term to facilitate phonation and benefit laryngeal functions for swallowing. Application of an external air source through the subglottic port of the tracheostomy can facilitate phonation with an inflated tracheostomy cuff. Airway patency should be confirmed *via* flexible nasendoscopy prior to trialling this method to avoid adverse complications.

Respiratory muscle loading (training) or unloading

A lower contractile activity of the diaphragm during invasive ventilation was associated with a reduction of diaphragm thickness. Additionally, patient–ventilator dyssynchrony and overloading the respiratory muscles during the weaning phase can also lead to prolonged weaning. This observation supports the idea that well-balanced, intermittent loading of the respiratory muscles during the process of invasive ventilation might be beneficial to prevent or ameliorate muscle atrophy. Indeed, modalities inducing (intermittent) loading of the respiratory muscles such as spontaneous breathing trials increase respiratory muscle strength. Surprisingly, little attention has been given to specific interventions to enhance strength and endurance of the respiratory muscles. Indeed, daily inspiratory muscle training (IMT) with six to eight contractions repeated in three to four series at moderate to high intensity was safe and improved both inspiratory muscle strength and weaning success in patients with

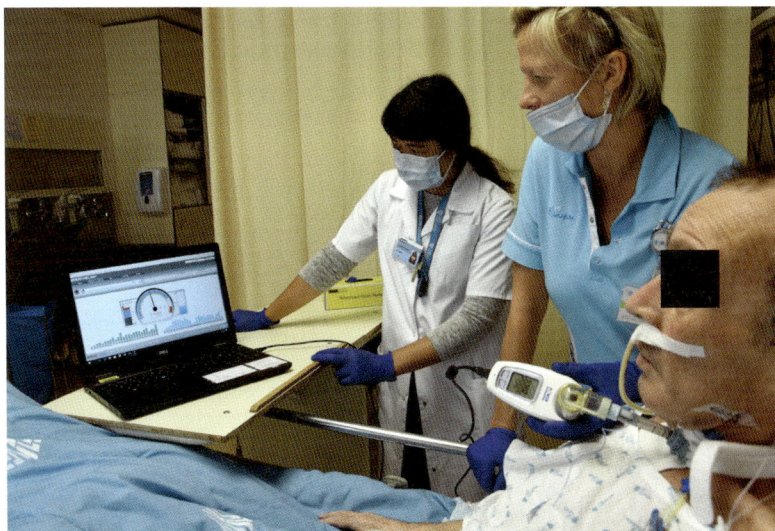

Figure 2. IMT with feedback as part of the weaning of a tracheotomised patient with difficult weaning from invasive ventilation.

difficult weaning. The studies performed so far on IMT in invasively ventilated patients were heterogeneous with regard to specific inclusion criteria, training modalities and evaluated outcomes. Specifically, patients with known weaning difficulties seem more likely to benefit from an IMT intervention during invasive ventilation. In addition, most of those RCTs used a mechanical threshold-loading device for IMT which might not offer the ideal loading characteristics in this specific setting. An alternative, potentially more optimal, way of loading the respiratory muscles is tapered flow resistive loading IMT. This isokinetic loading approach during tapered flow resistive loading is better adapted to the length-tension characteristics of the inspiratory muscles and visual feedback on the screen will allow larger V_T to be achieved during IMT (figure 2).

Alternatively, NIV has been applied to unload the respiratory muscles and allow extubation earlier in the weaning process and/or to prevent extubation failure. In selected (non-COPD) hypoxaemic ventilated patients, early extubation followed by immediate NIV application reduced the days spent on invasive ventilation without affecting ICU length of stay. Recent reviews demonstrated that the use of NIV in weaning from invasive ventilation, compared with ongoing invasive ventilation, reduces hospital mortality, the incidence of ventilator-associated pneumonia and length of ICU stay, particularly in patients with COPD.

Finally, biofeedback of the pattern of breathing to the patient can also enhance the weaning process of patients receiving long-term invasive ventilation. Voice and touch may be used to augment weaning success either by stimulation to improve ventilatory drive or by reducing anxiety.

Further reading

- Bissett B, *et al.* (2019). Inspiratory muscle training for intensive care patients: a multidisciplinary practical guide for clinicians. *Aust Crit Care*; 32: 249–255.

- Brodsky MB, *et al.* (2016). Screening accuracy for aspiration using bedside water swallow tests: a systematic review and meta-analysis. *Chest*; 150: 148–163.

- Brodsky MB, *et al.* (2018). Laryngeal injury and upper airway symptoms after oral endotracheal intubation with mechanical ventilation during critical care: a systematic review. *Crit Care Med*; 46: 2010–2017.

- Dubb R, *et al.* (2016). Barriers and strategies for early mobilization of patients in intensive care units. *Ann Am Thorac Soc*; 13: 724–730.

- Fernandez-Carmona A, *et al.* (2018). Ineffective cough and mechanical mucociliary clearance techniques. *Med Intensiva*; 42: 50–59.

- Freeman-Sanderson AL, *et al.* (2016). Return of voice for ventilated tracheostomy patients in ICU: a randomized controlled trial of early-targeted intervention. *Crit Care Med*; 44: 1075–1081.

- Goligher EC, *et al.* (2015). Evolution of diaphragm thickness during mechanical ventilation. impact of inspiratory effort. *Am J Respir Crit Care Med*; 192: 1080–1088.

- Gosselink R, *et al.* (2011). Physiotherapy in the intensive care unit. *Neth J Int Care*; 15: 9.

- Gosselink R, *et al.* (2008). Physiotherapy for adult patients with critical illness: recommendations of the European Respiratory Society and European Society of Intensive Care Medicine Task Force on Physiotherapy for Critically Ill Patients. *Intensive Care Med*; 34: 1188–1199.

- Hodgson C, *et al.* (2016). Recruitment manoeuvres for adults with acute respiratory distress syndrome receiving mechanical ventilation. *Cochrane Database Syst Rev*; 11: CD006667.

- Marini JJ, *et al.* (1986). Estimation of inspiratory muscle strength in mechanically ventilated patients: the measurement of maximal inspiratory pressure. *J Crit Care*; 1: 32–38.

- McGrath B, *et al.* (2016). Above cuff vocalisation: a novel technique for communication in the ventilator-dependent tracheostomy patient. *J Intensive Care Soc*; 17: 19–26.

- McGrath BA, *et al.* (2019). Safety and feasibility of above cuff vocalisation for ventilator-dependant patients with tracheostomies. *J Intensive Care Soc*; 20: 59–65.

- National Tracheostomy Safety Project (NTSP). Swallowing and communication (Adults). Speaking valve trial. http://tracheostomy.org.uk/healthcare-staff/vocalisation/speaking-valve-trials

- National Tracheostomy Safety Project (NTSP). Swallowing and communication (Adults). ACV – Above Cuff Vocalisation. http://tracheostomy.org.uk/healthcare-staff/vocalisation/acv-above-cuff-vocalisation

- Rose L, *et al.* (2017). Cough augmentation techniques for extubation or weaning critically ill patients from mechanical ventilation. *Cochrane Database Syst Rev*; 1: CD011833.

- Sutt AL, *et al.* (2016). Speaking valves in tracheostomised ICU patients weaning off mechanical ventilation – do they facilitate lung recruitment? *Crit Care*; 20: 91.

- Sutt AL, *et al.* (2015). The use of tracheostomy speaking valves in mechanically ventilated patients results in improved communication and does not prolong ventilation time in cardiothoracic intensive care unit patients. *J Crit Care*; 30: 491–494.

- Vorona S, *et al.* (2018). Inspiratory muscle rehabilitation in critically ill adults: a systematic review and meta-analysis. *Ann Am Thorac Soc*; 15: 735–744.

- Yeung J, *et al.* (2018). Non-invasive ventilation as a strategy for weaning from invasive mechanical ventilation: a systematic review and Bayesian meta-analysis. *Intensive Care Med*; 44: 2192–204.

Technical aspects of the ventilator

Frans de Jongh and Peter Somhorst

This chapter aims to explain and clarify the technical aspects of intensive care ventilators. Basic parameters such as pressure, flow, resistance and compliance as well as their relationships are described. Aspects of the ventilator, the tubing system and the patient are taken into consideration. Sensors to record parameters, modes of ventilation, and possibilities for algorithms to optimise ventilation are briefly mentioned. The chapter ends with the possible technical future of ventilators.

Basic principles of pressure and flow

Respiration is defined as transporting oxygen and carbon dioxide between cells and an external environment through the lung. Ventilation is the movement of air between the environment and the lungs *via* breathing. Movement of air is governed by a pressure difference: air flows from a high pressure to a low pressure. During spontaneous respiration, contraction of the diaphragm results in caudal movement of the diaphragm. Also the ribcage might be elevated by intercostal muscle contraction. As a result, the pressure around the lungs (the pressure in the pleural space) will decrease, in its turn lowering the pressure in the alveoli of the lungs. In this way, the pressure at the mouth (normally the atmospheric pressure)

Key points

- Ventilation is possible because of pressure differences between the outside and inside of the lungs. Ventilators aim to create these pressure differences, when a patient cannot create them for themselves.

- Almost all modern ventilators are designed to alter the pressure at the mouth, which is usually achieved with compressed gas. Valves control pressure and flow, and tubing systems are designed to minimise dead space.

- Sensors are used for control and feedback, which may be triggered by pressure and flow, as well as by electromyography signals.

- In the future, artificial intelligence systems may help to control increasingly complex ventilator settings.

will be higher than the pressure in the lungs so air will flow *via* the mouth to the alveoli. As soon as the pressure in the alveoli again is atmospheric, the airflow will cease and the patient is ready for expiration. Then the process is reversed: first the pressure in the pleural space is increased, after which alveolar pressure will become higher than the atmospheric pressure, after which airflow will start from the alveoli to the mouth.

This process can be mimicked by a ventilator that is able to change the pressure around the chest of the patient, like an iron lung/cuirass ventilator. The first ventilators were designed like this. However, an airtight seal around the body requires cumbersome equipment and in the 1970s it became clear that ventilation could be more easily achieved by changing the pressure at the mouth of a patient instead of changing the pressure around the chest. Increasing the pressure at the mouth (so raising it above atmospheric pressure) will again give a pressure difference between mouth and alveoli, so air will flow into the lungs. At the end of the inspiration, when alveolar pressure is the same as the pressure at the mouth (which was higher than atmospheric pressure), expiration can be initiated by lowering the pressure at the mouth (*e.g.* back to atmospheric pressure). In this way, positive pressure ventilation can achieve the same ventilation as spontaneous breathing. During positive pressure ventilation, the pressure in the alveoli is always the same as or higher than atmospheric pressure, while with spontaneous respiration the pressure in the lung is alternating between pressure higher and lower than atmospheric pressure. Nowadays, almost all ventilators are designed to alter the pressure at the mouth instead of that in the lungs/around the body of a patient.

Mathematically, the relationship between pressure and airflow is described by the equation of motion (based on Newton's third law) shown in equation (1), where P is the actual airway pressure, C_{rs} is the compliance of the respiratory system and R is the resistance between the mouth or mechanical ventilator and the alveoli. V_T represents the volume of the air above functional residual capacity in the lungs (the tidal volume), while $\dot{V}$ represents the change in volume, *i.e.* the flow of air. PEEP is the positive end-expiratory pressure.

$$P = \frac{V_T}{C_{rs}} + R \cdot \dot{V} + PEEP \tag{1}$$

From this equation, it becomes apparent that a change in pressure is required to both inflate the lung and overcome the resistance of the airways. The difference in pressure between the start and end of inspiration (ΔP) resulting in a change in volume during inspiration, *i.e.* the volume above functional residual capacity (V_T), is readily described by equation (2). Note that ΔP should be measured under static conditions (so with zero flow) and is known as the driving pressure.

$$\Delta P = \frac{V_T}{C_{rs}}, \text{ so } V_T = \Delta P \cdot C_{rs} \tag{2}$$

This implies that the V_T depends on the product of the static pressure difference (ΔP) between mouth and alveoli and the C_{rs}. The C_{rs} varies with sex, height, age and BMI and is a function of the lung volume and the disease state of the lungs and thorax.

During ventilation of a spontaneously breathing patient, the pressure governing the flow is composed of the pressure generated by the ventilator (P_{vent}) and the pressure generated by the muscles of the patient (P_{mus}), readily described by equation (3).

$$P_{vent} + P_{mus} = \frac{V_T}{C_{rs}} + R \cdot \dot{V} \tag{3}$$

Note that P_{mus} has an inward direction, *i.e.* inspiratory effort has a positive sign, and expiratory effort has a negative sign. If for instance the pressure of a ventilator increases during inspiration, but the patient tries to exhale at the same time, P_{mus} might equal P_{vent} and there will be no pressure difference, so no flow. If P_{vent} increases during inspiration while the patient inhales spontaneously at the same time, the transrespiratory pressure is increased and inspiratory flow will be increased. If the patient's muscles are not functioning, P_{mus} becomes zero and P_{vent} must be sufficient to achieve the correct V_T.

The technical demand for ventilation is therefore to have a device that is able to change the pressure at the mouth. There are several ways that air pressure can be changed. Most often, gas "out of the wall" of a hospital, compressed at 4–5 bar, is used. In fact this gas often comes from compressed gas stored in cylinders at high pressure (*e.g.* 150–200 bar). Luckily the respiratory system (lungs and chest wall) of a human is very compliant, requiring only around 2.5 cmH$_2$O of pressure change to inhale a normal V_T of 500 mL in a healthy situation. Knowing that 1 bar is approximately 1 atm and around 1000 cmH$_2$O, we see that increasing the pressure at the mouth from 1.0 atm to 1.0025 atm is enough to inspire 500 mL for healthy lungs. Even very sick/stiff lungs/respiratory systems are mostly not ventilated with more than 50 cmH$_2$O (1.050 atm), to reduce the chance of VILI, so the maximally needed pressure increase is limited. Reduction of the air pressure is achieved with pressure regulation valves.

Several other ways exist to create a changing air pressure, from oscillating pistons to oscillating membranes (*e.g.* loud speakers) or fast turbofans (blowers). Blowers are not able to achieve high pressures but require less energy and are therefore more often used for situations where transport is necessary, as the energy can be delivered for a long time by a battery or electrical connection.

Gas mixture and humidification

Pressurised air should have the correct gas mixture. The mixture is usually achieved using a blender that can mix compressed air with pure oxygen, thereby achieving oxygen concentrations between 21% and 100%. In special cases, other gas mixtures might be used (*e.g.* Heliox, which is a mixture of oxygen and helium) to reduce work of breathing but the clinical gain is mostly marginal. During normal respiration, inspired air is warmed and humified in the nose. During invasive ventilation this natural humidifier is bypassed. After passing the correct gas mixture through a heater/humidifier, the air is delivered to the patient through a tubing system.

Tubing system

The tubing system of a ventilator is not considered to be an integral part of a ventilator, since often several (disposable) tubing systems can be used. Considering their compliance, resistance, connectors and leakage was formerly important, since pressure and V_T reached depended on these factors. Nowadays, almost all ventilators use sensors, positioned in the ventilator as close to the patient's lungs as possible, to measure whether the intended target settings (for instance pressure and volume) are reached. The ventilator often fine-tunes the delivered pressure and volume to achieve the goals set by the clinician. If applicable, automatic compensation, *e.g.* for the tube resistance, can be incorporated. Knowing that, by the law of Poiseuille for laminar flow, resistance depends on the fourth power of the internal diameter of a tube, the tube is usually by far the highest resistive element in a patient–ventilator setting, so compensation might be obligatory. However, during the weaning phase, the respiratory muscles of a patient might need to be trained, so the work of breathing a patient should be able to deliver must increase. In that case, the compensatory setting to reduce work of breathing might be minimised.

Most often, the pressure, flow and thereby volume delivered to the patient are controlled by a valve located in the ventilator at the end of the expiration hose of the tubing system. By closing this expiratory valve in the machine, with an open valve at the inspiration hose, the air has no other route than going to the patient. Expiration can be made completely passive by closing the inspiration valve and opening the expiration valve so the lungs will deflate to the chosen PEEP level. The time constant of this deflation is mainly governed by the compliance and resistance of the complete system. This includes compliance and resistance of the lungs, chest wall and expiratory hose, and the settings and resistance of the expiratory valve.

Most tubing systems are designed to minimise the dead space. This is often the part from the Y-connector of the tubing system to the lungs of the patient. A small dead space minimises loss of gas exchange in the lungs but might increase resistance of the tubing system due to a smaller diameter. Another challenge is that most sensors are optimally placed so that they are able to measure the air that flows in and out of the endotracheal tube. However, placement of an airflow sensor between the Y-piece and the endotracheal tube increases the dead space of the system. The ongoing miniaturisation of sensors reduces this problem.

Sensors for control or feedback

The main sensors used are able to measure pressure, flow and the amount of oxygen (F_{IO_2}) in the inspired air. Volume is obtained by integrating the flow over time. To monitor the patient, capnography is used to measure the carbon dioxide content of the exhaled air. Pulse oximetry saturation, blood gas analyses and other signals may indicate how well the patient is ventilated. To minimise the chance of ventilator-induced diaphragmatic dysfunction and to increase comfort, patient triggers are used. The main goal is to synchronise the air delivered by the ventilator with the inspiratory effort of the patient. Pressure and flow triggers are most commonly used. These parameters inherently imply a delay in triggering. Inhalation starts with a neural signal of the patient's brain leading to contraction of the diaphragm. This contraction leads to a pressure drop in the lungs (which could be used as trigger). Due to this pressure drop, an inspiratory flow is induced (also used as a trigger), which finally leads to the patient's inspired volume. In recent decades, early signals of the spontaneous respiration of a patient have been investigated using electromyography of the diaphragm with a special oesophageal catheter (diaphragm electrical activity (EAdi) catheter), or using transcutaneous electromyography. This can be used to optimise triggering the ventilator. Not only might the time delay be minimised but also the amplitude of the EAdi can be used to give a proportional assist by the ventilator. Thus, a high EAdi might indicate that the patient wants to inhale a large V_T and the support of the ventilator can be increased for such a breath.

Over recent decades, closed loop ventilation has more often been used. This implies that several sensor signals are used in a predefined algorithm that might change the ventilator settings if the patient's condition changes. For instance, a lowering oxygen saturation might be automatically compensated by an increase of the F_{IO_2} delivered, an increase of the PEEP or a change in the combination of these parameters. In figure 1, an overview is given to show how ventilation can be controlled based on many parameters and how feedback loops are integrated in this process.

In summary, one can distinguish several sets of variables that can be used to optimise ventilation (table 1). The target variables/outcomes can often be reached in several ways and choosing the optimal combination (by an intensivist and/or computer) of control, cycle and trigger variables is mandatory for patient-tailored ventilation.

Modes of ventilation

Ventilators allow the clinician to choose different types of inspiratory support (modes). Early ventilators were limited to pressure-controlled or volume-controlled ventilators. Modern ventilators come with many mixed modes, most of which have some form of patient-triggered ventilation. The names of all these modes are not consistent and sometimes depend on the ventilator brand used. Chatburn tried to standardise this by describing ventilation as a combination of three elements:

1) a variable describing breath control (pressure-regulated or volume-regulated)
2) a breath sequence (intermittent mandatory ventilation, continuous mandatory ventilation and continuous spontaneous ventilation)
3) a "targeting" scheme (prescribing set-points, proportional or adaptive ventilation modes, bio-variability modes, intelligent ventilation schemes, *etc.*)

Instead of using trademarked product names, a worldwide standardisation in terminology would be a huge advantage. However, the fact that different clinical specialists (*e.g.* intensivist, pulmonologist, anaesthesiologist) all might have to ventilate patients hampers consensus statements. In table 2, an overview is given to show how ventilation modes have different names on different ventilators.

In recent decades, noninvasive ventilators have more often been implemented, since they do not require intubation but can deliver pressure (sometimes by high-flow systems with adequate moisturising) at the nose and/or mouth of the patient.

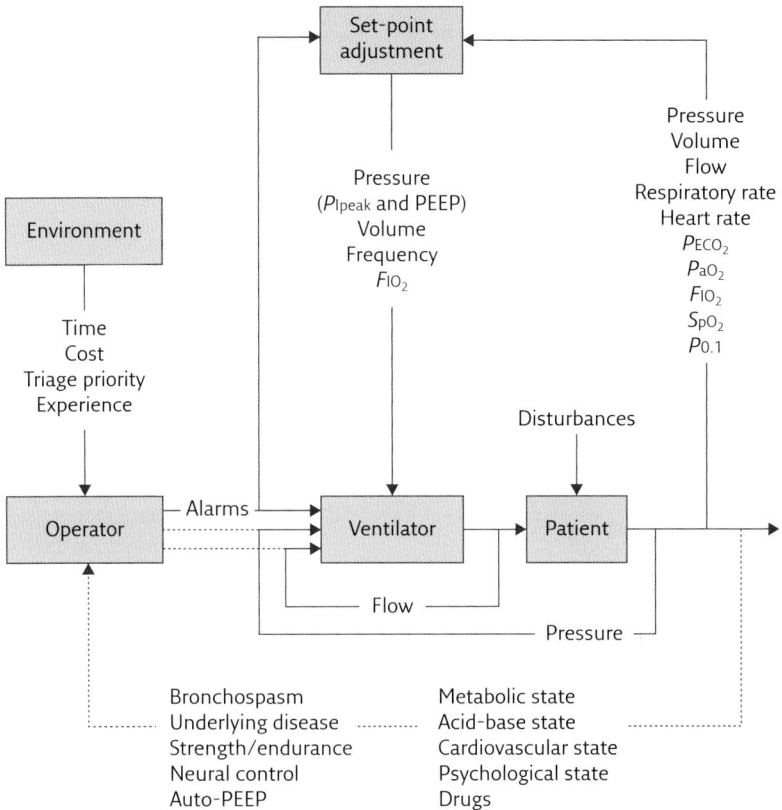

Figure 1. Computer control of mechanical ventilation. Solid arrows depict signals that have been used at least experimentally. Dotted arrows represent potential feedback signals. P$_{Ipeak}$: peak inspiratory pressure; P$_{ECO_2}$: expired carbon dioxide tension; P$_{0.1}$: airway occlusion pressure 0.1 s after the onset of inspiratory effort; auto-PEEP: intrinsic PEEP. Reproduced and modified from Chatburn (2004) with permission.

The equation of motion for flow without (or with negligible) energy loss is the law of Bernoulli, which states that:

$$P + \frac{1}{2}\rho v^2 = \text{constant} \tag{4}$$

In equation (4), P is the pressure (in Pascal), ρ the density (in kg·m^{-3}) of the air/gas mixture that is flowing, and v the velocity (in m·s^{-1}) of that air. In the absence of airflow (v=0 m·s^{-1}), the pressure is often atmospheric so the "constant" in that case becomes the atmospheric pressure. From this equation, one can see how the velocity of airflow can be converted to pressure.

Table 1. Variables that can be used to optimise ventilation

Control
    Pressure (P_{Ipeak} and PEEP)
    Volume
    Frequency
    F_{IO_2}
    Flow rate (determining how fast a pressure/volume is reached)
Phase
    Synchronised ventilation
    Delay time
Trigger
    Neural
    Pressure
    Flow
    Volume
Target
    Pressure
    Volume
    Respiratory rate
    Heart rate
    P_{aCO_2}, P_{ECO_2}, P_{ETCO_2}, P_{aO_2}, S_{pO_2}
Cycle
    Inspiratory time
    Respiratory rate
    $\dot{V}_{CO_2}$

P_{ETCO_2}: end-tidal carbon dioxide tension; $\dot{V}_{CO_2}$: carbon dioxide production.

One of the main differences from conventional ventilation is that NIV will almost certainly induce leakage of flow (and thereby pressure loss) at the nose and mouth. Thus, leak compensation is a very important feature for this mode of ventilation. For "classic" invasive ventilation, (tube) leakage can be quantified exactly as the difference between the amount of air entering the tube to the lungs of the patient and the amount that leaves the tube, so compensation by the ventilator can be easy. For NIV modes, leak compensation is much more challenging, since a high pressure at the nose/mouth might not result in adequate gas exchange in the lungs if, for instance, the upper airways are closed/blocked. A flow/pressure measurement might therefore be insufficient and other monitoring methods and feedback mechanisms to the noninvasive ventilator might be required.

The technical future of ventilators

More advanced algorithms can be built using artificial intelligence strategies, such as artificial neural networks or fuzzy logic. Although, theoretically, these systems (when well designed) should be better than the clinical expert (since if the clinical expert was better, they could incorporate their knowledge in such a system), a patient is such a complex multifactorial system that a clinician's view is expected to remain necessary. Chess computers are nowadays better than any human, and cars can almost drive independently, but these systems are less complex than a

Table 2. *Most common modes of ventilation sorted by tag and their equivalent mode names for four ventilators*

Tag	Covidien PB840	Dräger Evita XL	Hamilton GS	Maquet Servo-i
VC-CMVs	A/C volume control	CMV	Synchronised controlled mandatory ventilation	NA#
VC-IMVs,s	SIMV volume control with pressure support	SIMV	SIMV	NA¶
PC-CMVs	A/C pressure control	Pressure control ventilation plus assisted	Pressure control CMV	Pressure control
PC-CMVa	A/C volume control plus	CMV with AutoFlow	Adaptive pressure ventilation CMV	Pressure-regulated volume control
PC-IMVs,s	SIMV-pressure control with pressure support Bi-level with pressure support	Pressure control ventilation plus/pressure support APRV	Pressure SIMV NIV-spontaneous timed Nasal CPAP-pressure support APRV DuoPAP	SIMV (pressure control) BiVent Automode (pressure control to pressure support)
PC-IMVa,s	SIMV volume control plus with pressure support	Mandatory minute volume with AutoFlow SIMV with AutoFlow	Adaptive pressure ventilation SIMV	SIMV pressure-regulated volume control
PC-CSVs	Spontaneous pressure support	CPAP/pressure support	Spontaneous	Spontaneous/CPAP
PC-CSVa	Spontaneous volume support	NA	NA	Volume support

VC: volume control; CMV: continuous mandatory ventilation; IMV: intermittent mandatory ventilation; PC: pressure control; CSV: continuous spontaneous ventilation; s: set-point; a: adaptive; A/C: assist control; NA: not available; SIMV: synchronised IMV; APRV: airway pressure release ventilation; DuoPAP: dual positive airway pressure. #: VC-CMV is not available because the mode called volume control allows some breaths to be patient-triggered and patient-cycled; hence, they are spontaneous, making the breath sequence IMV rather than CMV. ¶: VC-IMV is available only with dual targeting, called SIMV (volume control) with the tag VC-IMVd,d. Reproduced and modified from Chatburn *et al.* (2014) with permission.

patient on a ventilator. For example, a developing infection may not be continuously monitored, while such a parameter might be critical for the optimisation of ventilator settings, medical treatment and life expectancy of that patient. Modern technology will allow the incorporation of more miniaturised sensors to measure many signals simultaneously. More complex monitoring modalities (*e.g.* forced oscillation technology to quantify the resistance and inertance of the respiratory system) can quantify changes in the airway mechanics of the patient's lungs (compliance and resistance). Intelligent ventilators might automatically adapt the setting based on the outcomes of parameters measured. Additionally, the natural variability of many signals is a sign of the disease state of a living organism and can be used/incorporated in artificially intelligent algorithms as extra parameters to optimise ventilation. Ventilators should not be sensitive to software alterations/updates, but technology incorporated demands highly complex hard- and software, which should be incorporated into highly complex information and communications technology systems. An extra challenge is that you cannot "reboot" your ventilator as easily as your computer, without consequences for the patient on that ventilator. As clinicians, we are in the lead to decide which signals have to be measured. Ventilator settings can be changed within the boundaries that we (still) do specify. Patients and their treatment are increasingly complex, so the field of the technical physician is becoming more and more important to be able to master the combination of engineering, (patho-)physiology and medicine.

Further reading

- Cairo JM (2016). Pilbeam's Mechanical Ventilation: Physiological and Clinical Applications. 6th Edn. St Louis, Elsevier.

- Chatburn RL (2003). Fundamentals of Mechanical Ventilation: A Short Course in the Theory and Application of Mechanical Ventilators. 1st Edn. Cleveland Heights, Mandu Press Ltd.

- Chatburn RL (2004). Computer control of mechanical ventilation. *Respir Care*; 49: 507–515.

- Chatburn RL, *et al.* (2014). A taxonomy for mechanical ventilation: 10 fundamental maxims. *Respir Care*; 59: 1747–1763.

- Dellaca' RL, *et al.* (2017). Trends in mechanical ventilation: are we ventilating our patients in the best possible way? *Breathe*; 13: 84–98.

- Pisani L, *et al.* (2012). Interfaces for noninvasive mechanical ventilation: technical aspects and efficiency. *Minerva Anestesiol*; 78: 1154–1161.

- Tobin MJ, ed. (2013). Principles and Practice of Mechanical Ventilation. 3rd Edn. New York, McGraw-Hill Medical.

Index

A

abdominal muscle wall, ultrasound 149, 151, 151f
absorbance ratio 101, 101f
ACURASYS trial 55–56, 86
acute lung injury, potentially recruitable lung 185–186
acute respiratory distress syndrome (ARDS)
    ACURASYS trial 55–56, 86
    airway closure 115
    airway opening pressure 115
    airway resistance 10t
    alveolar instability, collapse 185
    alveolar recruitment optimisation 109
    chest radiography 156f, 157
    controlled invasive ventilation 86
        vs partial ventilator support 55–56
    definition, modified (based on S_pO_2/F_{iO_2} ratio) 103
    driving pressure ($\triangle P$) 49, 86
        increase effect 22–23
    early phase
        prone position use 180
        ventilator settings 83–84, 85f
    extracorporeal lung support 84, 172, 173, 174f
    hypoxaemia
        mechanism 196
        refractory, almitrine in 199
    invasive ventilation 81–87, 172
        current considerations 86–87
        impact 16
        low V_T 83
        PEEP, setting 18, 83–84, 85f, 86, 133, 134f
        risks and aims 81–83, 82f
        settings 83–84, 85f
        strategies, aims 83
    late phase, ventilation 84
    lung collapse 185, 186f
        reversal, recruitment manoeuvre 187, 188, 190f
    lung compliance 10t, 117
    lung injury 172
    lung overdistension risk 83, 84, 172
    lung-protective ventilation protocol 17–18, 17f, 18t, 83
        best PEEP 18, 109
    lung ultrasound 139, 140t
    mechanical power, inflammation 14
    mild, controlled ventilation 86
    moderate-to-severe
        adjuvant therapies 84
        PEEP setting 83–84
        spontaneous breathing 86
    neuromuscular blocking agents 55–56, 86
    P_{aO_2}/F_{iO_2} 2
    pathophysiology 81–83, 82f, 185
    prognosis, dead space measurement 109
    prone position, use see prone positioning, in ARDS

recovery phase, spontaneous breathing 87
    recruitment manoeuvres 109, 185–186
        see also recruitment manoeuvres
    respiratory system compliance 10t
    ROSE trial 56
    severe
        ECMO, settings 84, 173, 174f
        ECMO and almitrine 199
        inhaled nitric oxide 197
        prone positioning see prone positioning
        right ventricular failure 178
    spontaneous breathing, ventilation considerations 86–87
    ultraprotective ventilation 86
    vasoconstrictors and vasodilators
        almitrine 198, 199
        nitric oxide 196–198, 197t
        rationale for 195–196
    ventilation/perfusion (V/Q') mismatch 81, 83, 172
    weaning, criteria for 84
acute respiratory failure (ARF)
    differential diagnosis 142, 143f
    inhalation therapy 201
    in interstitial lung disease 95, 97
    lung ultrasound 142, 143f
adaptive pressure-controlled ventilation 74
adaptive support ventilation (ASV) 74–80, 75f, 218t
    evidence and advantages 76
    INTELLiVENT-ASV see INTELLiVENT-ASV
    in passive patients 74, 75, 76t
    principles 74, 75, 75f
    settings, adjustments and monitoring 75, 76t
    in spontaneously breathing patients 74, 75, 76t
    for weaning 75–76
β_2-adrenergic agonists 203, 204–205
aerosol therapy see inhalation therapy (ventilated patients)
air
    humidification 202, 203f, 238, 254
    pressure, changing 254
    pressurised, mixture 254
    trapping 70
air bronchogram 140f
    dynamic 139
airflow 8–9, 252–254
    acute obstruction 40, 89
    airway resistance calculation 9
    breathing effort monitoring 121t, 122, 123f
    inspiratory, optimisation 163, 256
    inspiratory mismatching 161–162, 161f
    low, flow starvation 114
    measurement, ventilators 11
        proportional assist ventilation 68
    pressure difference governing 252
    pressure relationship, mathematical 253–254, 257

respiratory muscles, by ultrasound 30, 147-153
  see also diaphragm
  ventilation *see* ventilation
mortality
  interstitial lung disease 95, 96, 97, 98
  mechanical power association 14
  recruitment manoeuvres 190, 191f
mouth, pressure changes at, ventilator function 253, 254
mouth occlusion pressure 6
mucolytic drugs 205
multiorgan failure 29
  in ARDS 82f, 83
  in interstitial lung diseases 98
muscle fibres, atrophy, diaphragm weakness 27, 29
musculus transversus abdominis (TA) 149
myocardial ischaemia 224
myopathy, spontaneous breathing trial failure 224-225

N

nasal tubes 34
nasogastric tube 35
nasotracheal suctioning 248
NAVA *see* neurally adjusted ventilator assist (NAVA)
nebulisers 202, 203-204, 203f
  drugs used 204, 205
  jet 203f, 204
  performance, criteria affecting 204
  ultrasonic 203f, 204
  ventilator circuit with 202f
  vibrating mesh 203f, 204, 205
nephrotoxicity, nitric oxide 198
neurally adjusted ventilator assist (NAVA) 30, 63-67, 127, 218b, 219
  advantages 66
  contraindication 64
  conventional controlled ventilation *vs* 66
  diaphragm electromyography 165-166
  level 63, 64
    titration procedure/setting 64
  for monitoring patient-ventilator asynchronies 67
  practical use 64
  pressure support ventilation (PSV) *vs* 66
  previsualisation system 64
  principles 63-64, 65f
  use and limitations of 64, 66
neural respiratory drive (NRD) 3, 62, 63, 127, 255
  hypercapnia mechanism 6, 6f
  noninvasive marker 6
  physiological biomarker 6
  reverse trigger (entrainment phenomenon) 163
neuromuscular blocking agents (NMBAs) 55
  ACURASYS trial (ARDS) 55-56, 86

neutrophilic inflammation 14
nitric oxide, inhaled 196-198
  actions 196, 198
    evidence for 196-197
    mechanism 196
  administration 197
  adverse effects 198
  with almitrine 199
  dose, and monitoring 197
  indications 197, 197t
  nitric oxide production inhibition 198
  weaning from 197, 198
noninvasive ventilation (NIV) 256
  in COPD 88
  for decannulation (tracheostomy) 240
  differences from conventional ventilation 258
  early extubation, with 230, 250
  after extubation 209, 230
  in interstitial lung disease 97
  intolerance 231
  leak compensation 258
  prolonged weaning and 231
"normoxia," target, ECMO 173
nutrition, prolonged weaning approach 233

O

obesity, lung ultrasound limitation 145
obstructive lung disease 3
  airway resistance, hyperinflation 5
  dynamic pulmonary hyperinflation 88, 90, 92f, 93
  invasive ventilation 88-94
    goal 90
    pathophysiological basis 88-90
  passive invasive ventilation 90, 91f, 92f
    monitoring 90, 93
    settings 90, 93
  patient-ventilator asynchrony 93
  pressure-controlled ventilation 90
  pressure support ventilation 93-94
    monitoring 94
    settings 93
  volume-controlled ventilation 90
  see also chronic obstructive pulmonary disease (COPD)
occlusion pressure 6
oesophageal balloon 125, 126f, 127
oesophageal pressure (P_{oes}) 12, 18, 21, 22, 94
  breathing effort, monitoring 121t, 123f, 125-126
  changes during tidal breathing 116
  decrease, breathing effort physiological/excessive 126
  increase, breathing effort 126
  measurement 21, 113, 116
    advanced analysis 126
    method 125-126
  monitoring during passive ventilation 115-117, 115f